YOUR CONSCIOUS BRAIN
How It All Works and Why

Jan de Vinter

First paperback edition August 2022

Book design by Publishing Push

ISBN 978-1-80227-378-6 (pbk)
978-1-80227-379-3 (eBk)

A WIFE'S REVIEW

I obviously knew my husband was working on a book about how the whole conscious brain worked. He mentioned odd topics he was working on, but when he asked me to proofread it, <u>I didn't really know what to expect</u>!

I <u>*secretly*</u> thought "how can he write a book about this topic and ever engage most people's attention significantly enough for them not to become bored?"

I found it all fascinating, but, when I reached the section about the actual operation of the three different categories of departments that comprise the whole brain, as advised in the book, I focused not on their names and operation. Instead, I concentrated on the different roles and uses they crucially carry out for you every second and hour of your life. I continued through this section and just couldn't put it down during the whole of the rest of the book. I found it utterly riveting reading.

Be prepared to be amazed!

An introductory note from the author about how you will benefit from reading this book and hopefully gain significantly from the knowledge you will have learned. This book clearly explains the absolute and utter importance of why and how your consciousness's automatic creation and application of your consciousness is essential to every person who has ever lived on this planet of ours, who is alive today and who will live in the future.

NB These comments also apply basically to all other living creatures!

This book has clearly and with simplicity blown the cobwebs off the two-centuries-old mystery of how the whole of your brain actually works.

ACKNOWLEDGEMENTS

Firstly to my wonderfully supportive, loving, patient and intelligent wife, Ann. Particularly during the sometimes frenetic and long process of writing this book, Ann put up with me promising to do all kinds of the usual things, only to find me yet again at my laptop, sometimes into the late/early hours.

Ann also had to endure the numerous and regular shouts of exaltation when I thought that I had eventually found the answer of how a particular part of your brain's functionality worked, for which I had been searching, sometimes for a number of months. Usually, when I exploded with this discovery, I quite often attached the comment of, "As usual, it's a No-Brainer." The simpler the answer, the disproportionately more difficult it is to find it.

Latterly, after completing the book, Ann agreed to carry out the vitally important tough job of the first/initial proof reading, which she completed with the required tenacity, concentration and skill.

Secondly, I will be eternally grateful to the Emeritus Professor David Sanders with whom I met on a Fred Olsen cruise ship, following one of his absolutely brilliant lectures on the mind. We had a fascinating discussion about Consciousness which galvanised me into commencing writing this book.

EXTREMELY BASIC CONTENTS OF THE WHOLE BOOK

AN INTRODUCTION

About 40 years ago, through my work, I became increasingly fascinated by how our brains actually worked and the unbelievable power, capacity and capability they must have to accomplish what we each achieve as a consequence of them. I mentioned these thoughts occasionally to one or two people and continued to mull over how brains worked as an occasional background past time.

A few years ago, I mentioned this interest to our youngest son, and he bought me a huge book about the brain as a Christmas present. I started to avidly read this book, eagerly waiting to be enlightened about the **functionality of the whole brain system,** and I began making cryptic notes whenever I read anything of particular significance.

Very early on, I found that to date, no one has been able to define exactly what, in detail, our **consciousness, mind and soul** actually are, how the consciousness is created and how the three operate and interact.

I read this with disbelief and instinctively felt that I could do this. You may think what a cocky etc., person I must be, but please believe that I did not have these thoughts in that kind of way. It was as if these thoughts were driven by something I wasn't consciously fully aware of and I just had a deep-seated feeling. I suspect this was coming from an area in my brain as I had been considering this topic a lot more than I had been consciously aware of.

So please read on. I jotted down some basic notes for my definitions of each of these three aspects of our brain and continued reading the book to completion. Disappointingly, I made very few notes because I had expected to be given a **lot of information about the b**rain's actual processing functionality.

After more thoughts about the subject, and with my long-suffering wife Ann putting up with my increasingly frequent comments and saying, "For heaven's sake, do something rather than just talk about the subject," I decided to attend some large seminar or convention about the brain. I assumed that there might be an available option for me to get up and announce my thoughts on these three definitions.

Upon further reflection, I thought that if my ideas were judged to have any substance for useful consideration, they would have been broadcast on the internet before I had returned to my hotel for the evening, with others taking the credit. So I decided it would be best to write a book and make additional use of my retirement.

For the first time in my life, I commenced a process of great importance to me without initially mapping out any framework at all for this exercise. A week or two after I started, I began to realise that it felt as if I was the tool being used to carry out this process.

As the book progressed, this feeling was repeated at times, specifically after I had finally understood and developed a belief of how a particularly challenging part of the brain's functionality actually operated and what its detailed role was.

I felt so excited to be on a journey in which I just felt that the workings of our brain would gradually be uncovered to me. This may sound a tad naive or cocky or some other things, but it was just how I actually felt.

Such was my emotional drive with this project that I increasingly struggled <u>not</u> to work on the book continuously, throughout the day and too far into the early hours.

Basic ideas of principle, coupled with more and more details came flooding out of my brain. It was like before I retired and was at work again, producing a 150-page detailed engineering specification of production, performance, quality, design, manufacturing, testing, installation and commissioning for a very large multi-million pound, automated manufacturing process line. I was experiencing the same emotional buzz and sheer satisfaction all over again.

It felt as if all of this information and ideas had been gathering inside my brain. It had been waiting to burst out when tweaked, in an almost continuous flood of thoughts, ideas, questions and emotional energy about the topic.

As it was whilst at work, the more principles and details I received from my brain and placed on paper and on to my laptop screen, thus enabling me to look at them, study and consider them, the more they interacted, developed and blossomed.

My initial focus was on two of the three primary definitions I had very basically developed, with your consciousness having my main focus and attention, because I just felt it was so foundational to your brain's overall functionality.

I also worked equally on the individual development of your mind whilst at this stage, focussing on its' basic structure, because I also felt that it was the other key player in your brain's functioning capacities.

Over the following six months, l began popping down on paper various ideas, details, principles, questions, chapters and sub-chapters for my book. I did this during the day, evening and awakening during the night, out on our boat, walking in a thunderstorm, swimming, speaking to someone, driving the car, on an aeroplane: in absolutely every setting, everywhere. Even whilst sitting on a wall outside a museum on a Scottish island, I was intently studying a bird for an hour, perched on a guttering. I observed all of its actions, asking myself what they were for and what were its thoughts. My conclusion confirmed my initial diagnosis, which was that the bird was creating/updating its Consciousness. It was simply and continually looking all around, up and down, to look out for any danger to itself from birds or cats that it would have to take evasive action to avoid. It was also probably seeking any food or drink that may become available for it to stay alive. It was simply utilising the two primary objectives of its consciousness: to keep itself safe from danger and to have sufficient food and drink to provide sufficient sustenance to remain alive.

My wife is a professionally qualified dance teacher and, shortly after she and I retired, we began working on cruise ships. We taught the passengers how to dance and danced with them in the evenings. As happened fairly often whilst working on the cruise ships, when something out of the ordinary, extremely important or very unusual happened to me or someone else, I would note it down as something that warranted some detailed consideration, explanation and understanding. As soon as possible, I would type these notes, information and queries into the relevant section of my book to consider and expand in the future when appropriate.

Apart from the gradual and ultimate benefits for the knowledgeable development of my book, I began to realise that these notes and observations were also what felt like the organically evolving, primary objectives of what it was going to be used for. Therefore, they directed what its foci needed to be, in terms of benefiting people generally, which were:

a)   Writing it always with great clarity, for people who had absolutely no existing knowledge of how their brains functioned, and provide them with some understanding of their brain's principles of operation, along with some details.

My simple objective, particularly about each of my beliefs, was to explain them with the utmost clarity and state why I held them. Also, part of these objectives of clarity that I sincerely hope you will agree with, was my use of chapters, subchapters, numbering and lettering. This was to separate out information as I built up a topic to hopefully make the final understanding of it a gradual and, therefore, clearer process.

b)   Write to help individuals and their loved ones begin to have some degree of understanding of how their brains function, how their decision-making process and its resultant actions occur. Therefore, they will hopefully be able to help themselves deal with the trials and tribulations they suffer due to the increasingly and desperately challenging life we all lead, as a consequence of the combination of their financial, functional and generally life's difficulties and pressures.

c)   Write to propose a principle but simple suggestion of where people's physical ill health can possibly be better understood and therefore perhaps better treated.

d)   Write to hopefully be able to assist those who spend a lot of their lives trying to fathom the workings of our brain.

e)   Write to assist those who wish to improve their brain system's functionality of decision making that we all spend most of our lives carrying out.

f)   My beliefs and answers to a few ongoing day-to-day <u>Topical Questions</u> that I have noted within the media, about us, the human race and about the extraordinary functionality, power, depth and breadth of capability of our brains.

g)   Write to highlight and provide some principle suggestions for consideration and therefore some possible answers to a list of frequently posed questions within the media about the increasing percentage of the population suffering from serious mental and physical illnesses. I increasingly feel that, unless the current trends and common practices by a large percentage of the population, in some areas change for the better, there exists the potential to increasingly put at risk the good health and worse of our future human race.

FOREWORD

This is a potted history primarily relevant to the book of my life, up to the point and beyond when I started to write it.

NB At this point, I would like to explain why I have given such a lot of information about my dyslexia, so you can judge whether to continue and read all of this sub-chapter or not. This information is for those who have dyslexia, or someone they care for does, and they wish to help them.

Dyslexia affects a significant percentage of the population. It manifests itself in various ways or types of difficulties with different people. It has the potential to make dyslexic people's lives significantly operationally difficult. It can cause low self-esteem and for people to suffer from very high levels of anxiety with all of the resultant problems that follow.

1.0 My dyslexia – The extremely significant downsides

I contracted pneumonia when six months old and for three months, I was at death's door. Our GP visited my mother and me most evenings to normally say that I would probably not last the night, as my heart and breathing were extremely laboured. Every night I was administered a teaspoon of whisky to assist my heart's function. Penicillin was developed and literally saved my life.

During this time of my life, the periods of significant reduction of oxygen to my brain and the resultant damage to some of its departments caused me to suffer from extremely serious dyslexia dysfunctionalities which I continue to experience to this day.

The functional consequences of my dyslexia are that I struggle to spell, remember names, and so many other things which are all basics in life, like people's birthdays, including my wife's. I really struggle with learning, particularly new information, and more so if the information is delivered too fast for my brain to accept, causing it to shut down its consideration of the data. My memory retention and recall of even simple, basic information is extremely poor. However, one of my lifesavers is that when I receive or note something that I deem is very important to me, I will always remember it.

If I am calculating important data for a numerical solution, I have to progress at a relatively slow pace and check any calculations or considerations several times in succession to be confident in continuing the process to a successful conclusion.

Also, if I am simply reading a large paragraph of information listing four separate aspects, leading to some particular and important conclusion, I have to repeat this reading a number of times consecutively. This is the only way I can remember the collective effect of all of these separate aspects and therefore accept the final conclusion that they lead to or support.

These weaknesses made doing well at exams a particular struggle and when having to absorb new information at meetings etc., whilst at work. Outside work, it was, and still is, a challenge to recall people's names and most other categories of quite simple information, including learning new dance steps. I have to repeat them a hundred times or so over the few days after initially learning them to retain them in my memory.

Being dyslexic has been a significant factor throughout my life, particularly causing me to: Fail my eleven-plus which my dear mother told me many years later that my teachers were astounded when I failed it. I had nightmares for thirty-four years about the eleven-plus adjudicator announcing, "Fifteen minutes left," when I had only completed approximately 30% of the required questions. This caused an emotional and physical shudder that reverberates even today.

I only stopped experiencing nightmares about this exam experience after my mother informed me of my pneumonia and when I realised that I suffered from dyslexia. I started reading about it in order to help our eldest son, who suffered from it with different symptoms to mine and was unable to write correctly, even at fourteen. With my help and his utter determination to improve his writing, he developed the ability to write at a very respectable standard and now runs his own very successful business. The knowledge that I suffered from these dyslexia weaknesses and the understanding of why I struggled, enabled me to come to terms with it. Therefore, my eleven-plus failure and the nightmares disappeared.

Suffering from dyslexia also causes very significant lack of self-esteem difficulties due to feeling extremely awkward at struggling to learn in all types of environments, including when the information wasn't in itself difficult to understand. But, it is created by you feeling that other people who don't know you well, assume you are struggling due to being stupid, thick or lazy, etc., etc.

2.0 My dyslexia – The immense and extremely significant benefits

Approximately ten years ago, over breakfast, whilst working on the cruise ships, my wife and I got talking at length to a man about his profession. For twenty years, he worked with a vast number of people who were suffering from very serious dyslexia difficulties, helping and teaching them how to deal with it emotionally and operationally in their daily lives.

After listening to him for quite a while, I eventually told him I had suffered from dyslexia for the whole of my life, and was still suffering to this day. He asked me quite a few questions about my difficulties and he finally said to me, "I just can't believe what you have told me. I have met an enormous number of people who suffered far less severe symptoms than you have who experienced quite serious mental health difficulties caused by it. I have studied you very closely this last half an hour, and I can't detect any symptoms from your dyslexia that I would have expected to witness. To be honest with you, I would have expected you to quite possibly have ended up in some care scene as a consequence of them." This made me quite proud of the way I have dealt with it.

Although my dyslexia has caused very extreme difficulties operationally and emotionally, throughout my whole life, including today, I would not wish to change my life from how it has been. The **upside capabilities that dyslexia has given me far outweigh the downsides**. It is one of a number of factors that has enabled me to achieve many things at work and in my life and has assisted me in having, I believe, blown away all of the cobwebs that had shrouded the mysteries of consciousness.

Despite having no knowledge that I actually suffered from dyslexia until my mid-forties, as I became increasingly exposed to more exams, following my eleven-plus disaster, I realised I had particular learning difficulties generally and also certain problems with passing exams. As the exams featured more prominently in my life, I ensured that I developed more effective coping strategies to minimise my learning difficulties. I created a list of extremely crucial exam techniques for myself, finding and developing the optimum revision methods for each subject. The net benefits of all of these elements enabled me to obtain increasingly far better exam results and, ultimately, a magnificent final exam result.

I utilised some of the great strengths I inherited in my genes to achieve these objectives, which also obtained some consequential additional benefits. When I came to my Chartered Institution exams, I had to become an expert at learning a huge syllabus with literally hundreds of very complex formulae. Developing a long list of good exam techniques eventually enabled me to be able to complete all of the exam questions required.

I also forced my brain not to be as obstructive as it normally is, particularly whilst in live meetings. This was even more important following a very high-level promotion I achieved at work, which I had not really sought and decided to accept only after much consideration. I am convinced that because my brain is relatively uncluttered and devoid of not useless but unimportant data, it is relatively empty, compared with most people's, and this was a major benefit. It was refreshingly available to think about **anything** I put my mind to. I realised that I could see the framework of any system, throughout all of its complexity. When I put my mind to it, I could also see and home into any detail, when that view was required, in order to achieve whatever objectives prevailed.

Whilst at work, I supported my poor memory by developing an extremely large, extremely efficient, easy-to-use paper filing system. I used it for every single project, large and small, that was current and completed it from day one of my working life in engineering. I also found that I had the ability to focus on something I was working on that I deemed important, with an extreme, unbroken intensity for very long periods of time, if required.

I naturally seem to be able to study, understand and connect with people to quite a depth, particularly if I sense they have significant difficulties and require assistance, or when I am interviewing them. This sounds a bit self-congratulatory, but it is not meant to be like that. It's just the way I feel, how I see things and how I operate – always constructively and always to assist people and move towards the prevailing objective/s. I have utilised this ability of sensing what peoples' characters are, their prevailing attitudes and whether they are telling the truth etc., during crucial work meetings with people from many different countries and companies. This was to try and resolve complicated and very important situations within the many engineering projects I worked on, yet still retain our mutual respect afterwards, which is always an essential factor. I also used these skills within the day-to-day running of the company I worked at for nearly all of my working life after obtaining my engineering qualifications and the membership of the IEE that I was awarded.

3.0 My academic activities and achievements

I have had the absolute pleasure, joy and satisfaction of having benefitted from a wonderful academic and practical sandwich course-basis education in an extremely fulfilling Professional Engineering learning and working environment.

I obtained this education whilst being a student apprentice at the G.E.C. factory in Witton, Birmingham. I then went on to become accepted as a Chartered Engineer of the IEE (Institution of Electrical Engineers) after passing their IEE honours degree, part three membership requirement. With my erstwhile extreme difficulties with doing well in exams, I was so pleased with passing this particular exam because it was the most important and highest academic level exam that I had ever taken to date. It was also the last ever exam of its type for IEE membership. It was to be replaced with a different one, **and there were no re-sits as there always had been in the past.** It was also an exam that was sat throughout the whole of the country.

Because of this set of circumstances, all of our lecturers predicted that the standard of this particular last ever exam, which previously and normally had been a very high standard, would be relatively easy this time. I had never heard and seen so many gasps, with people struggling to stay on their chairs as they did their first read-through of the paper and were struggling to find any questions they could answer. One student did actually fall off his chair.

I received a lovely hand-written letter from our chief lecturer congratulating me on passing and saying that it was an extremely low pass rate of 25% over the whole country. I was on cloud nine for many days after this great news.

I rose to become Chief Electrical Engineer of my company, which was part of a global, highest technical specification, aluminium manufacturing and development organisation, and one of the world leaders in its field.

Due to a number of my successful and very challenging engineering projects and the position I eventually rose to, I was advised to apply for Fellowship Status of the IEE. I was so busy, that I didn't apply, which I now regret from a personal satisfaction perspective.

I have used the benefits of this education during all of my life, and not just within my working environment. I have now been fully retired for twelve years, having taken early retirement at sixty and returning immediately as a consultant until I finally fully retired at sixty-five years of age. I value beyond measure, being fortunate to be able to look back upon the whole of my education and working life and feel such an immense degree of satisfaction and pleasure. I feel privileged to have worked with all of the people at my factory and also all of the extremely capable engineers and research professionals at different laboratories, companies and countries. I worked on a vast number of engineering projects for forty years up to the day I retired, working for the last five years as a consultant.

It was not plain sailing at times, but the key is when your objectives are finally achieved and the manufacturing production, quality output, costs, timescales and reliability are all accomplished. You walk slowly for half an hour or more around the operating reality of the end product after five years of immense work from a large team of people from many different companies around Europe and beyond, starting from a totally blank piece of paper and imprinting a very large production line onto an empty area of the shop floor. No amount of money can buy that feeling of utter, immense achievement, just pure satisfaction, pleasure and joy.

4.0 My activities outside work

Playing sport all year-round from the age of five to my late forties was a very large part of my life outside work. I played tennis, squash, badminton, golf, hockey and did judo, all of which I took very seriously, but always with great satisfaction and enjoyment. The PE teacher at my senior school pestered the life out of me to take up boxing seriously. I kept refusing, saying that, with my big nose, it would get broken far too easily. In retrospect, I would have liked to have given it a shot! I played all sports at a very good level, with one played at a particularly high level. I carried out quite a lot of coaching. I eventually suffered from a very bad chronic lower back problem. I was forced to give up all of the sports I was playing at that time or risk ending up in a wheelchair for the rest of my life. This was the diagnosis from the surgeon upon studying MRI scans of my lower back.

Since retirement, I took up Ballroom, Latin and Sequence dancing a few years ago with my wife, who is a professionally qualified dance teacher. We worked on the cruise ships teaching and dancing with the passengers, which was extremely hard work, but we enjoyed it enormously. It kept our brains and bodies extremely fit, learning new dances, steps and routines whilst visiting a lot of the wonderful places in this fascinating world we are so fortunate to inhabit. Regular exercise is also extremely beneficial for de-stressing your mind, minimising any anxieties of the day that may have built up from a particularly tough day at work and therefore contributing significantly to keeping your mental health in good order.

Boating has been another big part of our lives since our mid-twenties. We had an estuary cruiser then, in which we and our family had many great adventures. We travelled many thousands of miles along the canals and, latterly, the inland tidal rivers of

England, which was an enormous change from the canals in so many exciting but extremely challenging ways.

We then moved on to a twin inboard engine seagoing/coastal boat in which we had many years of great fun out at sea and inland, cruising with the local yacht club and, at times, on our own. Again, this represented another major change from cruising on the inland tidal waters with many exciting and highly challenging differences.

In order to knowledgeably and therefore safely, be able to do our excursions, particularly on our own, on sometimes over sixty continuous miles of seagoing trips, in periodically pretty awful weather which was not predicted, I passed a two year, one day per week course examination and qualified with a Yacht Master's Certificate of which I was very proud and pleased to have been awarded. You have to have achieved an extremely high level of marks over the two-hour exam, but it provided an immense amount of vitally important knowledge of what to be aware of whilst at sea and very much more.

Because of my difficulties with exams and the amount of questions, a lot of which required mathematical calculations that needed careful thought, knowledge and concentration, I took time off work as a consultant during that period. I needed to work out a system for maximising my chances of passing the exam, as you did not pass if you failed to reach the very high pass level. I set out a very detailed revision schedule to embed the required knowledge, and I carried out this revision process daily.

I also got hold of four of the most recent two-hour exam papers. I sat down and, as fast as I could, worked all the way through the first paper and took four hours and fifteen minutes – **a big fail**. I analysed why I had taken so long, and it was the usual, old dyslexic-caused weaknesses. I listed out each of these weaknesses and wrote down how I would force my brain to operate differently, pressurised by my objective of – I had to pass!! I sat each of the other exam papers whilst consciously forcing myself to follow better procedures. The last practice exam I did was the day before the actual exam, so I could maximise the objective of overriding my brain's natural instincts. I completed this last test paper with five minutes to spare!

We currently have a medium sized motorhome which we use for holidays, visiting friends and our family.

5.0 Me as a human being

Throughout my life, I have always tried to do the best that I can in everything that I do, whilst adhering to the rules and obtaining as much enjoyment, satisfaction and fun as is possible. I have also tried to live a life based on the Ten Commandments, which, when I heard them for the first time at senior school, just struck me as a very simple guide of how to lead your life whilst on this planet of ours.

Throughout my life, at work and outside work, I have always tried to help anyone I have met if they have been struggling with whatever. This has never been for any reason other than if they needed help, and I thought that I could assist them, I would do my best, in an unobtrusive way, to aid them if they wished.

My wife and I have the pleasure of having two wonderful sons and their wonderful five grandchildren, all of whom we have quite a lot of enjoyable and interesting contact with.

I have inherited some very powerfully positive genes, which I have utilised to their maximum, but also some negatively powerful ones, which I have had to learn how to manage as I have passed along my life's journey. Fortunately, I have been able to step outside myself when necessary and also step inside myself to see what was going on. This has been a part of the process of managing my own difficulties and strengths. It has meant I can participate in a productive and acceptable manner in my personal life, my family life and within my work and the whole of my life's package.

I am able to experience a number of emotional views, senses and insights, which are:

a) To see an aura around the head of several people I have known over the years, who were about to die relatively soon after my having this experience. This was a completely unplanned and unsought after occurrence, and I gradually realised the significance of what I was experiencing.

b) Commencing whilst still a teenager and for a number of years, before retiring to bed, two nights out of three, when sitting in front of my bedroom mirror, I would go into a type of trance-like state for around an hour. I thought about many things in relation to my current and earlier life experiences and the consequence of this was to learn things of significance. This sounds extremely vague, but I will explain it as I experienced and responded to it at the time.

c) When someone is emotionally depressed, to at least, an unhealthy degree, without them speaking, I can see the aura and smell the depression emanating from around them.

These capabilities and my experiences have, I believe, enabled me to be able to help others who are struggling with their lives. It allows them to be completely open and comfortable about informing me of their difficulties and to being helped.

If I were to ask of you just one thing, it would simply be to please continue and read all of the book in the *order it is written.* It covers the functionality of the whole of your brain which. Because I believe that it is an inherently interconnected and interrelated processing system, it is easier to understand it all by reading it in this way. I have attempted to write the book in what I hope is the best order to achieve the easiest clarity of understanding of all of my beliefs and proposals. I very much hope that you will find it interesting.

At the end of the book, there is a description of the process through which I developed a significant percentage of my beliefs and proposals about the role and functionality of your brain, all as presented in this book.

Also, quite a few areas of functionality and key parts of roles that your brain satisfies have been described in more than one section. They are usually described slightly differently and with other uses or activities to assist with clarity of understanding.

So, please, let my book commence.

CHAPTER 1.0 – AN OVERVIEW OF YOUR BRAIN AND BODY

SUBCHAPTER 1.1: Your incredible, wonderful, wonderous brain

OVERVIEW: *I believe that The Grand Creator had a 10-out-of-10 day when he/she/it began the creation and* **continued evolution of your brain.**

I consider your brain to probably be the most powerful, capable, flexible, continually self-learning, potentially continually developing/ improving, system processing controller, SINGLE UNIT FACILITY that exists in, quite possibly, the whole of our Universe.

That, in my opinion, is the degree of breadth and depth of capability, capacity and power that it has.

NB If other human-type civilisations are found to exist – and I believe that this may not be the case, some of these will inevitably have a more advanced brain than ours, particularly those that visit us, rather than we visit them.

I first became interested in the functionality of our brains 40 years ago. This was when I began to become increasingly involved with the specification, project control of design, manufacture, installation, commissioning and management of extremely large and complex computer-controlled automatic equipment and processing lines in my industry.

I was swimming during my tri-weekly session and, as often was the case, my brain had been working on some important work-related problem that required solving, when I had this flash of judgement:

THE CAPABILITY AND CAPACITY OF <u>ONE</u> AVERAGE HUMAN BRAIN WAS EQUAL TO ALL OF THE COMPUTERS THAT EXISTED IN THE WORLD <u>AT THAT TIME.</u>

Since then, I have been interested to note that in some people's view, this relationship was in the correct ballpark, which supports the assessment of just how incredible your brain is.

AN EXTREMELY IMPORTANT POINTER TO NOTE:

With the **exception of all** these chapters/subchapters: **6.9** & **8.0** & **9.0** & **10.0, and the exception of a little** of subchapters **6.10** & **7.15, the following is applicable.**

I would like to say at this point that **all of my beliefs and proposals about the topics and factual details contained throughout this book (with the exceptions listed above)** are based on my beliefs of how **your consciousness** is created. I have studied its **role** and **purpose**, plus how and why all of the rest of **your brain's** basic rules, objectives, methods and activities of operating **all relate to and are governed by your consciousness.**

After I arrived at this immensely important juncture of having this vast amount of understanding and knowledge as described above, I found that it inevitably opened up **other avenues of your brain's activities** that were not part of my book's originally-planned primary contents and topics of investigation.

Everything you do emanates from your brain with a related what, how and why. These **other avenues** took me into **mental health, physical health** and **why we have pain, etc.** I explored perhaps how better, or in different ways, we can deal with certainly not all but some of these aspects, all of which are of immense importance to everyone alive today.

Your brain is **always** trying to help you. The trick is for you to let it.

<u>All details in the book, with the exceptions outlined above originate from the foundational knowledge I have created and gained.</u> A few of my beliefs may surprise you and others.

I recommend that you buckle up for the ride. I hope you will enjoy it all.

a) A basic overall view and description of your brain.

The organ that is your brain is comprised of approximately three pounds of corrugated, organic matter. It lives inside the physically protective shield of your skull. It is located in a position where it can function with excellent operational efficiency and effect. Your brain deals with crucially required incoming information that I will refer to as data, from your five senses, your Body's Health Status Monitoring System (B.H.S.M.S.) and your internal thoughts. It is protected from physical harm as far as is realistically possible, given its elevated position. This is required to receive the extremely important range of high quality, useful data which your senses can gather at this elevation and transmit into your brain.

NB Your Body's Health Status Monitoring System (B.H.S.M.S.) is the name I give to the part of your brain that has the dedicated job of automatically monitoring your whole body's physical and mental health. It alerts the appropriate Data Input Department if it notes you have a problem. This data will be process in the next update of your consciousness.

Your brain exists in an extremely dark and very quiet place, with almost the only sounds coming from your Data Scanning System. I believe this emits a significantly high pitched yet almost silent noise. Sounds also come from your blood coursing through your brain to help keep it cool, healthy and supplied with oxygen and sugar to satisfy its required needs.

Your Data Scanning System is the name I give to that part of your brain with the dedicated role of automatically scanning the data coming in from your five senses: sound, sight, smell, taste and touch, your B.H.S.M.S. and from your internally created thoughts.

b) What would be the consequences if all brains throughout our world stopped operating NOW?!!

To put into perspective the importance of brains to all of our lives, just imagine the fundamental consequences if NOW, **THIS VERY MOMENT,** the *BRAIN of every single human, animal and living creature and the brain equivalent of every single, living* entity **STOPPED FUNCTIONING.**

All humans, animals and creatures would very rapidly begin to die and fall to the ground, etc. All living entities would also enter into a process of dying. All human-driven cars would begin to crash; all flying aircraft would eventually crash land; all moving boats and ships would ultimately collide into something. All of the electrical and gas national power supplies would sooner or later cease and the whole of our planet would be in blackness during the night.

There would be no moving and operating machines or facilities apart from the solar, tidal, river, dammed and wind-powered systems. However, these too would eventually shutdown, if they rely to a degree on nationally supplied electrical supplies outside their own supply, plus operating systems and ongoing maintenance.

The whole of our planet would gradually revert to Mother Nature's basics and natural elements – devoid of its populations, their activities and barren of the moving and static creations of living beings.

SUBCHAPTER 1.2: Your wonderfully magnificent body

OVERVIEW: I believe that The Grand Creator had a 10-out-of-10 day when he/she/it began the creation and continued evolution of your body. This includes the senses, the muscles and sinews, the skeletal structure, the touch sensitivity of your fingers and skin. Other evolutionary tasks involved developing the extraordinarily high-speed coordination between (and within) your brain, and the sensors in your fingertips and toe ends. Another objective was to fix the exact locations of the various physical aspects and muscles of your body positions and the precise balances required to execute all of the ongoing physical objectives you will have.

Also, developing the incredible multiplicity of highly-complex and combinational sequences of movement that you can adopt to achieve the almost unlimited range and sets of positions and postures that your ordinary day-to-day and second-by-second objectives require. If you participate in more demanding physical activities, such as sports, your degree of required movement range and other aspects increase significantly.

When you see what *world-class, professional, specialising humans* in gymnastics, athletics, ballet and all other forms of dancing, music and sports in general achieve, it is utterly breathtaking to behold.

CHAPTER 2.0 – A MORE DETAILED VIEW OF YOUR BODY AND BRAIN'S FUNCTIONALITY

SUBCHAPTER 2.1: How does your *body function*?

OVERVIEW: To keep physically safe and function safely, effectively and healthily, as is necessary for a human being, all of the information, conditions and data inside and outside your body, in your immediate vicinity and beyond (as related to your current situation), including through your five senses (sight, sound, smell, touch and taste), must reach your brain. There it will be analysed, processed and its relevance to you fully understood. This is the case for every waking second (and parts of every second yet to a much reduced degree whilst asleep) during the whole of your life.

NB Your internally created thoughts are already in your brain, as is the data from your Body's Health Status Monitoring System (B.H.S.M.S.). These two sets of data are included in the above processing activities.

In addition to keeping you physically safe, all of these ongoing activities will enable you to make the best decisions and take action appropriate to the prevailing conditions affecting you and concerning your objectives and best interests.

This is a lifelong, ongoing, monumentally major task, which is at the core of you being able to experience a daily, healthy, safe, satisfying and enjoyable life on this earth.

Imagine your body and brain, in simplistic terms.

You, the whole and complete you, are fundamentally comprised of two different types of parts. To use computer parlance, which is understood by increasingly more people, these are called your **hardware parts** and your **software parts.**

AN EXTREMELY IMPORTANT OVERVIEW: The information to follow is of the utmost importance in terms of understanding the very basics of how nearly all of your brain's functionality is derived.

The first key part to take on board is the concept that: a) I believe that there are only three different categories of departments used throughout the whole of your brain, which I choose to name Category 1, Category 1A and Category 1B.

b) Each department category has a particular and very different type of role to play within your brain.

c) The functional operation of these departments is highly complex and can be extremely difficult to grasp for some people unless they have prior familiarity with this type of knowledge. With this in mind, I strongly suggest that you don't focus on their complex names or complexity of operation. Instead, focus on the different roles, jobs and uses they crucially carry out for you every second, hour and day of your whole life.

NB *I have left the complex operational details in the book for those who wish to study them in the immediacy or later.*

SUBCHAPTER 2.1.1: Your Software Parts

As they are not physical, your **software parts** can't be seen. They comprise of data items, information and processing routines, algorithms contained within circuits and sets of circuits, which themselves can <u>reside in groups. They have a common purpose</u> or role to play, normally as a relatively small part of the required, huge amount of overall processing functionality that your brain continually carries out throughout your whole life.

Each of these software groups, and sometimes with possibly other software groups if required, reside <u>within what I call departments.</u> There are an absolute vast number of these groups in total, all of them residing <u>entirely within your brain.</u>

There are only a total of ***three different categories of departments*** *used throughout the vastness of your brain. Each category has a different, specific and particular role to play within the whole set of functional requirements of your brain.*

The role each department is selected for is based upon its particular category. It needs to fully satisfy the particular and precise <u>operational</u> demands of the part of your body or your brain's processing/operational requirements it is dedicated to looking after for the whole of your life.

Each of these different categories and individual departments will contain the appropriate, detailed *design* of circuits of software to enable them to carry out their specific role required of them.

So that each of these different departments can achieve their required objectives and related functionality within the operation of your brain, they have to be able to receive incoming information (which I shall call inputs). These inputs come from their associated (and in some cases, not directly associated) items of sensing hardware – from one or more of your eyes, your ears, or via smell, touch and taste. They can also possibly come through internal inputs from other departments within your brain.

These different sources receive data inputs and pass information into your brain via the appropriate parts of your body's data transfer system. Your internally created thoughts are already in your brain, as is the data from your B.H.S.M.S., and these two sets of data are included in the above processing activities *when required*.

En route to your brain, the data goes through a data format change via a converter. This means it is in a format that your brain can recognise and therefore work with. This allows your brain to be able to analyse the data, identify what it is and what it means to you. It is then able to process it throughout your brain successfully. Data and commands are also passed between circuits within departments and between departments within your brain.

The data describing your brain's internally initiated thoughts is automatically passed into your brain's consciousness creation process. Your B.H.S.M.S. also automatically passes data about any concerns regarding your body's health into your consciousness creation process logic. Both form part of the set of departments used to create and update your consciousness.

It is from this large source of information that, at any given moment, what I call your Master Conductor (your M.C.) knows what it has to do in its crucial duties: orchestrating, managing, controlling and arranging your life.

From within their dedicated departments (which also comprise of subdepartments), each of your software parts or systems also have to carry out a multitude of different detailed tasks. A small sample of these are:

a) Issuing operational commands or triggers (I shall call these outputs) when required. For example, to move or activate parts of your body, they are permanently dedicated to being available to control your body movement, speaking, etc.

b) Outputting or issuing instructions or information to process, communicate and service the requirements of your mind and many other departments within your brain.

c) Providing the functionality in all of its facets, which I will call operational control logic. This is required by each of the systems located in their appropriate different category departments of your brain. It is needed for the complete range of facilities regarding the operation, control, utilisation, processing, updating and generally satisfying the need as required.

NB Reminder: Each of these three different categories of departments are permanently dedicated to looking after and satisfying the needs of their part of your body or your brain's functional requirements they are connected to and associated with.

I guess that the page of details above is a lot to take in at first reading, for which I apologise. However, your brain's ongoing processing functionality is all happening simultaneously (parallel processing) and involves a gargantuan number of data items and communication signals. This means that it makes even a major simplification of what is happening still quite complex to describe and absorb. This is, of course, unless you are used to these types of systems that are used elsewhere in manufacturing and increasingly in modern life.

I would like to refer you back to **AN EXTREMELY IMPORTANT OVERVIEW** in Subchapter 2.1, **a) b)** and **c)** and particularly c) as a reminder upon what to focus on!

To move on then, here are some more details of each of the three different categories of departments that exist within the whole of your brain. For each one, there is a sample of the type of dedicated role they carry out to satisfy all of your ongoing needs and requirements.

A) Category 1 Departments

All of your Fully Automatic, P.I.D., Closed-Loop Measurement and Control Systems.

They exclusively and permanently provide the dedicated measurement, operational control, condition and status for each of your *core functions and facilities.* For example:

- Your heart and your related blood pressure and blood flow
- Your body's temperature
- Your body's blood sugar level
- Your body's breathing requirements
- Your body's chemical health
- Many more core functions and facilities

B) Category 1A Departments

All of your Semi-Automatic, Open Loop Measurement and Control Systems.

They exclusively and permanently set out to monitor and keep in healthy order each of your *core states and conditions.* For example:

- Your mind's emotional/mental health
- Your food consumption control
- Your maintaining a healthy state of your brain's physiological health
- Passing water and opening up your bowels
- Many more core states and conditions

C) Category 1B Departments

All of your Developed, Semi-Automatic, Open Loop (with a degree of measurement) and Control Systems. They exclusively and permanently set out to provide each of your core processes, professional skills, knowledge, understanding and functionalities. For example:

- All Category 1B departments which collectively enable your M.C. to conduct all of the processes required for the creation of your consciousness.
- All Category 1B departments which collectively enable you to carry out all of your considerations, decisions and resultant actions in response to your updated consciousness.
- Many more core processes, professional skills, knowledge, understanding and functionalities.

For more detail about the full functionality and benefits of the three categories of departments above, see Subchapter 2.2.3.

NB *I have laboured this considerable amount of detail about these three categories of departments simply because I believe they are the most commonly used component units used throughout your brain. As such, it is important that you have sufficient knowledge of them as part of your basic understanding of the whole of your brain's functionality. Also, as highlighted on Subchapter 1.1, I would remind you to focus particularly on what job and role each category is used for. Don't get too burdened about their name and complexity of functionality unless you wish to.*

SUBCHAPTER 2.1.2: Your Hardware Parts

Because your hardware parts all have a physical state of existence, they can each be seen. Some are easily visible because they are on the outside of your body, like your arms, legs, hands, eyes, ears, tongue and nose, etc. However, others are unseen, such as your organs, touch sensors and the circuits that carry the electrical signals from each touch sensor back into your brain. Similarly, your muscles, ligaments, tendons, bones and heart, etc., cannot be seen unless they are exposed by opening up the relevant parts of your body.

During your life, some of your *physical parts* are there to maintain your body's state of good health. Others carry out all of your brain and mind's physical, functional, operational and status objectives. This takes place under the power of your *control* systems located within your brain, inside each of their dedicated and appropriate categories: 1, 1A or 1B.

SUBCHAPTER 2.2: *How* does your brain function?

OVERVIEW: *As mentioned previously, but now with additional aspects and details, I believe that your fully developed brain comprises a vast number of individual areas. Due to their functionality and the very specific role they each have, I call them departments. Their processing capacity/size relates to their role and the amount of processing work they are each required to carry out.*

I also think that the whole of your brain provides a total package of facilities of almost indescribable complexity, capability and capacity. It operates as a fully integrated system, *satisfying all of your needs constantly.*

The <u>total functionality</u> of all of these departments and their subdepartments within your brain allows you to keep healthy physically and mentally. It also lets you deal with all of the decision-making you have to face and process, therefore satisfying all of your intellectual objectives and physical functionalities. This permits you to live the life you require every second throughout your lifetime, and it is particularly busy whilst you are awake.

To achieve all of its functionality with the incredible, mind-blowing speed and efficiency with which it functions, including the astronomical *rate* **of recall of data from memories, I believe that** *your brain operates with true parallel processing. I define this as most of its departments, most of the time, are carrying out their dedicated roles, functioning together simultaneously, whilst they are required to be active. Some departments will also be interacting with others, all of which is driven by your prevailing requirements, throughout your entire lifetime, albeit at a much lower level of activity whilst you are asleep.*

SUBCHAPTER 2.2.1:Your brain's Master Conductor (M.C.)

Question A – Why do I believe your brain has a Master Conductor (M.C.)?

Take a moment to consider what your brain actually does and the <u>lightning speed</u> it operates at. Think about the vast number of <u>complex, multi-faceted decisions</u> it makes regarding your aims, objectives and functionalities during <u>every part of every waking second of every day of your life</u>.

Consider the vast number of dedicated, role-specific departments within your brain, many of which will have their own automatic internal data processing activities and two-way communications with various other departments.

Think about the vast number of items of information, data and detail your brain processes from your five senses, your Body's Health Status Monitoring System (B.H.S.M.S.) and your internally created thoughts.

Contemplate the astronomical number of Memory Departments and subdepartments your brain searches to compile and update your ongoing consciousness.

Then, consider that, for every consciously considered decision and action you take, you make *maybe fifty times or more* subconsciously considered decisions and actions.

This is the ongoing total of all of your brain's processing activities, some of which will comprise a sequence of several individual sub-processing steps, whereas others will <u>occur in parallel, simultaneously</u>.

Despite this lifetime of enormous processing workload and its complexity, the <u>*excellent quality and reliability of each decision,*</u> plus the resultant, co-ordinated control with which you conduct yourself, leads me to strongly believe that your brain must have a dedicated, overall monitoring and conducting facility. This is your Master Conductor, which manages and oversees all of this processing, information and results from all departments and subdepartments. It ensures that you **never** suffer from periods of operating in a chaotic and sometimes an absolutely chaotic manner.

Imagine, if you will, if even a very small percentage, of your brain's vast number of departments had the ability, in <u>isolation to each other</u>, to do the following:

a) Decide which incoming data to select to process, from all of the data your brain received, before the vast majority was deleted and before your prevailing consciousness was updated with what warranted your consideration and actions, in order to keep you safe.

b) Decide what your overall objectives, considerations, decisions and related actions were, <u>independently</u> and in contradiction to some or all of your brain's other departments, which were active at that time.

Just imagine the consequences of such an uncoordinated regime.

Your body could be instructed to take a whole range of opposing movements, and your mind could be trying to follow a range of conflicting objectives, causing you to be physically and intellectually out of control. This could range from a small disabling degree to an extremely disabling extent, causing you physically and mentally to thrash around like someone who was completely and utterly out of control – which is precisely what would be the case!

BUT, with people who are mentally, emotionally and functionally healthy, within the bands considered normal, this chaotic, out of control scenario never occurs, thanks to the crucially important and permanent involvement of your Master Conductor.

Question A.2 – What is the fundamental relationship of your M.C. to the principle emotional characteristics we all have and, to a significant degree, need to have?

Admittedly, when your considerations and related actions are driven by too much emotion and too little cold logic, the quality of your actions are often degraded in proportion to the ratio of emotion over cold logic. This is one of the very prominent and potentially powerful traits and characteristics of us human beings.

Our emotions of enthusiasm enable us to ride upon them as we enter into battle to achieve things in our life. Our emotions allow us to experience the most wondrous extremes of joy, satisfaction and pleasure. At the other end of the emotional spectrum, we can experience sheer panic, fear and absolute anger.

At times, these feelings can be beneficial, enabling us to react in the face of danger, keep us safe and remain alive.

I firmly believe that your M.C. is very much involved in the process of the consideration, control and management of each of your subconscious (and conscious) thoughts and resultant actions. However, you are not consciously aware of being involved in all parts of these processes, simply due to the astronomically fast speed at which your subconscious thoughts and decision-making occur.

The exceptions to when your M.C. has no involvement are:

1) When you are acting with involuntary thoughts and actions.
2) With any of the fully automatic control systems of your brain's Category 1 departments.

The third potential exception is:

3) When your Category 1B department, which houses your character and soul, is automatically involved with each decision and related action you take.

You won't necessarily have your M.C.'s involvement with this department, but there is a time when this third exception won't prevail. For example, if, before a decision is made, your M.C., being aware of the developing emotionally charged situation in your mind, decides it is necessary, and it can, it will add some appropriate degree of conscious control. It will adjust the potential dominance that your Character and Soul Department has over your decision-making and particularly your emotional reaction part of the process. Your M.C. will then pre-damp down the degree of your emotional response, and you will be consciously aware of this involvement.

Question B – Where do I think your Master Conductor (M.C.) is located and why?

I propose that, because of the Grand Creator's sensible design influence, your M.C. will reside in as central an area of your brain as is practically possible because:

1) It will have the lowest risk of being damaged from exposure to physical risks external to your head and, therefore, brain. Hopefully it will also have zero risk from exposure to serious infections from contaminated food, etc.

2) For any given speed of data transmission, the shorter the communication pathways are for data to travel from A to B, the faster it will be received by the data recipient. There is also less risk of attenuation, loss of data detail and reduction of accurate resolution.

Therefore, it is beneficial for your M.C. to be as close and central as is possible to all of your different departments and subdepartments with which it has the most frequent need to communicate. This proximity means it can issue instructions to and receive information from each of them in the quickest time possible. This facilitates the completion of each decision-making process and the required, related action as quickly, efficiently, correctly and effectively as possible.

NB Your M.C. communicates literally non-stop with all of your five senses. For the majority of people, the sense that inputs by far the most amount of data is your vision, particularly in the moments when you require maximum visionary detail. Your vision data input location in your brain, along with your other senses data input location's data and their data decoding locations in relation to your M.C., will, I believe, be the optimum arrangement for the fastest data speed transmission.

With the exception of your Category 1 departments, your M.C. actively communicates with all of your brain's other departments, directly with some, and via a Communication Collector Department with others, as appropriate to its prevailing needs.

If your M.C. was damaged, you would be unable to update your consciousness. Therefore, you would be unaware of your surroundings and unable to participate and function as normal in relation to your surroundings and situation. You would be incapable of making any considerations or decisions and taking any actions. However, your core functions and facilities operate fully automatically and independently of your M.C., controlling your heart operation, breathing, blood sugar level, involuntary thoughts and actions etc. These would continue, thus keeping you alive but unable to participate and function in life as normal.

Question C – Who do I think is your Master Conductor?

I believe that Your M.C. exists at the core of your mind and **IT IS YOU!!**

Has this surprised you?!!

Yes, I certainly think you are the master of your ship as she sails the sometimes choppy waters of your seas of life!

In terms of managing, influencing, overseeing and affecting most of your brain's activities, I believe that your M.C.'s role is the most important and critical one of all of the activities throughout the whole of your brain, along with your intelligence, which is also part of your M.C.'s capabilities.

It has the task of being aware of all <u>significant conditions</u>, thoughts, events, data and objectives of all categories, which come from the following sources:

1) All of your brain's departments, all of the time.
2) Inside your body.
3) Outside your body and around your immediate area and beyond, where conditions and activities are affecting your current situation, and be aware of those that may affect you in the near future.
4) Your brain's internally instigated and created thoughts and also, your brain's internally reactivated (unresolved) thoughts.
5) Your brain's externally instigated thoughts, created as a consequence of incoming data.

23

NB Your M.C. is <u>not involved</u> in the actual operation of your Category 1 and 1A departments. However, it will assist in helping to achieve the objectives of these departments control systems if it sees that you/they are experiencing symptoms of difficulties it recognises. For example, if you are becoming extremely hot and/or physically exhausted, it will ensure you take appropriate, rapid measures to recover your healthy status for heart control and/or your body temperature control. Your M.C. will continue to monitor your condition until it has returned to a safe, healthy position.

Your Category 1B department's control systems have many different types of roles. For example, the control of all of your body's physical movements, with each department having a lifelong, dedicated role for operating a particular body part whenever it is called upon to function. Your M.C. will, when necessary, make individual adjustments to a particular Category 1B department's control system. This compensates for any prevailing ambient conditions that would otherwise prevent the Control System's target or positioning objectives from being achieved, e.g. slippery conditions, rough conditions underfoot, gusty winds, people pushing etc.

Your M.C. makes basic decisions on objectives and their related actions for you based on the information that it derives from its observational and conducting role, plus requests for information and what it is made aware of via the many automatic sources of information throughout your brain. All of the while, it keeps you operating and functioning in a balanced, controlled and efficiently achieving manner whilst also monitoring your degree of emotion and

any biases you may be employing as part of your decision-making/
considerations process.

Question D – What creates your level of intelligence, what form does it exist in, and does it change with age?

OVERVIEW: *I believe that, fundamentally, your prevailing level of intelligence is created from the interactive combination of all of your current, characteristics, capabilities, skills and knowledge, residing within the very many departments, groups and sections of which your M.C. comprises and is in control of. The source of some of these qualities is your inherited genes.*

I don't think that your intelligence exists as a single entity, residing in a particular location in one of your M.C.'s very many groups of departments.

In the OVERVIEW above, I say prevailing because I believe that your effective level of intelligence is variable due to a number of factors:

a) The topic or situation you are applying it to and how much detailed knowledge you have at that time, in relation to this particular subject.

b) The state of your emotional health at that time, can significantly influence how effective your Intelligence level is.

c) Your attitude and how keen you are (or otherwise) to help, assist or solve the situation you are applying your

25

intelligence to. Please note that this could also be part of point **b)** on occasion.

Very importantly, I also consider that your intelligence exists over a very wide range of capabilities in the same or similar cohorts. It can also manifest itself in many different forms and therefore be utilised in multiple varied situations and settings.

NB Your soul can exist within an extensive list of possible and very different types of souls. See Subchapter 6.1.3, Question 3.

Similarly, your Intelligence can manifest itself in many different forms or categories. Each of these can be optimally utilised in an expansive list of very different scenarios or settings, with some comprising several diverse and possibly combined basic scenarios.

A few classic examples of different forms or skills that are perceived as demonstrating intelligence are:

1) A person being able to solve a problem or successfully resolve a challenging situation that they had not faced or dealt with before and therefore not seen the solution or watched others solve it.

2) A person commonly perceived by others as generally being enlightened, having the faculty of excellent reasoning and a good, speedy understanding of many different topics.

3) A person who has a high IQ rating. Interestingly, though, I know a person who is very clearly in this category, yet they

always modestly insisted that it simply demonstrated they were good at taking IQ tests.

4) A person generally perceived by others as being gifted with some or all of the following traits: being mentally penetrating, discerning, practically wise, acute-minded, shrewd and demonstrating profound wisdom, proposing solutions to many situations.

I believe that probably, at least the majority of your characteristics, fundamental capabilities and skills are inherited from your genes and are therefore innate at your conception. The departments each begin developing after your birth from their foundational state. They will continue *to improve during the rest of your life*, **providing** your brain, mental, emotional health and physical health remain in good order. It is also essential to retain an ongoing energy and zest for life, and keep pushing and challenging yourself to learn and to improve.

I consider that your brain is probably the most powerful single processing unit in the Universe, and I also think it thrives on being kept usefully busy. So, in order to maintain its optimum organic, functional health and intelligence, it is crucially important to keep it usefully busy, at least, most of the time. This includes whilst you are asleep so it can have completed all of its required activities each night before you awake.

Again, with these ongoing requirements being fully satisfied, as your life continues, the remainder of your skills will continue to stay sharp. In some cases, they will improve, for example, the speed, efficiency, quality and the range and depth of aspects you perceive and review during your decision-making. All this will happen as you have more experiences and consequently develop knowledge and confidence from which to draw.

Also, again with the same proviso reasons as above, I most firmly believe that you are capable of learning new skills, despite your age. Learning gives your mental health, plus potentially, dependent upon these new skills, your physical health an additional boost, too. For all of these reasons, I consider that your level of Intelligence should at least be maintained, if not continue to improve as you grow older.

I don't prescribe to the very commonly stated view that your brain development reaches a peak at the age of 30 years or so, for the reasons I have mentioned. Additionally, I strongly feel that, because of the total of all of the different aspects and sub-aspects, knowledge and memories, etc., of which we each comprise, we are all unique human beings: currently, in the past and in the future!

I have seen many people retire in a very good state of physical and mental health, particularly from a job where their brain has been a key part of their work. They come back to work to simply visit every few months, desperately trying to recapture close contact with fellow workers and resume some of their old work experiences, pleasures and self-worth as human beings. Very sadly, you can see them ageing at an alarming rate because they have pretty much stopped challenging their brain. The consequences are that their brain's capability, intelligence, degree of daily satisfaction, etc., diminish rapidly. You are witnessing the decaying human spirit, which, particularly in someone you enjoyed a very close relationship with over many years, is a very sad experience to behold!

Question E – What are the locations within your brain of your mind, M.C. and your three different types of departments, Categories 1, 1A and 1B, and what are the interactions between them all?

OVERVIEW: I believe that this very basic organisation and the contents within this arrangement is the foundation of all of the areas of functionality within the whole of your brain.

Your involuntary thoughts and **actions and all of the** functionalities, facilities and outputs created by your Category 1 departments, all take place without any influence from your mind or its Master Conductor (M.C.). (There are nominally one or two minor exceptions, one of which is the normal, automatic control of your breathing which you can consciously control if you feel this is required.)

All of the functionalities, facilities and outputs created by your **Category 1A** *departments take place with regular assistance from your M.C.to achieve their objectives.*

Your mind, under the management and control of your M.C. controls, deals with:

a) All of the continuing creation, updating and responses to your consciousness.

b) Updating your Category 1B <u>Memory</u> Departments, along with updating all of your other Category 1B departments.

c) Processing all of your thoughts whilst awake and asleep throughout your whole life. These include your brain's internally created thoughts, thoughts you are consciously aware of and the ones below your conscious awareness, your reasoning, decision-making and related actions under all conditions.

Within the boundary of your total and complete mind, which is the only one you have, are the following two major departments collections in your brain:

Collection 1 – Many multiples of groups made up of the majority of your vast number of Category 1B departments.

Collection 2 – Your Master Conductor's family of many departments, comprising the remainder of your Category 1B departments that are located within your mind.

Outside the boundary of your mind but within your brain, reside the following two major collections:

Collection 3 – All of your Category 1 departments existing in a large number of groups.

Collection 4 – All of your multiples of groups comprising solely of your *Category 1A departments*.

I propose that within your mind, in order to be able manage the ongoing monumental workload required to process all of the extremely simplified activities described above, at the astronomical speed achieved, the following communications take place when required:

1.0 Two way communication occurs between your M.C. and most of the other departments within your mind. This communication comprises, for example, your M.C. requesting data from an appropriate Memory Department. Or, your M.C. automatically receives a warning from one of your Vision Departments that it had seen a dangerous activity whilst you are driving a car. Your M.C. is immediately directed to view it and responds as it deems necessary.

2.0 Each department can communicate directly with every other department.

3.0 Each department can communicate with its own sub⁻departments.

4.0 Your M.C. is automatically provided with information from several other dedicated departments regarding several different data categories. For example, it is notified about the identification of a situation that requires an immediate response from you, and your M.C. needs to instigate an appropriate reaction.

This communication structure reduces a significant percentage of the processing workload from your M.C. and distributes it out to the other departments in your mind where possible. This, crucially and importantly, results in speeding up your brain's processing times required to respond to and complete whatever urgent actions are necessary.

Question F – Do you have an unconscious mind, and what do you need to be aware of?

NB It appears to me that many people support the beliefs that I list below. I hasten to add that I DO NOT SUPPORT THEM AT ALL, but nevertheless, here they are for your consideration.

1.0 We each have a conscious mind and ostensibly, a separate, unconscious mind, with the Conscious Mind being by far the smaller of the two, in terms of capacity and total capability.

2.0 There exists only an elusive connection between your conscious and unconscious mind. Without a strong connection between your conscious and unconscious mind, you are unable to create great works of artistic beauty and sporting prowess in the arts and sports.

3.0 Your conscious mind carries out your basic decision-making, and you are aware of each detail.

4.0 Your unconscious mind is outside the managed reach, study and control of your conscious mind. This is despite the fact that your unconscious mind plays a major role in most of your decision-making and its related actions.

5.0 You are not in control of most of the deliberations and decisions that you make as a person.

6.0 People debate how they can best engage and utilise their unconscious mind's extreme positive powers and capabilities of for their benefit, i.e. how can they turn these features on when required?

7.0 Some people discuss how they can best manage and minimise the potential negative powers of their unconscious mind.

<u>My beliefs and</u> <u>why</u> <u>I don't agree with any of these philosophies above are</u>:

1.0 I do not believe that you have an unconscious mind at all. I think you have one complete mind, all of which your M.C. has total access to and ostensibly can manage and control.

I much prefer to use the word *subconscious* rather than *unconscious,* when referring to your mind's activities that take place below your conscious awareness at the times of these activities. They happen when thoughts and decisions are being processed so ultra-fast they are therefore below your conscious awareness.

2.0 With the exception of your Category 1 departments, during a weekly period of your life, for you to live the full life you desire, second-by-second, your mind communicates with and utilises, via other departments, the majority of all of the departments

33

throughout your mind and within your brain's Category 1A departments.

3.0 Your mind, under the management and control of your M.C., reviews and responds to your prevailing needs as presented to you by your current consciousness. This is continually being updated, and this process continues throughout your life.

4.0 This decision-making is, at times, extremely complex, and, by virtue of the situations you are experiencing, it sometimes requires ultrafast consideration and decision-making. Inherently, this means that you are not consciously aware of all of the details of this process, particularly during highly problematic, fast-changing situations. However, in my opinion, this does not mean that you are not managing or in control of it all.

NB I am aware that I have repeated many times in this book, the principle of you (your M.C.) being in control at all times. Please forgive me for having done this. I have deliberately done so because, I believe that it is perhaps one of the most fundamental aspects of how your brain functions. Therefore, mentioning this feature within different functional environments of your brain will hopefully allow you to become comfortable with this concept, achieving a clearer feeling and ultimately a better understanding of it.

5.0 The highly charged, emotionally-driven elements of your character are extremely beneficial when your life or physical wellbeing are endangered . They have the potential to give you more physical strength, enhanced emotional determination and focus, with your brain working significantly quicker, which assists in your resolving the situation successfully. However, the potentially negative aspects of your character and the emotionally-driven reactions to scenarios that are not life or death are, I believe, primary risk areas. This is when your decision-making and actions are potentially liable to range from bad to possibly terrible ones.

I consider the most effective way to manage the potentially harmful powers of your character and soul, both of which are embedded within your mind, is to strive to become aware of them (There are hopefully not too many, with the vast majority of elements being positive ones). Learn to be mindful of the decision-making situations and environments that these unfavourable aspects are liable to emotionally and automatically impact your decision-making and reactions.

In my opinion, the highest risk of you being negatively influenced emotionally is when you are in a situation where you have to respond *fairly quickly* to a set of conditions. These often include other people and their inherent emotional attitudes, which inevitably combine with yours, thus possibly producing an explosive and possible highly emotionally-charged, emotionally interactive environment. Having made yourself aware of these risks, you can hopefully avert or at least minimise the impact of these negative influences before considering, then making decisions and taking their related actions.

Despite recognition of the extreme difficulties of achieving it, in addition to the aspects mentioned above, you should ideally aspire to improve your character and soul where you honestly see improvements can be made, thus minimising their harmful elements.

From my personal experiences and observing others, it is possible, providing you have the will to do so. Try to progress by gradually making relatively small and realistically achievable changes each time. Additionally, do not lose sight of the benefits stated of these emotional elements when you are in danger and probably angry.

Sometimes only one of these other decision/reactive drivers of, say, <u>your extreme dislike of someone will prevail,</u> to the extent that this driver alone causes you to ignore all other elements of rational and logical consideration. When this occurs, it will normally happen so quickly and forcefully it is likely to swamp and override the other considerations you were reviewing or going to review.

Another aspect is that the person themselves will readily detect your extreme dislike of them. If this occurs where you both work and they are in a higher position, maybe a much higher role than you, whether you work for them or not, you are at extreme risk of causing you very serious work-related trouble. This is a situation where you benefit from being very mindful. It is also best to be aware of your particular characteristics, etc., and consciously attempt to control them by foreseeing their occurrences, therefore suppressing them before you allow something negative to happen, or at least minimise their effect.

You may realise or say to yourself – this advice of not falling foul of your emotional decision- making drivers is theoretically sound, yet extremely difficult to actually follow in real life at the height of the decision making process. This, I admit, is true, and it also has the added difficulty for you in the first instance of <u>recognising</u> and <u>confronting</u> your weaknesses. Nevertheless, the benefits of such actions are immense, and therefore it is worth working at developing these skills and applying them.

It is, once again, about harnessing and then utilising the awe-inspiring, immense power of your mind. If you have it working for you with intent, confidence and determined focus to succeed, you will eventually be successful. Remember, everything gained of any significant value usually only comes after relevant and sustained hard work and the firmly held belief that you will succeed *á* la your placebo effect.

6.0 I believe that you can't unlock and engage these incredibly powerful elements by consciously requesting them. The way to harness the extremely positive and beneficial powers embedded within your mind, where your character and soul reside, is by consciously reacting positively to the situation you find yourself in, even when it is extremely challenging. Once this positive, totally focused and constructive process begins, it will acquire a self-generating and continuing momentum of benefits to you and those connected to you or who are engaged in the process you are in. I don't believe you need to, or even more so, it is best not to force any of the prevailing conditions to achieve the best level of targets or objectives you are aspiring to.

EXAMPLE: Let me give you an example of how I see this process developing in the real world.

You are dancing with your wife, your dancing partner of many years. You have reached the Ballroom World Championships Final again, as for the last three years, but you have finished third each time previously.

You are both beginning to struggle a little with some physical issues, which become relevant at this level of performance and you both know this is probably your last chance to win. Also, a new, young couple have appeared on the scene, and everyone is expecting them to win.

You walk onto the floor to dance the last dance of the competition. As you prepare to take up hold, your absolute favourite Waltz called Papillion starts to flood the whole ballroom with its magical music. You both exchange the most intense eye contact. The twenty years of practice you have committed to each other wells up deep from within your souls and you say to your wife, "Let's do this, darling."

The napes of your necks and your bodies tingle with latent, controlled power, intensity, total and utter focused intention and control as you both simultaneously enter the zone. Despite your brains operating automatically at very high speeds, time appears to slow down.

You commence dancing with majestic, controlled, deep confidence at a level you have not quite reached before, other than for very fleeting moments, during a dance. This time, from start to finish, you are both on it. The sheer majesty of your dancing, your frames' poise, balance, edge of control, your sways, your constant and continuous flow of movement, the look of purpose and sheer enjoyment in your eyes and faces created wonderment in your souls. There was an aura around both of you that the judges and all of the 2000 knowledgeable audience can't fail to enjoy, appreciate, wonder at and be mesmerised by.

You obtain the highest marks ever achieved in this competition and are duly crowned World Ballroom Champions.

The experiences above can and do occur in real life. They are an example of how you connect to and utilise all of the best, most constructive and beneficial aspects of your characters and souls and also fully engage your placebo effect. The negative elements that we all have, to some degree, were swamped out by the positive aspects that you both were fired up by, culminating in the performance you achieved.

The unlocking and engagement of these required elements from your character and soul can be utilised to enhance many other activities, for example:

1) Composing and Conducting music and the choreography of all styles of dancing.

2) Writing books and other articles.

3) Playing music.

4) Delivering a speech, talk or lecture of major importance to you.

5) Participating in a whole range of sporting activities.

6) Participating in a whole range of the multitude of wondrous activities of life.

7) Painting, sculpting and crafting, etc.
8) Passing on your acquired wisdom in particular skills to others via formal and carefully constructed informal teaching, demonstrating and lecturing.

The sheer pleasure and satisfaction derived from your performance are so satisfying to enjoy, and money just can't buy experiences such as these. The achievement may be at a local pub, school venue, or it may be at the Olympic games. The higher the level of competition will normally bring greater strength, depth of satisfaction and a longer duration of strong remembrance. This is mainly due to you having spent disproportionately more time practising and training, so the worth and external quantity of recognition of your achievement is so much more.

What is of absolute, critical importance to produce your required best performance is not to let certain potentially damaging elements of your character emerge. For example, excessive raw, uncontrolled determination or anger, or too much focused pointed application. Each of these emotions can vitally contribute positively to your performance, providing that none of them rises to too high a level. When this occurs, your judgement becomes cloudy, and your clarity of thought becomes fuzzy, causing your performance to fall away. There is a corresponding drop in your confidence, creating a downward spiral of achievement and standard of execution.

During my life, I have played a tremendous amount of sport within teams and individually, from 5 to 47 years of age and reaching a high level, particularly in one of them. I have experienced being in the zone often and recognise the critical importance of having the correct and healthy psychological attitudes whilst training, especially when competing.

Getting all of these aspects right makes the difference from being an also-ran to a winner. Being able to feed off the pressure from competing and not succumb to its presence harnesses the tremendous power of your mind. It creates an incredible high-speed performance of your mind and body coordination and generates significant additional muscular power when required. It also produces an extreme determination to continue battling the challenging and difficult conditions, compete and eventually win, whatever winning means in the particular situation.

To preserve the full availability of these facilities, I found that you have to utilise the maximum level of this wondrous power in small packets, and when it really matters. So, when you are training and maybe performing at lower and less important occasions, you operate at a reduced level of performance. However, not too low, or you will develop mental and physical bad habits and too low a performance level from which you will struggle to rise from, when it really matters.

Also, in terms of achieving what you wish to achieve without upsetting someone else in the process, what I find extremely interesting is that all of my life, I have been interested in psychology. I have observed and studied a vast number of people, plus carried out a lot of self-observation, self-consideration and self-questioning. Over many years, I have met a lot of people from numerous walks of life and helped them with their difficulties and along the pathways of their life.

I worked in industry all of my life and, looking back with a detailed review, I realised that I had probably used psychology every day in my working life and also outside, in my social life, in an extremely long list of applications:

- Interviewing people to decide whether they were suitable candidates for a job.
- Selling my ideas to other people who had to approve them.
- Getting people to do what I wished them to do in a pleasant and effective manner, particularly when they palpably did not wish to do it.
- Playing sport to win.
- Coaching techniques and attitudes to use in sport.
- Understanding what makes an individual tick, to adopt the best tactics for success with them, but always without them realising what you were doing.
- The list goes on and on and on.

I have concluded that we all use and receive psychological tactics quite a lot more than we realise.

Question G – What determines the quality of your prevailing consciousness?

I believe that the quality of your prevailing consciousness is directly proportionate to your level of intelligence. However, this is based on the following being true:

The quality and functional conditions and performance of each of your senses, with all the hardware of which they comprise, in addition to your five senses' processing systems, your B.H.S.M.S. and your internal thoughts, are all in excellent working order

Essentially, this means that you have to be in an emotionally healthy, well-rested, totally focused state of mind to engage fully and therefore apply the maximum/potential level of Intelligence you have available.

For more details on answering this question, refer to Question D in Subchapter 2.2.1.

Question H – What separate sections, containing groups of departments, does your M.C. comprise, in terms of categories of departments, and what is the role of each of them?

OVERVIEW: The following are the 11 separate sections, numbered 1.0 to 11.0, each of which houses groups of their required departments. I propose that the details of these sections and their departments are what your M.C. is comprised of, and they reside entirely within your mind.

Section 1.0 – This is comprised of 1 x Group of 7 of the vitally important seven Category 1B departments for developing, housing and utilising your consciousness, which is the foundation upon which nearly all of your brain's activities are based.

I believe that you have your consciousness as a priority, to ensure you are aware of any situations and conditions that jeopardise your safety. It helps you make the appropriate decisions and actions to ensure that these dangers are dealt with or removed, thereby maintaining your ongoing physical and emotional health and safety.

Your consciousness is also to crucially provide you with all of the additional, current information you require to be aware of about all prevailing situations and conditions that affect you. These are not related to your safety but ones that require your immediate attention and consideration. This information enables you to make decisions and take related actions to each prevailing condition/s, thus resolving all issues requiring prompt resolution and catering for some with longer time scales to completion.

Your ongoing consciousness provides the catalysts and the primary window of information into your immediate, local world in which you live, plus the rest of the world when you are engaging with presented news. It continuously enables and assists you to aim to achieve all of your academic goals, your functional objectives and all other categories of aims and objectives throughout your life.

Section One comprises the following Category 1B departments:

One for each of your five senses, one for your internally created thoughts, one for your B.H.S.M.S., and one for your data scanning review system, which is where your prevailing updated consciousness resides.

With regards to warnings from your B.H.S.M.S., it is vitally important that they are recognised in the fastest possible time and that your M.C. is immediately made aware of the problem. This is particularly important with those that relate to your body's physical safety, vital services, fundamental health status or mental health status. Your M.C. will initiate and manage the required actions. It will then monitor the ongoing situation and instigate additional actions to help restore to normal your safety, the health of your vital service, your physical health or your mental health as is appropriate.

Section 2.0 – This is comprised of a number of Category 1B departments that are very important for communicating.

Your Category 1B departments are located within your M.C. and also located outside your M.C. but inside the boundary of your mind. These communicating departments are also for communicating with all of your Category 1A departments which are outside your mind and within your brain.

Section 3.0 – This is comprised of a vast number of very important Category 1B departments for the utilisation of all of the relevant memory, knowledge and information departments within your brain.

Their role is to *understand the current or immediate relevance* of all information received from your five senses, your Body's Health Status Monitoring System and all your internally created thoughts. All of these departments mentioned are located within your M.C., which is located within the boundary of your mind.

This aspect of your M.C.'s work is the primary source of data (information) from which your prevailing consciousness is derived and understood. Its current/updated version is being held as detailed in Section 1.0 above.

Section 4.0 – This is comprised of a very large number of Category 1B departments (all of which are located within your M.C.).

These departments utilise your relevant <u>developed semi-automatic skills</u> to carry out the particular physical and/or mental activities or skills required to achieve your <u>current objectives</u>.

Your M.C.'s relationship with each of your developed semi-automatic skills, when in use, is *absolutely vital* because these skills are based on a basic set of detailed bodily instructions, or, for other skills, as appropriate, stored within the relevant Category 1B department's control system/s software. These instructions are sent out from your brain to achieve your required bodily actions, required functionality, or skills. However, they *always* need detailed fine-tuning by your M.C. in the moment to accommodate the prevailing ambient conditions. This achieves the required end results from each of your developed semi-automatic skills when they are in use.

NB I believe that your M.C. is, as always, in control of your final decision making and resultant activities. However, due to the phenomenal speed at which it and your mind operate, most of its considerations and actions are subconscious, i.e. well below your conscious awareness. This makes it appear, albeit incorrectly, that you are not involved with each part of this process.

Section 5.0 – This is comprised of at least three very important Category 1B departments that house your <u>short, middle and longer-term memories.</u>

These are required for part of your quick, middle-term and longer-term decision-making objectives. Your M.C. enters relevant information it has gathered from your other departments into a section in one of these memory departments and uses this information as part of its coming to a conclusion about each prevailing decision to be made.

NB. If your M.C. has difficulty making a quick decision and has more time available, it will continue reviewing this pending choice. If it is still unresolved, this can also take place whilst you sleep. You will probably have found, at times, you have come to a very acceptable decision upon waking.

Section 6.0 – This is comprised of quite a number of Category 1B departments that house some extremely important parts of which your intelligence partly derives from: your overall chairmanship, management skills and the ability to review situations extremely quickly and clearly.

Your M.C. uses this department's ability to be able to see the <u>framework </u>of the problem or situation within a large and complex system clearly, and therefore know what actions are required to satisfy the prevailing objectives.

Your M.C. also utilises this department to decide what information and considerations must be obtained and reviewed in the best order (some reviews will create other aspects that also require consideration). The results are "comparison weighted" to decide which one or ones have the most worth, to make the appropriate judgement and take the actions required for each objective or decision made.

A vitally important part of an excellent decision-making process is to be able to realise the following:

a) When you struggle to make what you _feel_ is a good quality decision, yet don't resort to making any decision 'just to get it done.' However, sometimes, when a decision is time-critical, you may be forced to make one under the expediency of time pressure.

b) Why you are struggling due to insufficient data about some aspect, or maybe some of the data you have is not valid or correct, or perhaps you do not understanding some of the data correctly.

c) You know where to obtain the additional information you judge to be required.

d) You know when a second opinion is best obtained, and/or you carry out a review of some of the data again.

Section 7.0 – This is comprised of a large and particularly influential Category 1B department, which is your soul. Your soul contains all of the elements of your unique human characteristics – your character – with most of them influenced to a degree by your genes.

This department also houses your developed attitudes, biases and personal views, derived from all of your vast number of different types of experiences in your life to date, with probably some additional genetic influences. It is most important that you are aware of the consequences of being guided by some of these influences, particularly <u>during some situations</u>. A combination of these influences will have a bearing upon every consideration, decision and action you take. This can range from a minor degree to a potentially major one, when you may have excluded all sensible and related logic and knowledge from your decision-making process.

Your soul sits at the core of your existence as a unique human being, and ostensibly, you are unable to alter any creative aspect from which it comprises. Crucially though, I think that if you really wish to, believe you can, and make a determined effort to do so, you can modify the influences it has upon your decision-making process. I also believe that, the longer you consciously try to dominate these parts that sit at the core of your influencing existence and require control under certain situations, the more your character-driven influences become beneficial. This leads you to make the best or most pragmatic decisions along with their related actions.

Hopefully, your M.C. will have learnt to be aware of and foresee the types of situations and their consequential decisions and actions developing. It will know when these character traits and views are best suppressed or toned down and will therefore attempt to do this.

Unfortunately, some people are not very good at these aspects and, consequently, make many poor decisions, particularly when driven primarily, if not exclusively, by their emotional reactions to a situation they are dealing with. This part of your M.C.'s role is such an important one for you to be aware of and to continually work at improving by being constructively self-critical and able to accept constructive criticism from others.

I believe that your M.C. uses this department where your soul resides as part of your decision and action making process. Therefore, in addition to cold, logical reasoning (as <u>will only ever be the case</u> from man-made, man-programmed, decision-making machine systems, such as a computer or robot), a range of human elements is included which have a wide range of degrees of importance upon the finalised decision.

I believe that part of this department houses your intuitional decision-making tool, which is quite often referred to as your <u>gut instinct</u>. This is potentially a powerful and quick tool to employ. In the case of dealing with severe danger or when it is essential that a decision is made extremely quickly, it can be the best and most expedient decision-making method to employ. If you have more time available, it is always better to mull over your gut instinct action or solution to hopefully either feel even more confident or not that it is the best decision to action.

This decision-making tool is potentially incredibly powerful in its speed of obtaining an answer and the multitude of factors and items of considerations that we <u>presume</u> that your brain is utilising to arrive at a solution. We make this presumption because the incredible speed of the arrival of most of your answers means that most of its considerations are below your conscious awareness. I believe that this why you just *feel* that your gut instinct decision is the *correct* one. You are unaware of the majority of reasons which have combined to create your decision.

Section 8.0 – This is comprised of a very large and particularly important Category 1B department housing your <u>planning</u> and <u>forward-thinking abilities</u>.

It is used to foresee the possible future consequences and results of decisions being considered, upon their being implemented, to make better quality, final decisions.

NB This department works closely with Section 6.0.

Section 9.0 – This is comprised of a substantial and important Category 1B department for giving your M.C. the ability, whilst you are awake, to think and have conscious, creative thoughts, e.g. daydreaming about a lovely holiday experience. Alternatively, you may have significant, purposeful thoughts to solve a situation that requires a decision to be made about anything in your life.

The process for this may include your M.C. issuing a request to another department, say, a Memory Department, to find some information for you. These thoughts or instructions will be in words that are spoken silently within your mind, but you can hear them as if they are real spoken words. Because of this,

I believe that these thoughts are internally processed to be understood in the same way as physically spoken words that you hear via your hearing sense.

Section 10.0 – This is comprised of a significant, large number of Category 1B departments for assessing, managing and dealing with social interactions with other people directly – face-to-face, or indirectly – via E-mail, phone etc.

By judging what their reaction and influence in situations may be and relating them to conditions, you are making decisions or estimations upon several things, which include:

All social skills; all of the relevant characteristics of diverse types of people, good and bad; different sexes; nationalities, and data relating to all of the people you have met throughout your life. In some cases, you have not actually physically met, but have read about, observed, heard about, maybe formed opinions of and perhaps conversed with them over different types of media.

Particularly when you are interacting face-to-face with a large group of people about a wide range of important issues, I believe that these activities involve engaging an enormous amount of brain processing power at speed. They also engage a wide range of different departments' activities within your brain so that you conduct these social interactions in a skilful, efficient, effective, enjoyable and productive manner.

Section 11.0 – This is comprised of a large number of Category 1B departments that work in conjunction with your M.C. when you SLEEP, servicing <u>many activities within your brain to</u>:

a) Assist in achieving, as far as is practical, a healthy state of
    your body's functional and physical health.

b) Review, delete or process, as appropriate, all new data: new
    experiences data and new learned experiences and attitudes
    data; new semi-automatic skills and any other types of new
    data received since your last sleep. All of this will have been
    located in a temporary, new data Category 1B department.

c) Be able to install into memory, each item or new data set in
    its appropriate Category 1B department with its location
    within it. This includes the appropriate information
    about each item, set or sets of data within each Memory
    Department.

d) Be able to delete, refresh and update <u>all existing memories,
    data and information</u> of all the numerous categories, as
    required.

e) Create your dreams, as part of your brain dealing with
    reducing your prevailing anxiety and emotional stress.
    This is how it finds good solutions to the problems you
    are currently dealing with, or in some cases, not dealing
    sufficiently well with.

NB Whilst you are awake your brain is very active and, at times,
extremely busy, compared to whilst you are asleep when you
are busy but not nearly as much so. Whilst awake, your brain is
processing the vast amount of incoming data from your senses,
your <u>B.H.S.M.S.</u> and <u>your internal thoughts</u>. It is also dealing
with all of the physical and mental activities that emanate

from this continual process which is to create/update your consciousness and take its required actions.

Due to this ongoing high processing workload, I believe that your brain relies heavily upon your nightly sleep, when only a small percentage of these "whilst awake activities" require processing. This enables it to carry out extremely large amounts of processing work to achieve its objectives, as stated above.

The total amount of restorative and filing work it must be able and allowed to carry out during your sleep requires many different types of activities to occur. This places such critical importance upon you having sufficient hours of good quality sleep every night for your brain to complete its large workload, meaning it has put its house in order. Consequently, when you wake up, it is refreshed and raring to take on the challenge of the new day with great vigour.

This healthy situation will allow you to enjoy good, ongoing mental and physical health. The average human brain's continuous effective and basic actual workload whilst awake is awesomely immense. It varies during the day in relation to what you are doing and what emotional and climate of expectation prevails, particularly whilst carrying out your job at work. This is why it is so important to have a proper lunchtime break. It gives your brain sufficient recovery time to tackle the afternoon work period efficiently and effectively, with you enjoying an emotionally upbeat state of mind.

SUBCHAPTER 2.2.2: The different types or categories of thoughts.

OVERVIEW: All the thoughts detailed in this chapter, IN ADDITION to the data mentioned in the previous NB section, will have combined to create all the decisions you make. These decisions culminate in creating the related actions you take throughout your lifetime.

A) Whilst Awake – Your Conscious Thoughts

Your related and dedicated Category 1B departments provide the capabilities, with your M.C. managing their processing.

Whenever you make a decision, your M.C. formulates <u>all</u> your thoughts, but the category of your **conscious thoughts** would be the only ones you were consciously aware of. This means you were aware of their existence and, therefore, their contribution towards the final decision and subsequent action taken related to the situation you were dealing with.

An Example:

1.0 Your phone rings at home, and it is the local butcher, Tom, saying that your Christmas turkey has arrived. It has turned out 2 kg heavier than predicted. He asks, "Are you happy to pay £5.50 more and would you like to collect it on Monday or Tuesday of next week? This will be the last day for collection."

You decide that Tom is always fair and trustworthy, and Uncle Ted will probably come for Christmas lunch now. However, even if not, it is fresh and the leftovers will make nice sandwiches and/ or curry, so you say yes to the extra weight/cost.

You remember that you will be away on Monday and not back home until Tuesday, late afternoon, so you have to ask a pre-answer question of, "What time on Tuesday will you close?"

Tom answers, "5 pm sharp, due to numerous commitments."

You remember that Cousin Fred, who you are visiting on that day, makes it extremely difficult to get away and also, the traffic home on Tuesday is going to be extremely heavy. You explain these aspects to Tom and that you will aim to collect the turkey on Tuesday between 4 and 4.30pm. If you get stuck, you suggest you could ring to say you couldn't make it and would it be possible for you to collect it from his home very shortly afterwards.

Tom considers this question for a second and remembers that you have always been a very good customer. He judges you to be the type of person who wouldn't take advantage of and make a habit of expecting this type of service regularly, so although he doesn't want to set precedents of this type, he decides to say yes.

You say, "Many thanks, Tom. I very much appreciate your understanding and help."

This very simple processing of information, describes the straightforward steps of logic, memory, character assessment and the prevailing characters of both people involved in this interaction. It is a predominantly <u>consciously controlled and consciously aware decision-making process</u>, with the addition from Tom of a gut instinct-type decision-making element which will include quite a high percentage of Subconscious thoughts.

B) Whilst Awake – Your Subconscious Thoughts

Your related and dedicated Category 1B departments provide the capabilities, with your M.C. managing their processing.

If you were asked, from <u>all</u> of your thoughts your M.C. had formulated about a particular decision, to select and highlight <u>*only*</u> those in the category of subconscious thoughts, you would be unable to. This is because they were the ones that <u>your M.C. had been involved with processing</u>, but, you were not consciously aware of their existence (because they were *below* your consciousness due to the high speed at which they were processed). Therefore, you would not be aware of their contribution towards the final decision and action taken concerning the situation you had to deal with.

C) Whilst Asleep – Subconscious Thoughts and Imagined Actions

Your related and dedicated Category 1B departments provide the capabilities, with your M.C. managing their processing.

I believe that these are the very many subconscious thoughts and imagined actions taken by your M.C. whilst you are asleep. There are many departments and subdepartments in which there are multiple processing actions undertaken as you sleep.

During this time, your brain is extremely hard at work, reviewing and updating data within its departments. It is putting itself and your emotional, chemical and physical health in good order, ready for you to face the world on waking, in an operationally fit and emotionally healthy state.

D) Whilst Awake – Your Instinctive Thoughts

Your related and dedicated Category 1B departments provide the capabilities, with your M.C. managing their processing.

In my opinion, these are your thoughts with their resultant actions that are innate. You are born with in their basic form and they are developed and improved with learning and experience. They are normally a self-preservation response; to protect your or someone else's safety.

They are actions processed through your M.C. so that you maintain an overall managed, cohesive, interrelated, effective and safe set of actions and reactions at all times.

Please note in the **NB** just before Subchapter 2.2.2 that: in addition to your internal thoughts data, you receive data from your senses, <u>and B.H.S.M.S.</u>, plus when dealing with all of the physical and mental activities that emanate from this continual process, which is to create/update your consciousness and take its required actions.

It is commonly thought that instinctive thoughts and actions occur automatically, <u>outside of</u> your control. I do not hold with this view, particularly when an instinctive action happens to protect your safety or life or to protect someone else's. Due to the nature of the situation, your <u>extraordinary, high-speed</u> recognition of it and your resultant response/s they all occur well below your conscious awareness. Therefore, it <u>appears</u> that your

M.C. has not been involved in the sequence of events. However, I believe that it has. It has to have been involved so that whatever instinctively-driven actions you are pushed to take, they are done under your M.C.'s review. It will control the final triggering of actions considering other prevailing conditions and objectives. Your M.C. will also evaluate other additional possible actions required at that time, so you are always operating in an orderly, overviewing, safe, efficient, objective and effective manner.

NB If taken without consideration of other prevailing conditions and their related actions, instinctively driven actions may place you in even greater danger. This danger may oppose the objectives of the other instinctively-driven action you have been guided to take. Should you continue with further opposing decisions and actions, you will increasingly become stricken by a mess of conflicting and maybe dangerous activities. You will give the appearance of someone acting out of sensible control – which would be the case.

E) Whilst Awake and Asleep – Your Involuntary Actions

Your M.C. is involved, but only to check that, for example, after the pain, movement, muscle spasm, or extreme danger has arisen, you have responded appropriately. Your brain will not allow you to prevent taking these actions!

These are actions that have not been developed but are inherent within those processes that occur outside your conscious thought. Therefore, your M.C. is never able to prevent or modify the action, but it is involved to check you have taken appropriate corrective measures.

I believe that you are driven to carry out this type of action to protect one of your body's organs, limbs, or your skeletal structure that has become unhealthy and/or injured, or is under damaging strain. Your Body's Health Status Monitoring System automatically detects this and, in the fastest possible time, initiates the required involuntary protective response/s.

From its memory, your M.C. recognises the significance of these response symptoms. It monitors your condition and supports your corrective actions until you have re-established a satisfactory safer/healthier status or condition, and these body reactions have automatically reduced and finally ceased.

An example of an involuntary action would be:

Your back has finally come to experience a slipped disc-type of condition, or a condition less severe but nevertheless becoming significantly worse.

Your B.H.S.M.S. has immediately put your back into a spasm. There is a very high level of pain to prevent the general area of your spine, where the disc is located, from carrying out any more movement for the immediate future. Therefore, this prevents *further* damage and promotes longer-term recovery, if that remains a possibility, despite this recent straining of the area.

F) Your thoughts are different to what _initiates their_ _creation_.

I believe that all your thoughts are created within your mind, but they are instigated in response to one or a combination of up to three different types of sources. These are:

1) The first _instigating source/s_ is the data coming in from _outside your brain_ via your five senses. The types of instigating sources are multitudinous. One example could be a direct question you have read or heard spoken, which is directed at or related to you. Or, it may be that the sets of data you have received require you to consider/think about them before finalising your required responses and taking their related actions.

2) The second _instigating source_ originates within your _brain_, inside your mind. For example, this could be in response to your B.H.S.M.S. informing you that your body has a health condition that requires you to take some action. Or, it could be you daydreaming, leading your M.C. to create a _new_ _thought_ about questioning what to do to help one of your grandchildren deal better with her difficulties at school.

As soon as it is made, this thought automatically goes into the appropriate Category 1B department of the set of departments that your consciousness comprises. This question will be processed/considered during the next cycle of updating your consciousness.

3) The third <u>instigating source</u> occurs from within your brain, inside your mind from <u>an already existing unresolved question.</u> These reside in your mind's appropriate Category 1B department for any unanswered questions you have. For example, where do I wish to go on holiday next summer? You have a spare half an hour in which your M.C. reviews the contents of your Unresolved Questions Department and selects this questioning thought. It automatically goes into one of the cells in your Internal Thoughts Department, within your Consciousness Department. It will then be processed /considered during the next cycle of updating your consciousness.

G) General, fundamental aspects that your thoughts are created and governed by.

1) We all have thoughts nearly all of the time, including whilst asleep. <u>Without thoughts, we would not be able to take any actions</u> (apart from instinctive and involuntary actions). Everything we do is preceded by thoughts or considerations from which the required actions are initiated and concluded.

2) Your M.C. creates your thoughts or considerations. As they are developed, with more data coming into your brain and/or from memories gathered inside your brain, they are held in a dedicated Memory Department on a temporary or longer basis, dependent upon the objectives of each set of thoughts.

3) Your thoughts are created by your M.C. and, as such, they are original. They are made instead of being presented to your M.C. by something or someone. This can only be achieved by your M.C. having the required degree of intelligence to achieve this creative act.

You might say that most thoughts have been created many times before, and as such, your M.C. is just repeating or copying these particular thoughts. This may be true in a minimal number of cases, but for the vast majority of them, whilst some thoughts may be similar to some previous ones, there will normally be some differences. These distinctions require recognising and being reflected in the detail of these thoughts to achieve the objectives of these thoughts fully. This facet is another reason why machines cannot create *original thoughts* – simply because they have no intelligence.

4) I don't think that your thoughts exist within the ether of your mind, just floating around without a home, even for the shortest period of time. If this was the case, they couldn't be efficiently processed, if at all. Your brain does not do anything at all in this ad hoc, laissez-faire manner – far from it. I very firmly believe that your brain has been created and designed with continual development and improvement, to carry out all of its processing activities in the easiest, simplest and therefore most efficient ways that are available, given its basic objectives. These methods will achieve the fastest possible processing speeds, along with the most realistic faultless performances from your brain – two extremely important characteristics for it. Every

thought is created within a home in a dedicated Memory Department, and its contents exist for the time appropriate to its collective needs.

5) As you consider and develop your thoughts in your mind, they comprise of words, feelings, numbers and recollections of visual memories, etc. During this time, you will be silently saying and hearing what each of these words and information sounds like or, to some degree of accuracy, looks like, as if they are actually being spoken, heard, experienced or described in reality.

6) Therefore, I propose that the coding type/format that represents the details of your thoughts as depicted by words, is identical to the words of each thought as if they had been spoken aloud. They are coded and processed within your brain in the same way. This standardisation therefore enables different departments within your brain to very quickly understand and process the requirements of all of your thoughts.

7) Your thoughts generally comprise words held in a related collection of information and built up as a dedicated memory in one of your Category 1B Memory Departments (comprising very many subdepartments). They have many purposes, a few examples of which are:

7.1 Part of the process of developing your consciousness.

7.2 Answering questions.

7.3 Answering an unresolved question or situation.

7.4 Processing reading anything in the real world – a book, a letter, a sign, etc. As you continue to read and gather more related information, you add this data into the Memory Department that your brain has allocated for this particular task. This enables you to remember all of the information that you have received.

7.5 Noting or understanding aspects you are seeing with your vision.

7.6 Conducting a conversation with someone in the real world, face-to-face or over the phone.

7.7 You have a lot of thoughts whilst asleep in dreams, in imagined conversations, etc.

SUBCHAPTER 2.2.3: Your brain's different departments, their role, operation and relation to your M.C.

This subchapter covers the different categories of Automatic Control and Processing Systems within your brain, detailing their basic location, role, how they operate, how they develop and their operational relationship with your M.C.

NB Please forgive me for repeating this reminder yet again, for the last time.

This section builds on Subchapter 2.1.1 to present <u>a lot more detail</u> about the functionality of the three categories of departments: 1, 1A and 1B. It also gives additional information about what <u>roles they play</u> and the <u>benefits you derive from them</u>. So, if you find their functionality tough to follow, please focus not on their names *or functionality but solely on the roles they have and the benefits they bring to you.*

A) Your Fully-Automatic, P.I.D. Closed-Loop Measurement and Control Systems

(This is a **Category 1** department facility.)

    They each reside inside your brain but outside the boundaries of your mind. Your M.C., which resides within your mind, <u>is not</u> involved with their operation. Their location gives them good physical protection from being attacked by infections. Whatever your prevailing activities are, all of these departments are <u>continually operating</u> <u>throughout your life</u>.

    OVERVIEW: These are the many control systems that keep your brain and body's vital core services, organs, conditions and facilities permanently alive and functioning correctly. Some of these include:

1)   *Your heart and your related blood pressure and blood flow*
2)   *Your blood sugar level*
3)   *Your body's temperature*
4)   *Your body's breathing*
5)   *Your chemical health*
6)   *Many more core functions and facilities*

The letters P.I.D. stand for the type of the fully-automatic control logic used in the control systems' control philosophy. They mean **Proportional, Integral** and **Derivative**.

How close the target condition you are striving to achieve is to the prevailing condition determines which types of algorithms are utilised to adjust the control system outputs, closing in ever tighter to their target.

These control systems are innate and are potentially there at your conception. They fully develop in your mother's womb prior to birth, as required, and continue their fine-tuning improvement and development thereafter. I propose that this type of control system has a degree of ability to self-learn and improve the effectiveness of its role of looking after your status. Each system learns from its operational experiences with your unique body, its individual characteristics and requirements. They operate independently from each other, are dedicated to their designated facility and operate fully automatically, at extremely high speed at your subconscious level.

Your M.C. is not involved in the actual operation of these systems but, will assist in helping to achieve the objectives of a control system if it sees that you are experiencing symptoms of difficulties it recognises. For example, if you are becoming extremely hot or physically exhausted, it will ensure you take appropriate measures to recover your healthy status for heart control or body temperature control as soon as possible.

The basic principles of operation and control of this type of system are continually setting out to achieve a condition/s or status that are the prevailing target/s or setpoints of the control system. Each actual condition or status is automatically fed back to the control system. If there is a difference to what is required, it will automatically adjust the output to the heart or blood sugar condition etc. This alters its prevailing status to change towards the required condition or value in a smooth and controlled manner as soon as possible.

NB These types of control systems are used throughout all modern industries around the world to manufacture and process of a lot of different products.

A more detailed description of the operation and control of this type of system is, for example, for the control of your heart. I believe that your heart's primary controlling software resides within a dedicated set of neural networks within a dedicated Category 1 department in your brain. They receive many input signals of data <u>from your heart</u>, which travel along your nervous system and into data signal conversion networks in your brain. They then go into your brain's heart controlling software input area to inform it precisely what the current operational status of your heart actually is. This data <u>from</u> your heart is commonly called feedback data. It includes your blood pressure around your heart, your blood flows, your frequency of pumping, at what pumping position your heart is in, and other crucially important items of data. This information is required by your heart's extremely powerful operational software P.I.D. (Proportional, Integral, Derivative) neural networks of functional control loops. They are able to decide whether your heart is being overloaded and therefore is under strain, whether it should continue to operate exactly as it currently is, or whether its current functional state or states needs to change. If so, it knows what operational aspects should change and by how much.

Your heart's operational software achieves its required changes of functionality by transmitting output signals along your nervous system. These signals are received by your heart's local control system, where very minor adjustments may be carried out, and they are also received by your heart's autonomic nervous system. The combinational effect of these signals <u>from</u> your brain and their resultant operational responses from your heart's control and operating system results in the appropriate operation of your heart muscles, valves and other parts. This, at all times, produces the correct functionality and output of oxygenated *blood flow* from your heart, required for your prevailing physical activities, plus an *appropriate and healthy blood pressure level*.

Your heart's neural control loops, housed within your Category 1 department in your heart's Fully-Automatic, P.I.D. Measurement and Control Systems, operational philosophy is fundamentally based upon setting out to achieve:

a) A variable blood flow under all of your required physical activities to fully satisfy their needs.

b) At all times to ensure that, throughout your body, a nominally constant blood pressure prevails, with an additional target of a certain maximum value of blood pressure is not exceeded. This protects the physical health of your brain and arteries throughout your body from being over pressurised. Your heart also plays a major role in assisting in the vitally important removal of waste products from your body.

69

B) Your Semi-Automatic, Open-Loop Measurement and Control Systems

(This a **Category 1A** department facility.)

They each reside inside your brain, but outside the boundaries of your mind. Your M.C., which resides within your mind, whilst <u>not</u> being involved with their operation, assists these departments to achieve their objectives when required. Their location gives them good physical protection from being attacked by infections. Whatever your prevailing activities are, all of these departments <u>operate continuously throughout your life</u>.

OVERVIEW: These are the many control systems that keep in good order your body's core states and conditions in order to keep you in a robust state of health in regard to, for example:

1) Your mind's emotional/mental health
2) Your food intake
3) Maintaining your brain's physiological health
4) Passing water and opening up your bowels
5) **Many, many, more** core states and conditions

I believe that these control systems are innate and potentially there at your conception. They develop in your mother's womb prior to birth, with some being basically fully developed by the time you are born, yet with all continuing their fine-tuning development thereafter.

I propose that this type of control system has a degree of ability to self-learn and improve the effectiveness of its role of looking after your status. Each system learns from its operational experiences and thus makes the appropriate adjustments to its control systems. They operate independently from each other, are dedicated to their designated facility and operate semi-automatically, at extremely high speed at a subconscious level.

The basic principles of operation and control of this type of system are to continually set out to achieve a safe or healthy condition or status, which is the prevailing target or setpoint of each of these systems.

The actual condition or status is automatically fed back to the control system. If there is a difference to what it requires, related symptoms will be caused in the following ways:

a)   Automatically, by the control system itself.
b)   Naturally by your body, reacting to the unhealthy condition.

Your M.C. will recognise from its learned experiences the significance of your physical and/or functional symptoms and will also know what corrective actions are required. It will instigate corrective actions and monitor your status until you have re-established a safe/healthy vital service status or condition, by which time all of these symptoms will have gradually ceased.

Examples of these systems in operation are if you are becoming short of food, you will experience feeling hungry or being a little light-headed, etc. If you are becoming too emotionally stressed, you may experience headaches, feel emotionally agitated and have difficulty with clear decision-making etc. Your M.C. will recognise the significance of these symptoms. It will know the underlying cause or causes of the symptoms are and the required actions you must take to alleviate each of the causes. It will then ensure that you take appropriate actions to recover your healthy status as soon as possible, at which time the related symptoms will have ceased.

C) Your Developed, Semi-Automatic, Open-Loop (with a degree of measurement) Control Systems

(This is a **Category 1B** department facility.)

They all reside within the boundaries of your mind with the minority within the boundaries of your M.C., which is in your mind.

These departments are a mixture of some operating continually and others only operating when your prevailing activities, under the orchestration of your M.C., call upon them to do so.

Your M.C. will, when necessary, make adjustments individually to the Category 1B department's control systems to compensate for any prevailing ambient conditions that would otherwise prevent the control system's target or objectives being achieved. For example, slippery conditions, rough conditions underfoot, gusty winds, people pushing, etc.

OVERVIEW: These are the vast multitudes of control systems that provide your core processes, professional skills, knowledge, understanding and functionalities *required, to enable your mind and body to achieve part of their ongoing objectives and related actions throughout your life. Each of these control systems resides*

within their own dedicated, Category 1B department to provide,
for example:

1) All Category 1B departments, residing within groups of departments, within Sections which collectively enable your M.C. to be able to conduct all of the processes required for the creation of your consciousness.

2) All Category 1B departments which collectively enable you to carry out all of your considerations, decisions and resultant actions in response to your updated consciousness.

3) An enormous number of more core processes, professional skills, knowledge, understanding and functionalities, some of which are detailed as follows:

a) The set of departments contained within one very large group of departments which I call your M.C. (Master Conductor). This comprises a very large number of Category 1B departments, with each one dedicated to a particular role, normally as part of a larger process requirement.

b) All of the departments for housing, developing and utilising each of your vast number of Developed Semi-Automatic Skills. An example of this is for the movement of each of your limbs and their parts, all of your other body parts and their individual movements. For each primary body part with its separate set of required movements, there is a dedicated Category 1B department assigned.

c) All of the dedicated Category 1B departments regarding the Speed Estimation, closing time to you and to others, of selected moving objects in your locality and beyond when you are walking in crowds or driving in complex congestion.

d) All of the dedicated Category 1B departments for Reading, Writing, Speaking, Remembering, Hearing, Seeing, Tasting, Touching, Smelling and Problem-Solving skills.

e) All of the dedicated Category 1B departments related to your automatic Body's Health Status Monitoring System (B.H.S.M.S.).

f) The dedicated Category 1B department for processing any internal thoughts you have.

g) All of the dedicated Category 1B departments related to your senses. These departments _receive all_ current incoming data via each sense and be able to <u>convert</u> it from its original incoming analogue format into an analogue format suitable for genetic coding. I propose that, from then on, this is the format used for its transmission and processing within all of your brain's departments.

h) There will be a dedicated Category 1B department for adjusting each sense's dwell time percentage of the prevailing scan to the current requirements of your M.C. This allows it to study each of the required senses sufficiently long enough as it requires.

i) There is a dedicated Category 1B department with the ability to be able to _search for and match up_ each converted dataset as in g) above, with an existing set of data already stored in your Memory Department. You are then able to recognise and understand its meaning.

j) There will be dedicated Category 1B departments working as part of the creation/updating of your consciousness, with the combinational <u>intelligence</u> to be able to:

i) Decide whether any sets of data considered together contextually relate to the particular situations or conditions you have noted, create an immediate and/or near-future safety situation or risk to you.

ii) Decide which <u>other remaining details and conditions</u> are not safety-related ones, <u>but are ones you should address</u> by immediate consideration and then take the related and appropriate required actions to satisfy or solve each of them.

NB This process, when you are in settings which are extremely busy, will have selected perhaps only 20% or less of the total sets of data incoming from your senses, leaving the remaining 80% or more to be deleted in that moment of time as not being important to your needs. This filtering out process is absolutely crucial at times to prevent your brain from becoming overloaded with too much incoming data requiring processing. The consequences of this could be, at worst, emotional fear and confusion and, at best, leaving you in a state of significant confusion.

k) Departments with the ability to make readily available each of these relevant and required sets of data above to update your consciousness.

l) Whilst working in conjunction with your M.C. during your next sleeping period, the abilities of a number of Departments to:

i) Be able to review, delete or process as appropriate *all new data:* new experiences data, new learned experiences and attitudes data, new Semi-Automatic Skills and any other types of new data received since your last sleep. All of this information will have been located in a temporary, New Data Category 1B department.

ii) Be able to install into memory, each item or set of new data in its appropriate Category 1B department with its location within it. This includes the appropriate information about each item, set or sets of data within each memory cell.

iii) Be able to delete, refresh and update all existing memories, data and information of all the numerous categories, as required.

There are a great many more Category 1B departments required. The ones above just give an extremely small flavour of the kind of requirements to be satisfied.

I propose that this Category 1B type of control system has been programmed to automatically self-learn. It improves its role's operational efficiency and effectiveness in providing the processes and functionalities you require. Each system learns from its operational experiences, thus making the appropriate adjustments to its Semi-Automatic Control Systems.

I believe that these Category 1B Control Systems are innate – potentially there at your conception, passed on in your genes from your parents and their forefathers, with a few, developing in your mother's womb prior to birth. Some are more developed than others by the time you are born and with a few fully functioning as required before delivery in order to keep you alive following birth.

They all continue their development naturally from your life experiences and improved deliberately with practice during your lifetime. They each operate independently within their own department and are dedicated to a designated role, operating semi-automatically at extremely high speed at your subconscious level.

The basic principles of operation and control of this category of system are:

Your Control System provide the operation of the process, functionality or skill that you require, whilst your M.C. will crucially be monitoring the ongoing results and status of the process as needed. Your M.C. will make adjustments to the Control System to compensate for any prevailing ambient or other conditions that would otherwise prevent the target or objectives of each Control System from being fully achieved. The setpoint, target or objective of each particular system, could be a movement or position, processing of thoughts, understanding of data, or one of many other types of objectives.

SUBCHAPTER 2.3: Your brain's cycle of the creation of and acting on your consciousness

This subsection looks at your brain's detailed, ongoing cycle of the creation, updating and taking action upon the status

of your consciousness, which occurs at a frequency of <u>250 times every second</u>.

NB Please note that this first/introductory description is less detailed than subchapter 3.1.1.

OVERVIEW: I believe that this most crucial capability cycle of creating and updating of your consciousness emerges very slowly before your birth. Soon after birth, it gradually increases in its frequency of development. It continues developing at an increasing rate as your exposure to life's multitude of experiences evolves and grows all of your brain's capabilities.

This cycle of your consciousness continues throughout the whole of your lifetime, night and day, awake and asleep, and whilst healthy, until the moment you die.

This never-ending cycle imposes a stable, operational heartbeat and flow, over which all other of your brain's activities operate from and in relation to. I propose that any other processing system designed by humans, even with a one-thousandth of a percent capability and capacity as that of your brain, would be unable to acceptably operate at all with sufficient effectiveness, safety and reliability. Realistically, its design functionality would unfortunately, I believe, be riddled with ongoing, unsolvable faults of countless categories, each caused by super-fiendishly complex, interactive conditions. These would be compounded by ever-changing fault creating, multi-faceted combinational conditions. The worst-case fault condition would be caused by a combined number of separate fault conditions that follow a particular sequence of occurrences, thus creating the resultant fault.

To those of you who haven't had a taste of the experience of those such worst-case scenarios, you may think all of this is just make-believe, but given the scenario described above, I consider it to be within the bounds of reality.

I am making this point to further sing the praises of how awesome your brain is. Despite its power, capacity, capability and the range and depth of all it can do, it is incredibly reliable and therefore safely dependable and never makes mistakes.

It's always there, whenever you need it, ready, willing and able, with no fuss, no questions, to carry out your every need – no problem!

NB *The proposed rate of your brain's processing activities stem from and relate to, in my opinion, the data from your five Senses, B.H.S.M.S. and thoughts being scanned once every millisecond (ms) by your Data Review Scanning System throughout your lifetime. Your M.C. studies this data via your Data Review Scanning System as it wishes to.*

I propose that the other phases of your brain's related processing activities operating times, match this 1ms in terms of this length of time. When it occurs, the interaction between these different phases of each step of the process has a natural balance and flow of connection. This leads to your brain having a good overall processing operational efficiency resulting in a very high processing speed and, therefore, a very fast/quick response to satisfying your prevailing requirements. This is particularly important when responding to and dealing with imminent and very serious danger to yourself.

A) A basic description of the first phase of this ongoing cycle of the creation and updating of your consciousness.

1) <u>Data inputs</u> from your <u>five senses</u> automatically pass into their own dedicated Category 1B department in your brain as part of the analysis process. This includes utilising your vast array of knowledge to commence understanding what they each are and mean to you at that moment in time.

2) Any <u>data inputs</u> from your <u>B.H.S.M.S.</u> that are *already within your brain* will automatically pass into another Cat-1B dept, as part of the analysis process. This includes utilising your vast array of knowledge to commence the analysis to understand what they each are and mean to you at that moment in time.

3) Data inputs from the *active* thoughts you may have *already within your mind* automatically pass into another Cat-1B dept in your brain as part of the analysis process. As in the two previous points, this includes utilising your vast array of knowledge to commence the analysis to understand what they each are and mean to you in that moment in time.

   The <u>prevailing processing status</u> for each item of data for all of these activities in A) above will nominally have been reviewed after 1ms by the end of the first scan cycle.

NB On some occasions, not all data items will have completed their analysis process within this 1ms simply because they comprise data that requires more processing time than 1ms to understand them fully. If this is the case, it is vitally important that these data items continue to be analysed. When this analysis is complete, they then join in the next cycle of your consciousness update to be processed.

B) The second phase of this cycle.

1)   The second phase is for your M.C. to study all of the data that has completed its analysis process. With its innate and developed intelligence, it will decide what data in the current situational context indicates danger to you or indicates no danger but requires your consideration and resultant actions to deal with.

2)   *All other remaining data which has no importance to you at that moment in time will therefore be deleted by your M.C.* This deletion assessment activity is of prime importance to you to minimise the risk/difficulty you would otherwise encounter on occasions of being overloaded with too much data to analyse and process correctly.

3)   Thus far, you have established your **updated consciousness, **which is **all of the data that requires immediate processing and responding to nominally, which has been sent to your Data Review Scanning System for review.**

81

The total time for all of these activities in A) above will be over a subsequent Scan Cycle of 1ms.

C) The third and last phase of this cycle.

1) Once again, your M.C. uses its inherent and developed Intelligence to create the required and appropriate Thoughts of Consideration. It reviews all of the <u>remaining data</u> that has completed its analysis process to consider any data that indicates danger to you in order of priority of importance. From here, it will decide what actions you are required to take from your Thoughts of Consideration to deal with each of them individually or collectively as appropriate.

2) Your M.C. instigates each of the required actions to prevent or dispel the dangers. This could be, for example, by it sending instructions in software format to a number of your Cat-1B Developed, Semi-Automatic Skills Departments. This will operate your activity of walking, speaking, reading or fighting and maybe carrying out some more thinking and very many other possibilities.

3) Once again, your M.C. will engage its inherent and developed Intelligence by addressing your Non-Safety related issues and requirements but nonetheless important ones, whenever it has the time, in between keeping you safe. It will address these by giving each one their appropriate Thoughts of Consideration it has created and instigating the

fitting instructions required to achieve the related action/s it has decided are necessary.

The total time for all of these activities in C) above to be completed within 2 Scan Cycles = 2ms.

NB-X The total time from each of your Category 1B Developed, Semi-Automatic Skills receiving instructions to each of these instructions actually being carried out physically and operationally will vary greatly. This is due to several factors, for example, how long will it take for each particular instruction to be completed. These instructions could vary from looking at a particular person's face near you, shouting a warning to someone or walking towards the end of a wall to read a notice etc.

*The total time for all of these activities in **NB-X** to be completed nominally ranges from 2ms up to a possible wide span of a number of seconds.*

D) <u>**The next cycle**</u> **commences with its first phase exactly as A).**

1) It is for analysing the incoming data, which may *include* NB-X and one or two of the results and consequences of some of the instigated Actions in **C)ii)** above.

2) To note and address all other data inputs as **A)i)**, **ii)** and **iii)** above where, in each case, some data inputs have not yet completed their required processing.

83

3) To continue to deal with every data item that has completed its process of analysis to understand what they each are and mean to you. Therefore be able to move them along through this ongoing process of updating your Consciousness and dealing with all of its requirements.

And so your brain's complete processing cycle of the <u>creation of and ongoing updating and instigating actions from the data status of your consciousness</u> continues. Your reactions to its requirements also continue infinitely, as described above in each cycle (A to C), repeating itself throughout the whole of your life every 4ms. This means it will have been repeated 250 times every second, ad infinitum.

    This equates to your consciousness being created/updated and then processing all of the actions required to be taken = 21,600,000 times every 24 hours. For your brain to be permanently that busy, with all of its additional work and never make any mistakes, it must have an overall M.C. to achieve this staggering performance.

NB There appears to be a belief held by some that your consciousness shuts down whilst you are asleep. I do not hold to this belief at all, for reasons given several times within the book.

SUBCHAPTER 2.4: How is your intelligence created, and what is its relationship to your M.C.?

How is your intelligence created? What is the relationship between your M.C. and your intelligence?
OVERVIEW: I believe that fundamentally, your <u>prevailing</u> level of intelligence is created from the interactive combination of all of your current characteristics, capabilities, skills and knowledge that reside within your many Master Conductor's departments. The source of some of these qualities is your inherited genes.

NB I do not, for example, believe that your intelligence exists as a single entity, residing in a particular location in one of your M.C.'s very many departments.

As a human being, your Master Conductor (M.C.) is inherently blessed with being intelligent. It deploys this immensely important capability to the whole functionality of your brain, wherever and whenever it is required. So, whenever I say throughout my book that your <u>M.C. does this, that or the other</u>, it intrinsically means it will deploy its Intelligence, or its other skills, appropriate to the prevailing situation it is addressing.

To follow are a few, every day, detailed examples of the actual way in which your M.C. fully utilises your updated consciousness whilst engaging your appropriate Category 1B Department Control Facilities.

Example 1 – Basic walking in the underground

The Scene: *Let's say, over a 15-minute period during a hectic rush hour, negotiating the London Underground out of the tube station, along to and up one of the moving elevators and out through the turnstiles.*

Throughout this time, your M.C. has been constantly engaged and extremely busy updating your consciousness with the vast amount of information being received via your senses and around your immediate location. It has instigated and engaged the application of your very many Developed Cat-1B, Semi-Automatic Departments Skills required for all of your extremely complex walking movements for your entire body.

Additionally, your M.C. has been observing all of the related data from your updated consciousness, derived from your senses. It has fine-tuned each of your Semi-Automatic Control Systems, for their dedicated and detailed walking movements, for each of your detailed toe, leg, arm, foot, hand movements and your ongoing balance requirements, etc.

This fine-tuning has been required to accommodate and compensate for the prevailing, ambient and always unique details in each moment. This is due to all of the movements, the hustle and bustle from everyone rushing from A to B, with their cases, bags and the close proximity of them all around you. Additionally, you constantly have to take account of, in order to avoid, unrequired contact with so many people and the odd dog, wheelchairs, blind people with white sticks, children, out of control people on their mobile phones permanently, etc. You then have to negotiate the escalator due to the constant and detailed movement and the people pushing to walk past you. You focus on not losing your balance and, God forbid, falling down, and you breathe a sigh of relief when you reach the end of it and skip off.

Despite the potentially difficult conditions, with your mental and physical faculties being in good order, you walk in a safe, efficient and effective manner. This is thanks to the combined performance of your M.C. and your extensive team of Cat-1B departments that control all of your body movements. Other Cat-1B departments also provide their prior knowledge of all aspects of underground travel that require the appropriate care to avoid being injured or injuring others. Your ferocious frequency of thought processing required during this outing to satisfy all of your safety requirements is very demanding and tiring. It requires an awful lot of focused concentration.

NB Having personally studied the motion of limbs closely, it's surprising how many fine movements are required to take place. This is particularly the case when maintaining very good balance and compensating for conditions as above and a multitude of other details not mentioned so that you proceed safely without any significant difficulties.

Example 2 – Playing golf

The Scene: *You have successfully driven a golf ball from a soft, muddy and slippery tee on to a wet and uphill fairway over 250* *yards away into a strong, left to right, blustery wind whilst it's raining.*

The ball lands on the centre of the fairway, just to the left of a large oak tree. You are able to play the ball from this position and can see and reach the green – just the place that you had aimed for, despite the number of extremely challenging prevailing conditions your M.C. had to be aware of and correctly make compensations for. These include:

a) The way you hit the ball to neutralise the sideways movement of the wind and rain.
b) The power that was needed to hit the ball to achieve the required distance of travel, despite the wind and rain effects.
c) To stop the ball from running back down the hill after it landed by imparting the sufficient amount of topspin on the ball.

Despite the combination of all of these required compensating aspects, It is quite astounding what accuracy and performance the average human being's brain, their M.C., and all of their vast number of Category 1B departments working in unison, updating your consciousness, controlling all of their body parts, are collectively able to achieve.

The other very significant parts that contributed to this performance are:

1) Thousands of hours of hard, skilfully correct practice, over a number of years, to hone the numerous range of

finely detailed golfing strokes skills, stored in each of their Developed, Category 1B Semi-Automatic Departments, each of which controls their particular body movements required for hitting the ball in different situations.

2) For the other Developed, Category 1B Semi-Automatic Departments for providing their knowledge, acquired over the years of experience of how to apply these necessary compensating aspects. In order to successfully achieve such difficult success, the final and most crucial aspect that must prevail is that, just before the golfer hits the ball, he must believe and have an actual real belief that he will be successful. This is cemented if he is able to engage his Placebo Effect with the sufficient amount or degree of his belief.

And just to cap it all, the golfer managed to hit the ball to apply sufficient topspin on the ball to stop it from rolling down the hill upon landing.

Example 3 – Dealing with glasses unexpectedly falling out of a cupboard

The Scene: *You are putting some glasses high up in a wall-mounted cupboard, and completely unexpectedly, you knock one over, out of the cupboard.*

Before it lands on the hard kitchen floor (where it would have shattered), you realise that you have:

a) Instantly moved three other glasses with your left hand, which were about to also fall out of the cupboard, farther on to the shelf for their safety.

b) This is immediately followed by bending your upper body and knees a little.

c) You simultaneously turn and move your body to the right with a slight tilt backwards. At the same time, your right hand is rotating outwards, with your left hand touching the work surface edge to stabilise your body a little.

d) You instantly move all parts of your body downwards.

e) Additionally, you move slightly to the right to catch up with the falling glass. You catch it and place it on the work surface, with all of these quite complex activities executed with consummate ease.

It is at this point that you realize what you have just achieved. You think – how on earth did I react instantly to the completely unexpected situation? How did I go through such a complex set of decisions of movement of the whole of your body, and bodily parts, your mind and body coordination, speed and complexity to catch up with the very fast falling and tumbling glass? How did I slow down to the speed and position of the glass, then grasp it successfully and place it on the work surface all within the time of around half of a second without any fumbling or other difficulties? If you had deliberately created this situation and practised and practised it, you would not have achieved the same percentage and degree of success rate you just had and have had with similar situations over the last 20 years.

So, how exactly did your brain and body combine to achieve the almost unachievable?

Under the normal, automatic and continual updating of your consciousness, beginning at the start of this sequence of events, under the instructions of your M.C., your sight and touch senses were set to maximum dwell time. These are the two key senses of data required for the successful conclusion of this situation. Your Master Conductor, upon seeing the situation, immediately triggered this very broadly Developed, Semi-Automatic set of skills that have been refined and improved over your lifetime by similar situations before and partially related ones from playing sports, etc. Once triggered, the very basic routine semi-automatically functioned, with your M.C. firing off the required/relevant responses at each moment, to cater for the prevailing ambient conditions. It does this by fine-tuning each of the numerous, different Automatic Control Systems, each housed within their own dedicated Developed Category 1B Semi-Automatic Department for controlling the movements of a particular part of your body at each particular moment of time.

This process continued as described above, with the absolute, critical key part of the success being played as it does every single time until its successful conclusion. This is orchestrated by:

a)   Your M.C., under the feedback data from your vision and touch.

b)   Your M.C., seeing where the target glass is at every moment, and also seeing where your relevant body parts are.

c) Your M.C., predicting where the glass will be in the next moment of time.

d) Your M.C., finely adjusting your body movement departments, each of which uniquely controls part of your body position and crucially all of the components of your right hand's position.

e) Your M.C., eventually arranging for you to catch the falling glass and return it to the cupboard in one efficient, smooth and confident set of actions.

A significant part of the incredible success of such skills is because virtually all of your limbs, hands, fingers, feet and toes etc., are manipulated with such incredible speed and dexterity by the operation of your muscles and ligaments, under the even quicker, lightning-fast speed control of your brain, utilising what have become Developed, Semi-Automatic sets of skills and instructions to achieve standard type movements and operations, each one of which had been under the overseeing management, adjustment and fine-tuning of your M.C.

These adjustments by your M.C. are vitally important to compensate for the uniquely different prevailing conditions that these types of situations comprise, in order to reach a successful conclusion.

Most people refer to the electrifying speed, accuracy and precision of control and performance as described above as being due to your muscle memory performance. However, I don't subscribe to this explanation at all. I would state that my belief is that every single memory cell within the whole of your body volume is located inside your brain, with none of them located inside your muscles.

The above experience actually happened to me whilst I was writing the book. I have found that the whole of this type of occurrence is almost like an out of body experience. It's as if you were a witness to the functionality of the events (rather than carrying them out) and think – how on earth did I do that? It was over in the blink of an eye, and before I was really aware of what was happening. The major factor that created this feeling is due to the lightning speed of your brain's processing. All of your M.C.'s processing activities happened so fast they were each way below your conscious awareness in the moments they occurred, and therefore you were not aware of them.

Example 4 – Quick and accurate judgements required at a meeting

The Scene: *At the meeting, the C.E.O. very clearly stated that he wished everyone in attendance to keep all of the information he was about to present to themselves until he gave clearance otherwise.*

The C.E.O. outlined his broad-brush plans for the design, development, commissioning and ongoing manufacture of a totally different form of car seen anywhere in the world to date. He said he would ask me, Mr X, a number of questions about this project, requiring each answer in the accuracy range of +/- 15%.

Question 1 – *Can we successfully design, build and commission this new car within our existing new car design and build building I have outlined, ready for it to be mass-produced for the world market?*

a)   How long will this take?

b)   How much will it cost?

c)   When will you need to spend 50% of this total cost? When will you require the remainder?

Question 2 – *Can we successfully build a car-assembly line for this new car in the designated area of our factory, as outlined today?*

a)   How long will this take?

b)   How much will it cost?

c)   When will you need to spend 50% of this total cost? When will you require the remainder?

Question 3 – *How many of the types of cars specified in this meeting and built within the car assembly line at the limit of the space available could we produce per annum, at maximum output?*

These comments are to you, my reader:

You may read this and maybe think, or not: Why write this scenario? It is just too ridiculous to contemplate. BUT – the above scenario is, believe me or not, one that can and does occur in some places in the real world we inhabit. So, how on earth can any single human being be put in this position and deliver these detailed answers with the required degree of confidence?

It is simply due to the absolute utter power of the experienced human mind and its M.C., together with their accumulated worldly wealth of knowledge, understanding, experienced professional skills, stored within many of their brain's Developed, Category 1B Semi-Automatic Open-Loop Departments and also in many Memory Departments.

The process that unfolded was:

1) As the C.E.O. gradually delivered each item of information, Mr X wrote the salient points of information on his notepad, under various appropriate headings, including short questions and under-linings.

2) Mr X also obtained copies of each presentation page for his personal use that day.

3) Mr X wrote a list of questions as they cropped up, with a space for each answer.

4) Mr X noted various historical projects similar to this one regarding principles, basic costs and time scales.

At this point, Mr X spent one hour in deep thought, studying all of his notes, broken whilst asking 15 questions of the meeting. He spent another 30 minutes in reflection, then confidently gave estimated answers to each of the questions. Several answers include a qualifying statement that some investigatory work was required to obtain the necessary accuracy of response to that particular question. Mr X said he would come back at the end of the week with all completed answers – all of which he did with a good degree of confidence.

SUBCHAPTER 2.5: What are the basic requirements of your brain?

OVERVIEW: *It is my belief that the role of your brain can be split into a number of sets of functions, each of which has a primary objective. The results of all of these functions combine to enable you to keep alive, safe, able to exercise, plus maintain good physical, emotional and chemical health. You can operate safely, efficiently and effectively to play your part in the world as you know it, relate to and would aspire to throughout every second of your whole life. Your* **ongoing consciousness** *plays a key and foundational role in every one of your lifetime's activities, with* **your M.C. playing an absolutely vital role** *in creating your consciousness, responding to and satisfying its required thoughts, decisions and related actions.*

The requirements above are carried out <u>by one or combinations of</u> the following listed facilities, each of which are housed within the enormous number of different departments within your brain housing:

1) **Your Category 1**, Fully-Automatic, Closed-Loop Measurement and Control Systems.
2) **Your Category 1A,** Semi-Automatic Open-Loop Measurement and Control Systems.

3) **Your Category 1 B,** Developed, Semi-Automatic, Open-Loop Control Systems.

4) **Your Conscious Thoughts** (and subsequent actions).

5) **Your Subconscious Thoughts** (and subsequent actions).

6) **Your Instinctively-Driven Thoughts** (and subsequent actions).

7) **Involuntarily-Driven Thoughts** (and actions, with your M.C. checking that the end results are as required).

SUBCHAPTER 2.5.1: An introductory, simplified list of your *brain's fundamental roles*

ROLE A – I believe that your brain's first fundamentally important role is to look after you at all times throughout your whole life together, in your intrinsically connected living and functioning arrangement.

ROLE B – Your brain's second fundamentally important role is to keep your body's vital services, organs, conditions and facilities alive and functioning correctly. This is so your brain and body are kept alive with good exercise and in good physical, chemical, functional and emotional health.

ROLE C – Your brain's third fundamentally important role is to create and continually update your consciousness.

ROLE D – Your brain's fourth fundamentally important role is to ensure that your entire body (your skeletal structure, muscles, sinews, bones and limbs, etc.) remain in a physically healthy functional state at all times.

It also ensures that your body remains free of any disease or inflammation. If the health of any of these objectives is in jeopardy, your brain's role is to guarantee that the appropriate corrective action or actions occur immediately.

ROLE E – Your brain's fifth fundamentally important role is to, at all times, keep your emotional health in the best possible order.

This enables you to live the life you wish, with its related enjoyment, achievement and satisfaction.

ROLE F – Your brain's sixth fundamentally important role is the utilisation of the incredibly powerful, effective, indicative and corrective tools it has available, which include pain, discomfort and/or functional disabilities. Additionally, you brain can prompt and guide you to self-help and fully engage your placebo effect.

Your brain employs these tools individually and collectively as appropriate, given each set of circumstances. They assist you in recovering from physical ailments and also poor Mental Health.

ROLE G – Your brain's seventh fundamentally important role is to remember. It needs to retain and recall all of the required details from your experiences and data or information that comes in via your senses.

Your brain needs to remember all of the learned conclusions you have derived from your mind's internal thoughts and considerations related to all aspects of your past, present and future life at work, home and at leisure throughout the whole of your life.

SUBCHAPTER 2.5.2: An in-depth, detailed list of your *brain's fundamental roles*

ROLE A – Your brain's first fundamentally important role is to look after you, at all times, throughout your whole life together, in your intrinsically connected living and functioning arrangement.

OVERVIEW: *The principles of this, your brain's most crucial of roles, is to care for you at all times, throughout your lifetime together, with total commitment, trust, devotion, unconditional care and consideration. Also, it is to create and continually update your consciousness, <u>the foundation upon which you can:</u>*

1) Be kept safe.
2) Keep your emotional, physical and chemical health in the best possible order. At times, this includes your brain deliberately causing you to experience significant pain and/ or functional difficulties. This is because it cares for you,

and these are part of its strategies, along with promoting self-help and employing the placebo effect, for healing any physical or mental health difficulties you may have.

3) Make each one of your lifetime's multiples of trillions of appropriate <u>decisions</u> and take each of their <u>resultant</u> and required <u>actions</u> concerning the prevailing conditions and situations you are presented with every second, minute, hour and day.

NB These decisions and actions quite often demand incredibly fast response and reaction times from your brain. They also require multiple processing of different data, with various processing activities occurring at the same time. These operating features are all needed to keep you safe and/or to finalise very complex multi-faceted decisions and their actions. For example, responding to extremely fast-changing conditions whilst satisfying many prevailing objectives when driving your car in highly congested, ferociously challenging conditions. These functional features are also required whilst participating in many sporting activities with rapidly changing conditions involving numerous players with complex, ever-changing movements, etc.

On top of all of the attributes above, let's add the vast range of functional performances, control and balance coupled with the incredible speed of movement that your body is capable of. It seems like we have the creation of the virtually perfect machine of mind and body. What other than this would we expect from our Grand Creator?

What other job is permanent, from birth, nominally for three score years and ten, 24 hours per day, 7 days per week, with no pay, no holidays, no time off, no total sleep? On some occasions, **the almost immediate consequence of failure** in any of its fundamental duties is **your permanent demise!** No meetings, no judgements, no time for pondering your performance – you are dead!

Providing you give your brain sufficient good quality sleep every night so that it can get its house in good order, it thrives on being kept usefully busy. This keeps it organically healthy, functionally efficient and effective.

Yes, it's an awesome job, requiring a monumental range and depth of skills, capabilities, knowledge, flexibility, control and continual self-learning. All of this, I believe, is potentially available to you and your brain throughout your life if you really desire it.

The resultant benefits and abilities of all of the skills, detailed within ROLE A) above, is that when you become a mature, experienced adult, your body, with all of its incredible range of functionalities, under the control of your brain, is able to adapt to an almost unlimited range of highly complex conditions and situations. Sometimes, you have never experienced these before, and occasionally, they are presented to you completely unexpectedly.

However, despite all of this, in all weathers and conditions, and with all of the data coming into your brain in a clear and accurate condition to be processed by your brain, it is immediately able to respond appropriately. Finally, it will produce a safe

101

and acceptable resolution to any of the multitudes of different situations containing multifactorial, integrated and interrelated conditions you unexpectedly may find yourself facing.

Also, of the utmost importance, is something that I believe man-designed and man-made machines can't do now and never will be able to. Humans, who indisputably really do have intelligence, are able to suddenly be confronted with a complex set of interactive conditions, some of which they have never had to face before. By using their intelligence and assessing the consequences of the conditions in their present context, humans can understand the complexities they face. Consequently, they can find effective solutions to deal with all of these conditions successfully, normally within the extremely short periods of time required by the pressures of the prevailing situation.

ROLE B – Your brain's second fundamentally important role is to keep your body's vital services, organs, core states and facilities alive and functioning correctly and in healthy order.

This enables your brain and body to be kept alive with exercise, in good physical, chemical and functional health, and your consciousness to be continually updated throughout the whole of your life.

OVERVIEW: *The above role is basically accomplished by your mind and your M.C. utilising and benefiting from the operation, capabilities and achievements of all of your Category 1, 1A and 1B departments. The achievements of your Fully-Automatic, P.I.D. Closed-Loop Control Systems and your Semi-Automatic, Open-Loop*

Control Systems also play vital and dedicated parts in all of the above.

An example of your body automatically reacting to an unhealthy and Vital Service condition is snoring whilst you are asleep. I propose that this is caused because your Breathing Control System has detected that you are short of oxygen and automatically causes you to snore, the loudness being in proportion to the degree of lack of oxygen. The objective is to wake you up, to get you to solve or at least minimise the problem by getting you to alter your sleeping position, etc. Also, your sleeping partner or others hearing your snoring will inform you of your habit, hopefully encouraging you to get help to solve this condition if it regularly occurs.

The shortage of oxygen will, I believe, lower your sleep quality and reduce some of the activities and their intended health benefits which occur during your sleep. Eventually, this may result in you experiencing difficulties, including poor functional brain health.

ROLE B-1: A list of examples (with additional details) of some of these Vital Service's core functions and facilities your brain requires management of, as provided by one of your dedicated Category 1 departments.

Please note that this is not an exhaustive list – there are many more vital Core Functions and Facilities.

The first of these Vital Services is to maintain your *heart, blood pressure and blood flow* as required by your body. *This serves* to pump oxygenated blood from your lungs around your body and to carry waste produce*d by* core functions and facilities to other organs such as your lungs and kidneys to *be* remove*d*.

The second of these Vital Services is to keep your *blood sugar level* at the required and healthy level – not too high or not too low. It achieves this by altering the amount of insulin produced in your body which converts your sugar to energy. If you are diabetic, your blood sugar level automatic control system is faulty, so you have to measure and manage your sugar levels manually by medication and injections to suit.

The third of these Vital Services is maintaining your *body core temperature* close to 98.4 degrees Fahrenheit. If this temperature becomes too high or too low, your body's core temperature control system will automatically take measures to change your core temperature to the required 98.4°F value.

The fourth of these Vital Services is to keep you *breathing* at the necessary rate and depth to satisfy your body's required oxygen level in relation to your physical activities and other requirements.

NB You have the ability, when appropriate, to consciously regulate your breathing rate and depth in tandem with your underlying Semi-Automatic control system.

The fifth of these Vital Services is *your Body's Health Status Monitoring System (B.H.S.M.S.)* which automatically detects the following: whenever one or more of your vital organs, limbs, etc. has received an injury or developed an unhealthy condition; you are suffering from a mental health issue; an area of your body has become infected or diseased. Each condition requires an appropriate and immediate response by your body reacting in the most suitable, protective and/or healing way.

The sixth of these Vital Services is to maintain your chemical health in good healthy order.

ROLE B-2: A non-exhaustive list of some examples of the Vital Core States and conditions your brain requires the management of, each provided by one of your dedicated Category 1A departments.

The first of these Vital Core States is maintaining your emotional anxiety level in a healthy state to ensure that its ongoing day-to-day level is not too high.

The second of these Vital Core States is maintaining a healthy food intake and operating your Digestive System, basically converting your food to energy.

The third of these Vital Core States is passing water and managing your bowels.

The fourth of these Vital Core States is maintaining a healthy state of your brain's physiological health.

ROLE B-3: A list of examples (with additional details) of some Core Processes, Skills and knowledge that your brain requires service and management of. Each is provided by one of your dedicated Category 1B departments.

The first of these Vital Core Processes and Functionalities your brain requires is to provide the necessary Category 1B Departments that collectively enable your M.C. to conduct all of the processes needed to create your consciousness and carry out all of its required actions.

The second of these Vital Core Processes and Functionalities your brain requires is to provide an incoming and internal Data Review Scanning System. This continually gathers data from your five Senses, your B.H.S.M.S. and your internal thoughts, supplied from your seven Category 1B departments. This arrangement enables crucially important data items to be constantly available for viewing by your M.C. for its continual use in the creation and updating of your consciousness, upon which the whole of your Brain relates.

Part of the required functionality of this Data Scanning System is that it can receive instructions from your M.C. on its priorities. Therefore, before each scan cycle, it can set the percentage dwell time for each category of your five senses, your B.H.S.M.S. and your internal thoughts to suit the requirements of your M.C. at any one moment in time.

The third of these Vital Core Processes and Functionalities you require is maintaining a functioning and effective extensive list of your Developed Semi-Automatic Skills, with each one being satisfied and serviced by its own dedicated Category 1B department. For example: Reading, Writing, Speaking, Hearing, Seeing and executing the vast number of bodily movements you require to carry out.

ROLE C – Your brain's third fundamentally important role is to create and continually update your consciousness.

OVERVIEW: In my opinion, all humans, animals and living creatures have a consciousness. I also believe that all other living entities have a form of consciousness that, compared to humans, is at the other end of the scale of all-round capability. However, in all cases, its first priority is to keep its human or entity safe from harm and supplied with food or energy in order to stay alive.

After having a healthy body in all of its many aspects, I believe that the creation and constant updating of your consciousness are next in terms of importance. It is the absolute functional foundation upon which your mind, under the conductorship of your M.C. keeps you physically and emotionally safe and makes all of your considerations, decisions and their resultant actions in every living moment.

In my opinion, the fundamental benefit of the creation of your consciousness is that it provides the information to notify your M.C. of all of the situations and conditions that exist around and close to you, plus from within your own mind regarding what relates to and is of importance to you, in that moment in time.

Your consciousness provides the foundational part of the process. It enables you to make the most correct and appropriate choices and actions to each of your prevailing decisions required to be made. The goal is the achievement of your optimum intellectual and functional objectives during every moment within your world. This is the world that is sensed, detected, and decoded by you. Therefore, it is related to you and your specific needs concerning this world which is your reality in that moment of time.

I believe that your consciousness is created from the receipt of all raw data that enters your brain via your five senses and comes from within your brain, from your Body's Health Status Monitoring System and your internal thoughts. All of this data/information is converted and analysed and its full understanding and particular relevance to you is obtained in each moment.

A vitally important part of the detailed makeup that your consciousness comprises includes having an awareness of your emotional state and also an understanding of the emotional climate around you. This emotional climate relates to and connects with your prevailing situation and circumstances and is normally created by one or more individuals and yourself.

ROLE C-1 Your consciousness whilst asleep.

Many people believe that, when you go to sleep, your consciousness immediately shuts down and remains so whilst you are sleeping. I don't subscribe to this philosophy at all.

Whilst you are awake, I believe that your consciousness exists on an ongoing, continually updating, constant and *complete* basis. It continues to exist at a *very much reduced state of awareness whilst you are asleep*, mainly because your visionary senses are shut down. Whilst you are awake, they normally provide a vast percentage of the incoming data into your brain.

During this time of sleep, the primary and continuing purpose of your consciousness is to attempt to ensure the safety of yourself, your children and or others you care for who may also be there. As you sleep, the source of incoming data that your consciousness is derived from is primarily your hearing, with some lesser degree of sensitivity from your other three senses and zero from your vision.

ROLE C-2 *The crucial importance of making informed decisions.*

The importance of being able to make informed decisions can't be overstated. Without this ability, your body would be alive and exist, but you would be in a functionally vegetative state. You would be unaware of and unable to react to and take part in the world in which you currently exist and in which you hopefully play and enjoy an active and stimulating part.

You may feel that this continuous decision-making role is primarily one of making single and isolated choices. In reality, it is nearly always a case of making an ongoing set of interrelated decisions to satisfy objectives set up by you, plus by circumstances you find yourself in and also by other people, with some or all of these, on occasion, being interwoven.

Because the situations and conditions in which you are alive are continually changing to some degree or another, constant reviews are required. You have to reevaluate what you are doing and review some of the decisions you have made or about to make to take account of the prevailing conditions at each moment in time.

An example of an everyday experience of utilising your consciousness to make informed decisions and take the required actions to keep you safe and achieve your prevailing objectives.

Consider the following example to see how extensive a range of conditions and questions you can be faced with and the resultant decisions and related actions you have to make whilst carrying out everyday type activities and experience. This contains some life-threatening situations as well as some quite ordinary ones. However, each requires a significant amount from you of updating your Consciousness, data processing, thoughts of consideration, with their related decision-making and actions-taking.

Example – Walking around an extremely busy shopping high street, desperately trying to find someone.

What situations could you be faced with? What thoughts, related decisions and actions might you have to initiate during this activity which takes place over an hour?

You are walking along the pavements of an extremely crowded, busy road of a large city-centre shopping area on a Friday afternoon, just when the schools have closed for the day. You are desperately trying to find someone you wish to make very urgent contact with, who you suspect will be in this area at approximately this time.

Certain or likely activities you would be carrying out:

1) **On an *ongoing basis*,** you would be considering what safety situations existed and what appropriate actions you should take to keep you safe. You would be utilising, to the full, the immense amount of data coming in primarily from your eyes whilst straining to ensure you take notice of any sounds you receive, which must be dealt with appropriately. This

includes listening out for the extremely distinctive voice of the person you wish to meet.

2) **Your visual sense is *continually* straining extremely hard,** as you walk along the pavement on your side of the road, trying to spot the *particular person* you wish to speak with. Your vision desperately attempts to scan the faces of people coming towards you on your side and nominally coming towards you on the other side of the road. As best you can, you are scanning the faces of people going past you on both sides of the road. In an attempt not to miss this target person, your concentration is operating at the fiercest degree possible and burns up a lot of emotional energy.

3) **You notice a group of young school children** chatting away just in front of you. They are about to cross the road into the path of an oncoming lorry, oblivious to the oncoming danger. You warn them to be careful of the situation, which fortunately they take notice of.

4) **You are *constantly* manoeuvring** away from, around and past people, desperately attempting to physically avoid them whilst not wishing to miss sight of your target face. The difficulty of this activity is compounded, by the significant number of people engrossed in conversations with others. Also, with those who are walking along with headphones on whilst tapping into their handheld devices, oblivious to their surrounding world and all of the dangers and difficulties within it. This lack of awareness of potential dangers extends beyond their immediate zone, increasing the potential risks they are exposed to, none of which are

within their prevailing consciousness. This is a situation that is more prevalent today because of the incessant use of mobile phones whilst walking, etc.

5) **Your hearing sense is working extremely hard** by listening continually to all of the voices of anyone within your hearing range, trying to establish whether the person you wish to meet is near you. At the same time, it is listening out for any noises that may constitute dangers to you. Your thought processing activities are also working in overdrive as you are striving to remember what typical clothes this person would usually wear when you had been out shopping in the past. They also normally wore a particular and unusual hat, but you could not recall from memory what it looked like due to your state of anxiety.

Additionally, you may be faced with having to deal with one or two of the following possible situations, which your thought processing and your updating of your consciousness will be working actively upon:

6) **How to react to the sudden appearance** of a large, uncontrolled and extremely aggressive dog attempting to bite the leg of a small child near to you.

7) **How to react when you unexpectedly** see someone you know very well but do not wish to speak to them to at that particular moment, and your thought processes prepare you mentally for the worst if you are trapped into talking to them.

8) **How best to deal with** an oncoming very heavy rain squall you have predicted from observing the sky near you because

you have no waterproof clothes and you forgot to take an umbrella with you.

9)   **You suddenly realise** that your time in the prepaid car park is up in 5 minutes and you have an 8-minute walk to reach it, with an £80 fine at risk. What is the order of balance with this against your desperate need to speak to this person you seek? You decide to continue trying to find this person.

10) **How to react to the audible information** coming in from your ears of an alarming noise from behind you and to your right-hand side, of a car seemingly travelling above the speed limit, with squealing tyres and pedestrians shouting and screaming with fear. Your hearing and visionary data have been computed by your M.C. to judge that this car will be colliding with you in a few seconds. You turn round to assess the danger to yourself more accurately.

Your M.C. has been working at breakneck speed, preparing and commencing with self-preservation actions when a very old lady who knows you very well and who can only walk extremely slowly and has a white stick suddenly shouts to you for help. You instantly see everyone else is travelling away from her for self-preservation, leaving her stationery and in the danger zone. This means you have to backtrack into the danger zone if you go to her aid. Your wife just had your first child a week ago. This has transformed your life's priorities and has therefore had a significant bearing upon your decision making, particularly when it involves you entering into danger that you can avoid if you decide you should.

All of these many but vitally important internal thoughts have flooded into your updated consciousness to be considered by you, in addition to all of the others mentioned. What a continuous and ever-changing cauldron of consideration and decision making to process by your brain, with the compounding difficulty of having so little time available to finalise each of your decision making and action-taking activities.

What option do you decide upon?
It is very unlikely that you will be faced with all of these conditions and situations requiring your decisions, actions and involvement. However, you may well have to deal with a significant number from this list or ones that are similar in their degree of difficulty.

The net result of all of these multi-faceted set of conditions prevailing is that:

a) Your mind will be working furiously fast to keep pace with and understand the meaning and relevance of each item of the vast quantity of speedily changing incoming data, flooding in from your senses and internal thoughts, updating your consciousness 250 times every second.

b) Your mind will additionally have to process many different questions, considerations and actions, nominally at the same time. It will be utilising most of your senses, internal thoughts, several of your learned skills and lots of your memories from some of your Category 1B departments. All will be working individually and collectively during the whole process under the management of your Master Conductor.

All this gives an appreciation of just how busy your mind is without you being fully aware of this being the case. It highlights just how much your consciousness has to be continually updated so that your M.C. can hopefully make all of the best, correct, expedient decisions and actions to keep you safe from danger successfully. This is also necessary so your M.C. can successfully deal with all of your other, non-safety related ongoing decisions and related actions, all of which your consciousness presents to you, continually, all of the time.

ROLE D – Your brain's fourth fundamentally important role is to ensure that all of your body (your skeletal structure, muscles, sinews, bones and limbs, etc.) remain in a physically healthy functional state at all times.
It also ensures that your body remains free of any disease or inflammation. If the health of any of these objectives is in jeopardy, your brain's role is to ensure that the appropriate corrective action or actions occur immediately.

OVERVIEW:I Believe that your brain uses incredibly powerful, effective, indicative and corrective tools to help you achieve your objectives above. These are pain, discomfort etc. and/or functional disabilities, depression numb ness etc. and prompting and guiding you to self- help and inherently engaging your placebo effect.

*I believe that these objectives are **also** achieved by your Body's Health Status Monitoring System (B.H.S.M.S.). This is the system* *that automatically detects if you have a mental health problem, whether one or more of your vital organs or limbs, etc., has received an injury or developed an unhealthy condition, or if an area of your body has become infected or diseased. Each condition that is identified requires an appropriate response.*

The related Category 1A department of your brain will immediately, in the fastest possible time, report this unhealthy condition into your appropriate internal data input department so it will be processed in the next update of your consciousness. This will cause your body to react in an appropriate, protective and/or healing way. Your M.C. will recognise the meaning of these reactions. It will monitor your condition and support your corrective actions until you have re-established a safe/healthy status or condition. By then, these body reactions will have gradually ceased.

NB All of your Category 1A departments are located outside your mind and in the same general area where your Category 1 departments reside. This position affords them very good protection from physical injury and attack from infections because if your Category 1 departments, in particular, are damaged, your body will be unable to survive.

An example of your body reacting to an injury or damaged condition is in the case of a back injury. The appropriate part of your back will, as an involuntary action, automatically go into a spasm with associated constant pain. This ensures that you don't attempt any movement in the damaged part of your back in the immediate period.

From your learned memories and experiences, your M.C. will recognise the meaning of these symptoms. This will result in you visiting your doctor, taking the appropriate medication and carrying out the appropriate physical activities with the proper care for your back to return to its previously healthy state.

An example of your body reacting to an unhealthy condition that has developed is in the case of your heart becoming unhealthy. You will usually automatically experience regular aches or pains (of an appropriate level in relation to the degree of how unhealthy it is), in your chest, left arm or upper back and plus possibly other areas.

From your learned memories and experiences, your M.C. will ensure that you visit your doctor and take the appropriate medication and/or surgery. It will consciously work to reduce your emotional stress level, if applicable, until, hopefully, your heart has returned to its previously healthy state, and all of your aches will gradually have ceased.

ROLE E – Your brain's fifth fundamentally important role is to, at all times, keep your emotional health in the best possible order, thus enabling you to live the life CHANGE you wish, with its related enjoyment, achievement and satisfaction.

OVERVIEW: It is important to be aware that although you may have superb physical fitness and all of your bodily functions, conditions, facilities, and senses are in the best of order, if your emotional health is poor, with too much ongoing anxiety, you will suffer from unhealthy levels of Emotional Stress. This could lead to possible periods of depression, depending on a number of factors.

117

NB Regular physical exercise is recognised as an excellent way of de-stressing and helping to deal with mental illness. However, there are many cases of super-fit professional sportspersons who suffer severe mental health issues. One causal factor could be that skilled athletes are exercising in a far more emotionally and physically intense manner compared to those exercising recreationally. Thus the professionals derive less anxiety reduction benefits from exercising than recreational sportspersons.

If you are experiencing an ongoing poor state of mental ill-health, this will cause you to suffer increasingly from poor quality and quantity of sleep. This is due to your mind being full of negative aspects that continue to worry you, thus causing you difficulties getting to sleep in the first place. Also, during your fractured sleep, your brain is desperately trying to resolve your anxieties and worries by using your dreams to search and find solutions for you.

Your ongoing sleep problems cause you to wake up in the morning with elements of the work that your brain had planned to carry out being incomplete, proportionate to the degree of your sleep issues. The direct consequences of this are that your brain has not completed and fully tidied up all of its processing activities of the day. It is not refreshed, reset and ready to face the rigours of a new day. This means that most of the time, you will have to force yourself out of bed to go to work, school or wherever you are committed to being. You will not feel mentally sharp, with the emotional energy and vigour that we all need to operate as well as we are capable of and would like. You will not be able to concentrate effectively and not be mentally able to function clearly, efficiently and enjoyably.

At times, your decision making will be driven by too much emotion or fuzzy headedness and illogical thinking. You are at increased risk of your flaky emotional state and the consequential, fluctuating, high level of your Ongoing Tower of Emotional Stress emotionally over-reacting to a co-worker who you dislike quite intensely and who is not too keen on you either. You will therefore be in danger of saying the wrong things inappropriately to your boss, in front of the C.E.O. and some board members, then feeling forced to apologise, leading to all sorts of potential and avoidable difficulties for you.

The combinational consequences of all of these factors are that you will be increasingly unhappy. Your life will be difficult at work, at home with your family and no doubt socially. It will be an all-round struggle and strife life for you – not enjoyable most of the time.

Continued high levels of Ongoing Emotional Stress contribute to your related ineffective responses to dealing with your life's difficulties. This creates more poor quality and quantity of sleep problems and, therefore, even greater emotional stress. Consequently, you experience more episodes of anxiety, leading to a degree of depression. And so, the wheel of interconnected psychological and emotional difficulties turns faster and stronger, as it gathers its inherent momentum, becoming increasingly unstable and difficult to slow down and gain control of. You will no doubt, and not surprisingly, to some degree, feel that your life is increasingly falling apart.

It is my belief that your brain, mind and body are fully inter-meshed, intertwined, closely coupled entities, comprising of the ultimate and most coordinated team of three units that probably exist in our Universe.

If you are ever suffering from the conditions above, **IT IS VITALLY IMPORTANT THAT YOU SEEK HELP AND VISIT YOUR GP AS SOON AS POSSIBLE.** If the preceding conditions continue for too long, you will develop increasingly significant mental health illnesses, which will likely lead to substantial physical ill-health.

Full recovery from these conditions could be extremely difficult. It may take a long time to achieve, resulting in possibly having to accept expedient degrees of recovery improvements along the way.

ROLE E-1: Three required conditions or states your brain seeks to keep in good order to enjoy good emotional health.

1-a) The **first** is for your brain to maintain your Ongoing Emotional Anxiety Stress Condition at a nominally low, healthy level and understand how to achieve this.

One of your Category 1A departments in your B.H.S.M.S. is continually working to achieve this objective by automatically monitoring and evaluating your body's Ongoing Emotional Stress Level. It is reviewing its overall rise and fall rate, plus analysing your Emotional Stress Instantaneous Peak Levels when they occur.

Inside your mind, I believe everyone has what I refer to as a Tower of Emotional Stress, the prevailing height of which I call your Ongoing Emotional Stress Level. Each condition or situation that makes you feel unhappy and uncomfortable creates its own individual block of Emotional Stress that adds to your ongoing Tower's total.

The height of these blocks of stress varies, depending on what you are currently thinking about each of them. The total height CHANGE of this Ongoing Tower of Stress fluctuates as you progress through your day, dealing with all of the situations that life brings, with some of them having a degree of Emotional Stress attached. Unfortunately, some of these blocks of stress will be caused by situations that are ongoing in your life simply because you have not solved them to date.

If you experience an *Emotional Stress Instantaneous Peak Level* which is unhealthily high, your brain's appropriate Category 1A department will automatically initiate an increased level of adrenalin. It will open up your arteries to increase the blood flow to your brain, thus helping you think and respond as clearly, quickly and effectively as possible to deal with the difficulty. This peak is normally caused by sudden, unexpected exposure to bad, dangerous or deeply worrying news or a situation that causes a high level of anger and/or Emotional Stress. In addition to these actions stated above, your M.C. will, from Learned Memories relating to your state and the actual prevailing condition it is witnessing, initiate other activities that deal with the difficulties. This consequently lowers your Emotional Peak Stress Level as the crisis becomes resolved.

NB Your spike of Emotional Stress Instantaneous Peak Level will sit on top of your pre-existing/prevailing Tower of Stress. If this is already at an unhealthy height, it will probably push the total height of your Tower of Stress over the threshold. It will enter into the band where you are increasingly at risk of seriously uncontrolled and unacceptable/unhealthy decision making and resultant actions/behaviour. The higher your Tower of Stress grows, the more your decisions and related actions become driven by raw emotions and less by cold logic.

If your Ongoing Tower of Average Emotional Stress Level has become unhealthily elevated, this will likely have been caused by the <u>cumulative effect</u> of some of the following Underlying Causes. They have probably existed for too long a period, thus causing you disproportionate stress.

This is a list of the Underlying Causes of Emotional Stress that prevail in our modern life. It is vitally important that your brain is aware of these causes and monitors your Emotional State at all times to take the necessary action required to protect you.

1) Your lifestyle and activities at work, home and socially.
2) A significant and frequent shortage of good quality and quantity sleep.
3) The lack of job security, with ongoing worrying about whether you will keep your job.
4) Pushing to keep up with your workload and targets at work, therefore having to work harder, more efficiently and typically additional hours.

5) A new boss, with all of the numerous possibilities relating to consequential stresses.

6) Trying too hard to get promoted.

7) Being expected to, and eventually taking, fewer and shorter break periods at work.

8) Being contactable via emails and your mobile phone after hours and whilst on holidays.

9) Worrying when your next pay rise will be.

10) Being unexpectedly made redundant from your work.

11) Relationship difficulties at work, within your family and beyond.

12) Ongoing problems with paying bills, particularly the essential bills for gas, electricity, heating and food.

13) Trying to keep up with the Joneses.

14) Feeling that your life has become a daily battle for survival.

15) Worrying where the next order is coming from to keep your company afloat.

16) Worrying about the poor quality of competence and attitude of your employees.

17) Worrying about your children and your grandchildren.

18) Worrying about your health and your family's health.

19) Doing insufficient regular exercise, creating a lack of physical fitness, being overweight and the resultant anxieties.

20) Bereavement caused by:

a) The unexpected death of someone extremely close to you, particularly when you had no time to prepare.

b) The death of your last parent.

c)   The death of a long-lived and much-loved animal.

21) Finally retiring from work that you absolutely loved and enjoyed the whole of your life can create many difficulties. These include a significant loss or reduction of self-esteem and self-worth, the lack of a reason to get up each day, and not having a clear purpose for your life. This applies particularly to men, with the loss of the majority of their acquaintances and friends.

NB Notably, for some men who spend most of their life being extremely busy at work and at home, rushing here and there, the consequences can be that their hectic life is covering up or putting a lid on a mental health issue or issues. When they retire, these issues are cruelly exposed when they surface and cause significant mental ill-health. This adds to the very significant emotional stress created by stopping work forever.

22) In children or young adults, significant Emotional Stress can be caused by their increasing and health-damaging excessive use of their mobile phones. They are constantly used for communicating with their vast number of social media friends. They are compared and voted upon regarding their facial beauty, figure, the number of so-called friends they have, their attractiveness to the opposite sex, etc.

NB Making contact via screens rather than face-to-face is not developing their brains in the previously normal healthy way as they are not evolving crucially important social skills. Using phones virtually at all times whilst awake is damaging and interferes with maturing their physical and mental health. It also negatively affects the quality and quantity of their sleep, which, in itself, causes a raft of physical and mental ill-health. Many parts of young people's brains are not being developed as they should be to lead an emotional and functionally healthy, effective and normal life.

23) On top of the existing ones, there are an increasing number of new/additional facets to modern life that may add Emotional Stress to young people, if they are affected by them. These include:

a) Deciding what sex you are, compared to what sex you are born with. This, I believe, is a situation that, if not handled with extreme care, has the potential to destroy a person's future. There can be fundamental and so far unknown difficulties resulting from the decisions made and the consequences of each of them.

b) The frequent and intense pressure imposed upon each of them, with the importance of academic learning, taking tests, exams, assessments. All of which is added to the pressure life puts them under, during the natural process of growing up.

c) The ever-increasing use of the internet to communicate with so many so-called friends can lead to a serious level of internet usage addiction.

d) The ever-increasing use of social websites and games via the internet, which were, by instruction within the software company in which they were originally created, designed to be powerfully emotionally addictive. Thus, the users became emotionally addicted and therefore unable to stop using them, as alcoholics become unable to stop drinking excessively. These users attempt to satiate their addictions at every opportunity, usually every day.

I have unfortunately noticed that more and more older people are also carrying out these practices. The overall emotionally addictive effect of all of these devices that an increasing percentage of people suffer from makes me very concerned for their future mental health and the general health of a growing portion of our human race.

Under the extreme stranglehold of addiction that these practices impose, people seem to switch off their brains when you attempt to warn them of the damage they are doing to themselves. If you advise them to throw them away, you can immediately see a panic attack flickering.

24) The role that women increasingly play is moving away from their previously natural yet absolutely fundamental female and motherly-type priorities. Many are now striving to live the life of a part-time mother whilst working in a full-time job, with the belief that they should look upon their working life objectives as being identical to men. Some (I suspect the majority of) girls-only schools, adopt this extremely high profile with focussed, strident encouragement for all of their girls.

However, I believe that this vision and objective presented to their students should include the vitally important and, for the majority of them, inevitably connected aspect of them having children, because therein lies the potentially conflicting difficulty.

I consider that this "have it all" goal and, in many ways, adopting a manly attitude to an increasing number of aspects of life places many functional and emotional stresses upon women that, for the vast majority of them, did not previously exist. A significant amount of this additional emotional stress is caused by acting out emotionally, mentally, verbally and physically, masculine rather than feminine attitudes and actions. As this can be rather unnatural, it causes, in itself, a significant amount of additional stress and anxiety in women's everyday lives.

All of these unnatural objectives, attitudes and lifestyles inherently create the majority of unachievable goals, thus generating even more functional and emotional stresses. This leads to poorer quality and less quantity of sleep, reduced self-esteem, feelings of inadequacy and failure. There is an inevitable increasing resentment and, in many cases, anger towards their husbands and men in general, creating a growing rate of sliding into a pit of deepening despair.

NB At this point, <u>I must firmly point out</u> that I do not hold any of these views from an anti-women stance at all – <u>far from it</u>. <u>Nothing could be further from the truth.</u> I am, and always have been, a great admirer of women and champion the wonderful emotional and physical differences between males and females. I believe with my whole being that neither men nor women are inferior or superior – they are simply different, emotionally, physically and with a varied skillset (at times).

These differences make our world go round in the most interesting and enjoyable way that I believe it certainly does. I see the cornerstones of the whole of our lives on this planet earth are that we human beings inhabit it, in both male and female format, each of which is wonderfully different and was formed as such by the marvellous Grand Creator.

If the human form morphed into a non-male and non-female form, I honestly believe that the majority of life's fundamental, basic and sheer pleasures would have totally disappeared.

I feel I must repeat that these views I am expressing are driven purely by one singular objective, which is my increasing concern for the worsening mental health of women. This is linked to the increasingly sloping downwards path they are taking or being driven down by high profile ladies in a few instances. Most of them have a totally different and potentially easier lifestyle, compared with the vast majority of the non-high profile, typical women of our world.

ROLE E-1b) How your brain deals with an extremely unhealthily high Ongoing Tower of Emotional Stress, with one particular causal scenario of suffering from migraines.

I believe that the condition of an unhealthily high Ongoing Tower of Emotional Stress will be the **functional cause** of your mental health difficulties. It will probably have caused you to suffer from increasingly poor quality and quantity of sleep, leading to becoming increasingly mentally unwell. You are likely to experience making more and more poor quality decisions, plus having more relationship difficulties at home, work, and in life generally.

This unhealthy state of your Average Ongoing Emotional Stress Level will automatically have been detected by your appropriate Category 1A department. It will most likely cause you to experience at least <u>one</u> of many different types of <u>headache</u>. The location and type of headache depend upon your character profile, your physiological and related genetic makeup.

The severity and frequency of these headaches, will relate to the level of unhealthy emotional anxiety and stress you are suffering from and, to a degree, how long this condition has existed for.

You may also experience functional difficulties and discomforts (pins and needles, numbness, poor clarity of vision, muzzy thinking and speaking) at a level proportionate to the degree of unhealthy Average Emotional Stress you are experiencing and suffering from.

From its learned experiences and memories, your M.C. will notice and recognise the significance of each of these symptoms. It knows they are your brain's attempts to warn you and help you, get you to slow down functionally and emotionally, lead an emotionally healthier lifestyle and get more good quality sleep. Your M.C. will review what it thinks are the individual **Underlying Causes** behind your anxiety. It will work tirelessly to try and get you to drive down the degree of each of these from which you are currently suffering. Ideally, it aims to stop you from carrying out as many of these causes of your anxiety as possible.

NB At this stage, it is also extremely worthwhile assessing whether the state of your **physical health** is a significant contributory factor in the creation of your mental health difficulties. This is particularly the case if you have previously been very fit for many years and, for whatever reasons, your physical fitness has gradually evaporated. If true to some degree, this situation will cause you significant additional anxiety in your life due to having lost a good level of physical fitness and the related loss of wellbeing that being in good physical condition always creates. The additional and significant loss you will have suffered is being unable to benefit from one of the best ways of reducing your anxiety – going out and having a great four-mile run on your own or with some mates, playing in a match of football, rugby, hockey, or having a swim, etc.

Whilst you are carrying out these types of physical activities, you are creating feel-good chemicals, and crucially, you forget about your worries of the day from work etc., as you focus upon entirely different and emotionally healthy objectives. A shower afterwards, and then a drink with your mates is enjoyable contact with other human beings. Your world has taken on an entirely different hue and is a pleasure to be part of.

To continue from above: If this process proves successful, as these Underlying Causes of each of your blocks of Emotional Stress are either eliminated or reduced, the total height of your Ongoing Tower of Emotional Stress will proportionately reduce.

This will cause your headaches and other symptoms to gradually decrease until you recover to an emotionally healthy state when they are all hopefully gone. By this stage of the process, you will have progressively become significantly calmer and less stressed, as if you have been emotionally cleansed.

If, at **any time**, you are not making good progress and your state of emotional health has not improved much, if at all, **it is imperative that you seek the urgent help of an experienced counsellor through your GP. Enlist their guidance** to focus upon identifying and dealing with the **underlying root causes** of your anxieties and why you react so much to each of these ongoing, unresolved difficulties in your life. This aspect of consideration and change of your dealing with each of the Underlying Causes of anxiety, recognising **why** you are so stressed and unable to resolve or even minimise them, are very likely to be the areas you didn't deal with well enough or possibly at all.

I would like to leave you with this extremely important message: try to help yourself, initially by working with your brain as above and talking to your best buddy and/or partner. **Please don't tackle it all on your own, and crucially, don't leave it long before you visit your GP.**

ROLE E-1c) How your brain ensures that you develop and maintain good quality people relationships at home, work and play during your whole life.

*OVERVIEW: To achieve this objective, I believe there are several **Category 1B departments** in your brain for assessing, managing* *and dealing with all of your social interactions with all other people. This data includes all social skills, relevant characteristics of diverse types of people, good and bad, different sexes, nationalities and information relating to all of the people you have met **throughout your life**.*

As you continually interact with people, these departments work particularly hard to update all of their relevant subdepartments of detailed data concerning each person and general information about people. I believe that details about each person or type of person are related to and triggered with an image in your memory of that individual or kind of person. When you are socially interacting with other people, your brain is working at an **extremely high level of Data Processing activity**. It utilises a very wide range of skills, facilities observations and memories within your brain, which are reflected in many factors:

1) The total number of different departments in your brain that it is using.

2) The total range of emotions, experiences and the skills it is employing.

3) The total number of new and repetitive observations, decisions and actions it makes per update of your consciousness.

4) The degree of concentration it is employing.

5) If you are playing a team sport or other physical activity involving a lot of other people, the total number of new observations, decisions and actions your brain is making per

consciousness update involves it operating at an extremely fast and busy processing speed.

6) The range of your own, Developed, Category 1B departments, Semi-Automatic Skills employed by your M.C. needed for the application and coordination of your physical actions and in relation to other people's actions and reactions is immense. In addition, the application of a number of Category 1B departments to utilise their contained data of particular knowledge is necessary during your sporting activities.

Although, nearly all of your life's difficulties and negatives are caused by the frailty and damaging characteristics of people's decisions and actions, almost all the good and satisfying aspects of your life are also created by people, some of whom are the same. Life without people would be lifeless, and life with people who were 100% perfect all of the time would be utterly boring and unfulfilling, in my opinion. Unless you live the life of a recluse, all of our lives revolve around people. They are involved directly, indirectly, immediately and remotely with every aspect of every day of your lives. For your emotional health to be in good order, I believe it is so vitally important to have friends who:

Firstly, give you help in your difficult times and value the support you offer them in their difficult times. Secondly, have an involvement in the life around you and have a varied range of interests in their own life. Thirdly, have a good number of healthy relationships that they enjoy on a regular basis.

To achieve all of this requires you to have developed the necessary range of interpersonal skills and have a significant and healthy degree of self-respect and liking of yourself, without which you will find that you can't like and respect others, at least sufficiently so. A very significant factor in having an emotionally balanced and happy life is to regularly enjoy several healthy relationships with various types of people throughout your life.

ROLE E-1d) How your brain ensures you obtain sufficient good quality sleep every night.

Question 1 – Why does your brain require you to *sleep* *well on a nightly basis?*

***OVERVIEW:** Throughout your life, I believe that it is crucially important to ensure that you have sufficient, excellent quality sleep, ideally every night. This is the foundation of being best able to live an emotionally and physically healthy life. Without this very solid foundation to live upon, your life is inevitably going to be a big struggle!* After a hard day's activities, sleep is for your tired body to rest and recover physically. It allows your body's system's chemical health/statuses to be re-optimised as far as possible. Your emotional health can be improved, and your brain's functional health status and operational efficiency brought up to date. It also gives time for updating all of your Memory Experiences and Knowledge subdepartments, plus attempting to resolve any unanswered, important questions and difficulties you have.

In order for your brain to keep in an optimum state of functional and cellular health, it requires sufficient, good quality sleep every night. However, *not too much sleep*, particularly dozing, semi- waking and dozing, etc., because I believe that your brain, once refreshed, **needs** to be fully awake and begin working in the new day.

Providing you have had enough good quality sleep during a night, hopefully, all of the primary objectives of your brain will have been achieved. Therefore, you will be very well-rested and refreshed, with your emotional, chemical and physical health being in very good healthy order, thus meaning that your overall health will also be in excellent order. So, on waking, this will be an optimum time to take medicines or drugs with any particularly important objectives, as I would surmise your body will react to them in the most beneficial way.

Question 2 – What happens to your consciousness when you are asleep?

OVERVIEW: Some people believe that when you go to sleep, your consciousness is immediately shut down and remains shut down whilst you remain asleep.

<u>I don't believe this at all.</u> I believe that, during your sleep, your consciousness continues to be updated non-stop as it does whilst you are awake for exactly the same reasons as when you are awake. Data from your five senses is sent <u>into your brain</u> for immediate processing. Data sets from your B.H.S.M.S. and internal thoughts are passed <u>internally from within your brain</u>

where they already exist and again are processed immediately
into the next update of your consciousness.

Obviously, with your eyes closed, your brain will not be
receiving any Visionary Data. However, your data processing
systems will still automatically check for Visionary Data and
will continue if some does arrive. Therefore, they are not caught
out and lose valuable response time, particularly with respect to
keeping you safe at all times.

All of the data from these sources is continually processed,
night and day, within your brain to create and update your
consciousness. Your M.C. studies the information contained
within your consciousness. It selects any data that relates to your
safety being in jeopardy, plus other data that does not relate to
your safety but requires you to consider and take appropriate
actions in all cases.

The degree of ability of your senses to protect you whilst you
are sleeping is obviously significantly reduced, particularly from
the perspective of a loss of vision. This is also dependent upon
the sensitivity of detection your senses have at any time, due to
bedclothes and pillows, etc. I believe that if danger is detected,
your response to it will be categorised at the highest attainable
level of importance, and your decision making will be engaged
in the fastest possible time.

However, despite all of the above considerations and
conditions, whilst you are asleep, I propose that your brain
continues, as best it can, with creating and updating your
consciousness and dealing with any conditions that it deems a
priority to keep you safe and for other objectives.

NB During sleep, the frequency of data changing and conditions changing coming into your brain will generally be extremely minimal compared to whilst awake. I believe that for most different types of living entities, the location of where they sleep, the pattern, length and frequency of their sleeping all relates to minimising the prevailing dangers they face. Typically, these are from their natural enemies, predators and also from environmental and terrain-related difficulties and risks to them.

If you are asleep in your own bed at home and you do not have any unusual or particular reasons to be unsure of your safety, your average level of consciousness will nominally be 5% of the norm of when you are awake. However, if you are sleeping in a strange bed in a foreign room and an unfamiliar location, the degree of your consciousness will be elevated, proportionately to the degree of your being emotionally uncomfortable, particularly during your first night. All this will result in you not having your normal good quality sleep, meaning you wake the next morning not feeling sharp and refreshed or ready to tackle the new day.

Question 3 – What detailed activities take place in your brain during your sleep?

I believe that you have many Category 1B departments, each with many subdepartments, for managing the various activities within your brain **whilst you are sleeping every night.** The principles of these activities are for:

1) Your M.C. to review all information in your short, medium and longer-term Memory Departments, related to your brain's recent decision making, deleting any information that has become redundant, retaining and updating information for future use as required.

2) Logging all relevant data related to carrying out further thinking about very important, current decisions your brain has yet to make, which, during your waking hours, you have not been able to come to a conclusion on. Quite often, this further deliberation whilst asleep will result in you making an acceptable and sometimes a remarkably good decision. However, if not, your M.C. will hopefully have become aware that a very likely reason you have not been able to make a decision about some situation may simply be caused by there being too long a list of considerations, with some items having their own list of considerations. This will result in you wheeling around the list of aspects to consider, changing from one decision then to another, never really feeling confident of any of your possible solutions.

I have found the best way to resolve this is to carry out the following written exercise.

- Whilst awake, compile a table containing a list of each of the objectives you require to be fulfilled by your decision or solution.
- Rate from 1 to 10 (10 = the best) the weight of importance to you that each of these objectives has.
- List all of the possible solutions you can think of.

- For each of these possible solutions, note on the table how many of the objectives are satisfied and for each one, add its rate weight value.
- Then finally, note which solution gives you the highest accumulated weight. This is the one that is, on balance, the best solution.

3) Reviewing all new data: new experiences data, new learned experiences and attitudes data, new learned Automatic Skills and any other type of new data received since your last sleep. All of this information will have been located in a temporary, New Data, Category 1B department and goes through the following process:

   Firstly: Deleting what is not required to be retained.

   Secondly: Sending that which is to be retained to its appropriate, permanent department. Here, each item of data or sets of items of experience data will be reviewed by the department's Processing Neural Networks system, to update existing data or store new data as required. The above process will involve reviewing, deleting, updating and adding new data to all Memory Departments and all other types of departments, covering Categories 1A and 1B.

   Thirdly: Refreshing any memories to support their continuing retention, located in their appropriately labelled Memory Category 1B Department Memory Cell.

4) As far as possible, ensuring that all **unfinished activities** within all of your brain's departments are completed.

5) Utilising your dreams – see Question 4 below.

6) **Rapid Eye Movement** – It has been found that, during your sleep, whilst you are dreaming, your eyes move with rapid movement, referred to as **R.E.M.** I understand that there is speculation why this movement occurs, particularly when your bodily motion is automatically inhibited during dreaming. When you are awake, and with your eyes open, as you look around and take in the vision of your surroundings and general visionary information, your eyes are moving here and there most of the time, looking at different and particular visual details. Therefore, I believe that this R.E.M. is simply your eyes moving in relation to the changing visions that you imagine during your dreams, as they would do in your real life, waking situations.

Question 4 – Why does your brain cause you to have dreams?

1) One of your brain's priorities during your sleep is to work very hard to reduce your ongoing prevailing Tower of Emotional Stress by addressing the most stressful issues currently affecting your life. It uses dreams as the primary tool to achieve this objective. This is achieved by acting out your worries in your dreams, either in the principles and/or details of the actual worry itself or via a coded set of actions and situations.

   The benefits of this activity are for you to be able to face up to and confront your difficulties a lot easier than in reality. You can also reduce the stress you feel in real life, and it can lead you to form solutions to your concern or requirements. All of these benefits may not be achieved immediately, but potentially, eventually, dependent upon the emotionally related degree of each item of stress creator plus other items and conditions that contribute to your current, ongoing Emotional Anxiety Stress Level.

2) A certain number of blocks of stress that continue to circulate in your mind regularly and have done for many years may relate to awful experiences that date back to your early life at school, etc. Each of these created an extremely high level of emotional damage to you, which is retained in your memories and continues to hurt you because a) you simply haven't attempted to deal with them or b) you have attempted to, but without success. It will be beneficial to you if you try to gradually minimise/run them down by facing up to them, accepting they occurred and moving on from them in the ways most appropriate to their details. It will take quite a number of cycles of this process, but you should gradually reduce their emotional sting.

A few of your dreams may relate to some of these, and it is so important to face them one at a time. Relive them, learn from them where appropriate, reduce their emotional level of hurt, banish them forever and mean it. The cumulative damage they cause to your ongoing Tower of Stress is no doubt very significant and is added to your day-to-day blocks of stress.

3) During your dreams, I believe that one of your brain's objectives is that you're required to experience them as if

they are emotionally real. However, to protect you and anyone near you from harm, your ability for physical movement to replicate the physicality of your dream movements is automatically disabled. I also think that, from your caveman era, your motion during dreams is disabled to protect you from exposure to harm from your enemies, both in human and animal form.

I propose that the people who, whilst still in some depth of sleep and dreaming, walk and carry out other activities, or sit up in bed and talk for some reason, have not had their movement and talking capability disabled as usual. This is because they are extremely emotionally stressed about something, and their brain makes them act in this manner to further attempt to help them become de-stressed about their difficulties. In my opinion, everyone dreams at times during their sleep, over a range of frequency of occurrence. Some people remember their dreams easily and others not so readily, with some even insisting that they don't dream much at all.

4) During sleep, with your body in a physically at-rest state and your brain having minimal external data to respond to, it is relatively free to tidy itself up. Therefore, it can maintain and optimise the chemical health status of your many systems and facilities, each of which is so crucial to the quality of your emotional, chemical and physical health. I believe that your brain works tirelessly, in conjunction with particular Category 1A and 1B departments, trying

to keep your physical, chemical and emotional health in the best of order.

I also propose that, as you sleep, when your brain is in a period of relatively inactive state, it undergoes a kind of cleansing process. The objective of this is to physically cleanse and refresh all of the physical constituents that it comprises to keep them in as optimum a state of cellular health as possible.

Question 5 – What are the consequences for your brain of having insufficient, good quality sleep?

1) I believe that if all of these activities listed above are not fully achieved each night due to a lack of sufficiently good quality sleep, you will feel emotionally and mentally sluggish the following day and will be unable to function at maximum efficiency.

2) If you continue to have insufficient good quality sleep on an ongoing basis, your emotional, physical and chemical health will suffer. This will be proportionate to how many nights of ongoing poor quality sleep you have suffered and to what degree of poor quality sleep you have suffered.

3) If your lack of sleep continues, it can approach becoming critical, for example, when you have suffered a significant amount of jet lag when flying and had virtually no good quality sleep, but continue to keep going when returning home. If this is the case, your brain will suddenly virtually try to shut you down. It will quickly make you feel

exhausted, forcing you to stop doing what you are doing and get sleep as soon as possible/straight away, so it can commence the processes listed above.

4) Because your brain is such a highly complex and busy facility, if it does not have its daily period of sufficient, good quality sleep, it will very soon, dependent upon its workload and current functional health, gradually become increasingly functionally unhealthy. If deprived of insufficient sleep for too many successive days, it will become unable to function healthily and effectively at all, and you will begin to go out of sensible control in an increasingly alarming manner.

Question 6 – What are all of the actions your brain can ensure that you take to keep itself in the best of condition and functionality whilst warding off dementia and other diseases?

For a detailed list of the answer to this question, refer to Subchapter 7.11.

ROLE F – Your brain's sixth fundamentally important role and activity is the utilisation of the incredibly powerful, effective, indicative and corrective tools it has available.

They include pain, discomfort and/or functional disabilities – depression, numbness, etc. Additionally, your brain can prompt and guide you to self-help and inherently engage your placebo effect.

Your brain employs these tools above, individually and collectively, as appropriate to each of your individual circumstances to **HELP and ASSIST** you in recovering from physical ailments and poor mental health, with your B.H.S.M.S. and M.C. being crucially involved.

ROLE F-1 The types of and reasons for pain.

Your brain causes you to experience two types of pain for different possible reasons. It also causes you to experience many diverse forms of dysfunctionalities, mainly for one common reason – a very high level of ongoing Emotional Stress. Additionally, your brain takes every opportunity to prompt and guide you towards self-help and inherently engage your placebo effect.

ROLE F-1a) Suffering from pain

a) **Suffering a continuous type of pain:**

Reason/Cause 1.0 – You can experience **continuous pain** at any time, caused by any part of your body being damaged. For example, where you are cut, burnt, suffering from physical injuries or damage caused by diseases. In each of these cases, your sensors will detect that you have a problem in their area and send your brain **continuous** pain data signals to inform it of the situation. Your brain will then give you constant pain in the appropriate area.

Solution 1.0 – Your M.C. will deal with the situation by arranging for you to take immediate and appropriate actions to address whatever the problem is by contacting your GP or phoning for an ambulance, etc.

Reason/Cause 2.0 – You can experience **continuous headache pain** from a list of various types, each with different names and locations when experiencing **migraine** difficulties. I believe the reason for this pain is your brain noticing that you have a very high level of daily, ongoing anxiety and are extremely stressed. Therefore, your brain is deliberately giving you these bad headache pains to try and get you to slow down. It wants you to de-stress yourself by making you less able to continue doing what is contributing to your elevated level of Ongoing Emotional Anxiety and Stress.

Solution 2.0 – Your M.C. deals with the situation by making you contact your GP to arrange help from a counsellor to deal with all of the separate causes which are contributing to your **high Tower of Emotional Stress**. This is causing you to suffer from a prevailing consciousness dominated by suffocating Anxiety, Emotional Stress and resultant negativity.

b) **Suffering from a very short sharp stabbing type of pain:**
Reason/Cause 1.0 – If you have a chronic back problem, you may experience **very short stabs of pain** at any time, as arranged/created by your brain. For example, when you are overloading your back beyond its prevailing

capability, your brain will give you a sharp **stab of pain** in the appropriate area to remind you, don't do this. You have a bad back, and as soon as you have removed the load on your back, the pain will go.

Reason/Cause 2.0 – If you have a chronic knee problem, and you are overloading your knee by hauling/pulling a lady around the dance floor who is resisting you leading them, which, as a man, is your role, your brain will protect you with a warning stab of pain. You will immediately stop the pulling action, and the pain will immediately disappear. You will also experience the same helpful type of pain with any other joint problems.

I believe that if you suffer from a chronic joint problem, the very worst thing to do is not move it at all and just take medication. You must move it as often as possible with an effective exercising activity that stimulates blood flow which promotes healing and, crucially, reduces inflammation. If you have been carrying out some activity that employed moving your chronic joint, and you experience only slight ache-type conditions, don't worry. Carry on the good work.

ROLE F-1b) Suffering from dysfunctionalities

OVERVIEW: *These dysfunctionalities can be very variable in their existence in their location and intensity. They take the form of a few examples of one or more of a selection from a very long list of possibilities: numbness or pins and needles; experiencing Brain Fog/ not thinking clearly and not speaking very clearly; not being able to see clearly with flashing lights; shimmering vision; feeling extremely drained of physical and emotional energy; having aches and pains in various locations, etc.*

NB A patient can suffer symptoms and difficulties both with their mental and physical health. Often, no direct root cause of many of these dysfunctionalities a person is experiencing is found. Specialist opinions they are given quite often include the questioning statement of – is the cause in the patient's mind, or is it in their body? I believe that it is in both, but you have to understand why, in order to be able to start to treat them effectively. If you don't know and fully understand the principal causes of any illness, how are you able to know what to do to affect a cure? In fact, it is potentially dangerous to commence any treatment, in my opinion.

You can suffer from a very long list of different types of dysfunctionalities.

Reason/Cause 1.0 – Migraine – You can experience various forms of dysfunctionalities when experiencing migraines, which can be an extremely serious and debilitating illness. Your brain is subjecting you to these symptoms because it has noticed the degree of your daily/ongoing Anxiety and Emotional Stress has become damagingly high for a long period of time. Your brain is desperately trying to slow you down and de-stress you by making you unable to continue doing what is contributing to your **elevated level of ongoing Emotional Stress** and therefore causing you significant mental ill-health.

Solution 1.0 – Your M.C. must get you to immediately deal with the situation by contacting your GP, ideally to arrange help from a counsellor. This is to unearth and then deal with all of the separate causes contributing to your high Tower of Emotional Anxiety, which is the underlying Functional Cause of your Illness.

Reason/Cause 2.0 – Depression – You can experience this one most common form of dysfunctionality. The degree or depth of depression can be a very light level all the way up to that of an extremely serious and debilitating degree when the patient is incapable of or wants to do anything at all.

Solution 2.0 – If this dysfunctionality has returned or is new and has been prevailing for too long a time and is not showing signs of getting better, **you must visit your GP as soon as possible.** This is to ideally arrange for you to get help from a counsellor to unearth and then deal with all of the separate causes which are causing you a **significantly elevated level of ongoing Emotional Stress** causing your depression.

Reason/Cause 3.0 – A Mental Breakdown – Apart from one other, I would describe this as the ultimate dysfunctionality of them all. Anyone suffering, or who has suffered, particularly for a long time, from a persistent, ever-growing, **very high Ongoing Tower of Anxiety and Emotional Stress** is at risk. Your brain could become so worried about your state of mind, poor-quality decision-making and increasingly frequent loss of control and relationships with others it takes the ultimate action left in its toolbox to stop this downwards spiral into the pit of despond or worse. It makes you have a mental breakdown.

Solution 3.0 – You must deal with potentially the most crucial of all mental health situations by contacting your GP immediately. They need to very carefully decide what best to do in the first instance, by asking a number of questions appropriate to your life situation, for example: Are you able to immediately take two months off from work? Ideally, the GP would arrange for help from a counsellor when you have sufficiently recovered to unearth and then deal with all of the separate causes which are contributing to their depression. It is potentially an extremely tricky decision regarding how best to deal with it, and every case is inherently unique in all of its relevant details.

Reason/Cause 4.0 – A Low level of Emotional energy – I believe that you achieve things in life – anything you have as an objective – by riding to it on a steed of emotional energy which carries you along through difficult times. During wondrous periods, when all is rosy, you just flow along with the greatest of ease. Like everything in life, emotional energy exists in various degrees, from virtually nil to bursting to the brim.

If you wake up one morning and realise you have no or very minimal emotional energy, you don't really feel like doing anything at all. This condition, in my opinion, is subtly and importantly different to depression. You don't feel down, in a pit of some depth of despair as with depression. With low emotional energy, you feel emotionally flat.

Solution 4.0 – Again, if this condition has persisted for an extended period, without a fairly upward improvement trend, **you must see your GP.** One very important aspect to investigate is whether you are getting a good number of hours of good quality sleep, including going to bed at least not later than midnight? The other question is, are you emotionally addicted to playing games on your computer, including gambling, which comprises two intertwined serious addictions. This typically entails playing against people around the world until the early hours of the following day. If people are gaming in this manner, they will undoubtedly have awful sleep quality.

If someone is getting good quality sleep, confirmed by feeling well-rested shortly after waking, this low emotional energy condition requires additional investigation. It will be worth exploring if the patient does anything in their life which stirs their emotional juices, like playing any or all sports, going dancing, playing an instrument or any form of connecting with other people. The more they participate in activities that provoke their emotional juices the more they will hopefully improve their condition. Also, investigating experiences that have happened in their life or are happening now may throw up combinational or contributory causes.

If at any time you realise you are suffering from poor mental health and you are aware that, despite trying to help yourself, with hopefully, additional support from your partner or someone else who cares, you are not getting better or, perhaps, getting worse, **you must seek professional help from your GP.** The longer your difficulties continue, the more likely they are to become deeper rooted and therefore more challenging to cure.

ROLE F-2 In recent years, both in public and in private, why have we increasingly lost the right to have a

151

personal opinion about anything? Also, why, effectively, have we lost the right to have free speech on anything?

My beliefs of the contributory factors that answer these two questions are:

1) Increasingly looking inwards towards ourselves and not looking outwards to consider others. This leads to a lack of respect and regard for others, plus too much focus on ourselves.

2) Occasionally, religious fanaticism.

3) Daily arguing, on one side or the other, about Brexit for such a long time had a major contribution. As this went on for so long, it embedded new, extreme, frightening permanent attitudes and bad habits. Animosity, hate, high levels of emotionally driven tone, depth of feeling, all became the standard and norm of every discussion or, more often, every rant from people in all walks and levels of life, including politicians.

4) The other regular debate of climate change prevailed, along with Brexit, and additionally, COVID-19 was added. Each of these different and extremely important topics created very fervently held views on one side or the other of the debate which collectively continued the worsening habits referred to in point 3.0 above.

5) The increasing use of the internet, with each of its facilities being deliberately designed to be highly emotionally addicted, such that once you start using them, you are

unable to stop. The internet gives each technically clever and savvy user an immensely powerful platform, virtually connecting them to everywhere they wish, to express their views to increasingly more people. These users very cleverly create hordes of worshipping followers who, in many cases, come to idolise their platform leader.

6) I believe that some of these platform users inherently encourage a specific type of person to increasingly become narcissistic, which can further increase their usage and effectiveness of whatever campaign or objectives they may have.

7) These forums allow everyone to communicate with everyone else without a direct and live physical connection. Therefore, as there is never the risk of upsetting someone so much they immediately punch you, or worse, it encourages people, particularly some types, to adopt extremely bad manners. They show no respect to the other person's view and argue, shout, offend, etc., with safe abandon. It also moves people towards adopting this unacceptable behaviour when they actually meet someone in person.

8) More so than previously, politically motivated and driven objectives are dictated for the greater benefit of a particular party above all else. All members have to follow the party line. This situation can also prevail within privately run companies.

9) Forums very frequently impart/embed views or beliefs, particularly about a very important topic that affects most people and which someone in high office or from some

other platform wishes to implant into everyone's lives. They achieve this, not by encouraging open public debate presented by acceptably knowledgeable honest people, but by constant repetition within various settings, carried out over a long period of time. It is an obvious brainwashing technique, but despite that, it can normally and eventually be very effective.

A FRIGHTENING COLLECTION OF CONTRIBUTORY CAUSES!

ROLE F-3 Despite the increasing talk from more and more people, from more and more walks of life, about mental health illness, the list of prevailing concerns and difficulties about the topic remains worryingly extensive.

OVERVIEW: I strongly believe that the effective treatment of mental health illnesses requires a lot of frequent treatment and guidance sessions from an extremely capable and experienced professional counsellor in order to obtain and maintain acceptable progress. This is particularly applicable, where, as in many cases, the ongoing degree and height of the patient's Tower of Emotional Stress has been so disruptive for such a long time.

Mental health illnesses can be by far the most difficult to treat of all medical health illnesses. There are increasingly frequent and worrying conditions in our prevailing mental health system with a growing shortage of sufficient numbers of people capable of dispensing help and treatment.

1) A significant amount of mental ill-health could have been avoided.

2) A significant amount of mental ill-health costs could have been avoided.

3) The extremely worrying continuing escalation of mental health illnesses in modern life, particularly in the younger generation, more specifically among young women. Also in men, most of whom struggle to be able to ask for help.

4) The continuing and worsening lack of resources to treat mental ill-health.

5) The patient's **functional cause symptoms** of their ill-health are primarily treated medically, not their **underlying causes**, nor the **underlying root causes** of their symptoms.

6) The patient is normally prescribed anti-depressants for depression, instead of investigating and confirming the functional cause of their difficulties. It would be beneficial to create a detailed list of each of the underlying causes of their difficulties and decide how to deal with them. This includes investigating their underlying root causes and discussing addressing these.

7) Ideally, I believe that patients should only be put on anti-depressants if they are so severely depressed they are difficult to connect with emotionally and therefore difficult to be able to begin helping. If this is the case, they should be put on the weakest dosage to enable effective Cognitive

Behavioural Therapy to commence. As soon as possible in their treatment programme, they should be carefully weaned off them, and their treatment continued to nominal completion.

Patients can become hooked on anti-depressants with extremely disruptive side effects and can't get off them. Also, some remain permanently on anti-depressants thinking they are cured, but they are not. They gradually return to their old mental Health damaging ways and require another round of treatment, probably with stronger medicine. Consequently, so the continual cycle repeats itself with ongoing medication expenses, use of the already overstretched mental health treatment resources and their costs, and patients who live in a world that is to some degree removed from reality.

8) Usually, it is significantly easier, quicker and cheaper to successfully diagnose, treat and permanently repair the ill health of the physical parts of your body, compared to treating and attempting to rectify illnesses of your mind forever.

9) Unless we fundamentally change and improve the ways we treat mental ill-health, I strongly believe it will become, at an ever-increasing rate, the most debilitating health concern in current and future life.

10) More people becoming mentally ill will be additionally debilitating to the efficient functionality of companies, organisations, and therefore profits and, more generally, to a growing number of families and people's lives within them.

11) The list of the Emotional Stress Creator conditions is growing, particularly over the last fifteen years. See ROLE E-1a) list, earlier in this Subchapter.

12) It is crucially important that we all become aware of and address each of these underlying causes in **11**), where they occur within our everyday life at work and outside work. The goal is to remove and minimise each one of them wherever possible, thus assisting in maintaining the good quality of our mental health states.

ROLE F-4 The consequences and their related symptoms when suffering from a persistently high level of anxiety, creating an ongoing unhealthy Tower of Emotional Stress in your mind, including the risk of a mental breakdown.

*OVERVIEW: A **critical point** to highlight at this stage, when presenting the crucially important and complex topic of mental illness is, I believe, that a significant percentage of people who unfortunately have experienced periods of very damaging mental illness will have suffered from fundamentally the same condition as mentioned in the section description above – **an ongoing, unhealthy Tower of Emotional Stress**. This part will be the same for everyone, but the rest of their experiences will be different and unique to each person. These variations include their history of difficulties, timescales, their list of **underlying causes** and **underlying root causes,** and so much more.*

157

For this reason, over the remainder of this section on Role F, whenever I set the scene and describe someone having mental health difficulties, I will describe their overall situation. This may include their detailed symptoms, involvement with treatment or not, and other details. I will describe what actions they should take etc., so that each time I do this, I will present a different picture compared to the others I have given on this topic. In doing this, at least one example I share may be fairly similar to the situation some of my readers are familiar with, either personally or with someone they dearly care for. Therefore, they can make an easier connection and hopefully derive more understanding and benefit from the information. To those readers who may find this a little tedious, please accept my apologies.

Let's turn our attention back to responding to the section description in ROLE F-4 above.

If your ongoing Tower of Emotional Stress has been unhealthily elevated over a long period, you run the risk of suffering from:

a) Your Tower of Stress rising to an even higher peak level during times of additional stress. Should this happen, you are liable to display the **symptoms** of high levels of emotionally unhealthy states. You will make increasingly troublesome and bad quality decisions, leading to their related actions. You will come across as a person who is struggling to control their temper and other emotional reactions and, generally, unable to hold themselves together emotionally.

b)   Some **symptoms** from a list of various types of significant headaches and/or from several different dysfunctionalities. Examples include vision problems, difficulties thinking and talking clearly, numbness in parts of your body and feeling sick, all of which could be named migraine attacks.

c)   Some **symptoms** such as self-harming, panic attacks, suicidal thoughts, attempted suicide, having periods of a complete lack of mental and physical energy and suffering periods of pain over different parts of your body. Sometimes, doctors question whether the patient is imagining these extremely debilitating symptoms and ask, is the cause in the body or the mind?

d)   Gradually have problems with your heart and other organs that eventually become damaged, leading to possible **symptoms** of aches and pains.

e)   This significantly debilitating state will also create the extremely serious and worsening condition of inferior quality and quantity of sleep. This leads to deterioration and an increase in the symptoms above, plus several other serious problems.

f)   The poor functionality of your brain displays **symptoms** of difficulty in making any decisions at all, and if any are made, they are of very poor quality.

g)   Inadequate chemical conditions within your body create a number of different **symptoms**.

h)   An growing height of your Tower of Emotional Stress, leading to even worse degrees of **symptoms** than above.

i) Sliding into an emotional pit of depression and possible obesity.

j) Creating Increasingly low emotional and physical energy displaying the **symptoms** of mental and physical lethargy. **If your mind becomes unhealthy, then your body ultimately does the same.**

k) You are liable to move towards experiencing a mental breakdown of some degree of severity. This, I believe, is the inevitable consequence of your brain, after having attempted to force you to significantly slow down by subjecting you to some of the symptoms described above, to get you to stop carrying out some of your day-to-day activities, which are creating a lot of anxiety for you. IT wants you to reduce the pace of your whole life functionally and emotionally, but you have not done it sufficiently enough. Additionally, the consequences of you not dealing adequately with the underlying causes of your anxiety are that your Ongoing Tower of Emotional Stress has remained far too high and maybe, in the worst case, has risen even higher.

Causing you to have a mental breakdown is your brain's ultimate/ last tool for helping you to de-stress yourself. It puts your working and social life into stop mode, simply by making you unable to and unable to want to do anything. However, hopefully this is the start of the process of you beginning a slow but optimistically sure rebuilding of a healthier life for yourself with, crucially this time, the assistance and guidance of therapy from an experienced mental health counsellor, arranged by your GP.

The counsellor will guide you in reducing your emotionally damaging Ongoing High Tower of Emotional Stress and guide you in how to start to **begin helping yourself** and take increasing degrees of control and management of your life. This time around, you will hopefully fully engage your M.C. and your placebo effect, and gradually, your mental health will steadily and securely recover.

ROLE F-5 What actions would you take if you were suffering a significant physical injury?

As your injury was significant, your corrective actions would no doubt not be to seek professional medical help from your GP because they are not set up to treat significant physical injuries. Therefore, you would go immediately to your nearest A & E department for treatment, or possibly call an ambulance if it was more serious.

The primary point in this situation is that there would be no doubt in your mind that you must take **immediate action** to get the appropriate treatment to become physically well again.

ROLE F-6 What actions would you take if you were suffering from significantly poor mental health?

The likelihood is that you would **continue to suffer this condition for a relatively long time before you took any action at all**, particularly if you were a man and, to a much lesser extent, if you were a woman. There are multiple, combinational factors for this troublesome lack of response to fairly quickly seeking help from the professionals, which include:

a) I believe that it is perfectly normal and potentially healthy and beneficial to suffer from a certain amount of anxiety and emotional stress. At times, maybe this will turn into a degree of feeling down/slightly depressed. Typically, we all have day-to-day situations and conditions in our lives that are important to us. They each require we give our appropriate consideration to and take the related actions to solve them to our benefit. Some of these situations can easily and quickly be dealt with, but others take longer.

Initially, you will experience a degree of these emotions in order to remind you they require resolving. Your brain may become concerned that you are not tackling some of these situations with the appropriate degree of application, and too much time is passing with possibly a worsening situation. Therefore, it will increase the degree of these emotions you are experiencing to attempt to remind you of them and push you into action.

b) Because it is normal to experience these emotions, as mentioned above, quite regularly, you have to decide whether the degree and type of the feelings you are currently experiencing are in the range of you being mentally ill or not. This requires you to separate, analyse, and evaluate what you are reacting to. This is not easy to do with any high degree of accuracy, particularly because it requires you to analyse yourself. For most people, this is extremely difficult to do with precision and objectivity.

c) In the past, there were far fewer facets to most people's lives that created significant Anxiety and Emotional Stress compared to these times. Previously, when people became stressed, they tended to live in closer family and neighbour groups, so they sought help and advice from family members and friends. That aspect of everyday life meant that any troubling issue was dealt with soon after coming into existence, therefore preventing it from becoming the monster growing way out of proportion. These days, however, even when, after a long time, they eventually accept that they have become mentally ill, most people are not comfortable broadcasting it. This is particularly true for men, because they feel like a failure for being unable to cope. They worry that their family and friends will also see them as a male failure, which further delays them seeking help.

d) Most men are extremely concerned about informing their boss that they have a mental health illness. A significant percentage of bosses in the private business world would not employ someone who has had, and more so, currently suffers from mental health issues. They feel they have a business to run at a profit and can't functionally cope with people off long-term sick with mental health issues. There is additionally the risk of someone with this propensity to make costly/poor business decisions, particularly when embroiled in stressful situations at work.

e) Another thing that prevents people from accessing professional help is being worried about their long term state of mind. Will they ever get better? Are they becoming mad? Will they become mad? Will they suffer the terrible side effects that they have heard that mental health treatment medications can create?

ROLE F-7 My understanding and description of the current medication regimes for treating what I describe as Physical Health Illnesses and Mental Health Illnesses.

Physical Health Illnesses:

Symptoms of discomfort and/or pain, with physical injuries or damage identified.

If you are unhealthy and found to have a physical injury or physical damage to your body, the injury is inspected, the damage is medically treated by repair or replacement. Drugs are used to kill infections, etc., with the appropriate type and strength of pain killers administered, if necessary, until no longer required. Your injuries are re-assessed at regular appointments until you are finally cleared when your treatment is deemed successfully completed.

The consequences of this medical treatment regime are normally extremely successful, with the patient having medication and reviews as required, during one continuous period, <u>treating the root causes of their pain</u> and functional <u>difficulties.</u> Recover occurs as soon as is possible, depending on the injuries, etc., and they return to and remain in good health.

The above regime is to identify the root cause or causes of the symptoms being suffered and treat these, the usual results of which are that the patient is cured and remains cured. Throughout the process, the patient immediately, readily and happily divulges their injury, etc., to anyone who is interested, typically, without any embarrassment at all.

Mental Health Illnesses:

Symptoms of discomfort and/or pain and/or functional disabilities, with no physical injuries or physical damage identified.

You **eventually go to the doctor** with some of the following symptoms: a type of painful headache and/or functional difficulties of vision, speaking, and reasoning and/or feel emotionally unwell and have low emotional and physical energy, coupled with periods of significant depression, numbness, poor quality and quantity of sleep, to mention a few. If the doctor can find no physical ailments and suspects none, they will usually ask a few questions about your well-being, current life situation, family and history. You will generally be primarily treated with medication for pain suppression and possibly medication for depression and advised to return in a short time for a review.

There are some crucially important points that I feel should be made here that need taking into account.

165

a) The GP's extremely short consultation time that is available.

b) The GP's knowledge that the complexity of the multiplicity of the combinational causes that led this patient to them requires an in-depth consultation. A review of their life situation, currently and to an appropriate degree, their history is necessary even to begin to help them correctly and safely along the road to hopefully a nominal full recovery.

c) The GP, knowing that the waiting times for offering this type of help of Cognitive Behavioural Therapy are growing worryingly longer, takes the expediency of the moment and administers some helpful advice, along with possibly some pain relief and possibly/probably some anti-depressants. You are asked to return to see them again in a few weeks for a review.

After some time, which may have involved your medication being altered to obtain greater improvements for your conditions, with varying degrees of success, the eventual consequences are that the symptoms disappear or they become more tolerable. However, some months later or even sooner, they reappear as before, or even worse. Another period of basically the same treatment regime will possibly be repeated.

This semi-continuous, repeating regime can persist for a long time with the following possible consequences:

1) Having a reasonable percentage of patients leading a life which, although in principle is not perfect, allows them to have their symptoms suppressed sufficiently, without

suffering noticeably from any adverse reactions to their combination of medicines. Therefore, the regime allows them to lead a life which is emotionally stable enough, enjoyable enough and hopefully involves taking relatively low-strength medicines. This means the patient's sensitivities of emotions and other awareness are not dulled to diminish the pure emotional joys of their life too much.

NB If the Functional Cause, Underlying Causes and Root Causes of their difficulties are not identified and addressed, there are several risks. The reactive and resultant combination of the patient's medicines, their unique ongoing chemical balances and states, personality traits, genes, functionalities and outputs of their brain's departments that affect their emotional health and decision-making, all may alter. All of these aspects, combined with the patient experiencing new root causes, can result in significant and possibly even more adverse changes to the patient's mental health.

2) No real improvement in the patient's health.

3) Costing an escalating amount of money to the taxpayer.

4) Causing the patient a large amount of pain, discomfort and time off work.

5) Adverse reactions to the prescribed medications, sometimes to an extreme degree.

6) The patient becomes increasingly disillusioned by still being ill, probably becoming more ill due to the additional related Emotional Stress and despair they feel as a consequence.

7) After suffering the above for an extended period and, due to a combination of some of the points above, plus worsening quality and quantity of sleep problems, the patient's body begins to experience high blood pressure, heart and other organ problems, in addition to the symptoms above.

In conclusion, I would propose that, for a significant percentage of the patients, the fundamental flaws with the regime above for treating mental health illness are that:

a) The **functional cause** of the patient's symptoms (their high Ongoing Tower of Emotional Stress) was not discussed with and accepted by the patient.

b) A list of the **underlying causes** of the patient's high level of anxiety and stress was not sufficiently if at all, searched for with the patient. Therefore, a solution plan for each item on the list was not agreed upon and enacted by the patient.

c) A list of the **underlying root causes** was not searched for and dealt with appropriately by the patient.

This flawed process inevitably leads to the symptoms and not their multiple level causes being treated. In turn, this leads to the patient never being able to become completely cured.

The solution to this is that the patient must return to their GP and request urgent help from an experienced counsellor.

I believe there should be three stages to this intervention.

1) <u>**The first stage**</u> is that the **Functional Cause** that causes the vast majority of mental illnesses is the patient suffering from **far too High an Ongoing level of Emotional Stress**. The symptoms of this condition are one or more from a long list of possible symptoms we have covered previously. One or more types of painful headaches and/or one or more dysfunctionalities such as numbness, vision problems, brain fog, lethargy etc. See ROLE F-1 earlier in this Subchapter for more details.

   In discussions between the patient and their therapist, who hopefully support my view, the patient must accept and buy into this basic diagnosis. Consequently, they will enter into the subsequent treatment process with solid belief, commitment and will also, therefore, fully engage their placebo effect. They benefit from this additional and extremely powerful healing agent, thus standing the best chance of a successful treatment outcome.

2) <u>**The second stage**</u> is that the many and usually separate, **underlying causes** of each of their blocks of Emotional Stress need to be clearly identified and put on a list by their professional counsellor working with the patient.

3) <u>**The third stage**</u> is for the counsellor to assist the patient to help themselves by facing up to these underlying causes and addressing the way they are failing to manage them and their life sufficiently. With some underlying causes, there might even be the possibility of completely resolving them. A crucial part of this stage is to investigate and understand why the patient reacts so anxiously to these situations. This

involves searching for the **underlying root causes** that create these strong, anxious reactions. This phase of the process can involve quite a lot of very hard work by both parties.

All this sounds easy, which it is in principle. However, in practice, it requires an awful lot of consistent hard work and honesty by the patient, supported by their ideally unchanged, ongoing, professional counsellor.

ROLE F-8 A more detailed description of the process for identifying and tackling the Underlying Causes and Underlying Root causes of your Anxiety and Ongoing High Tower Of Emotional Stress.

The aim is to gradually reduce your ongoing Tower of Emotional Stress to a relatively low and healthy level from being a VERY HIGH LEVEL FOR A LONG TIME.

OVERVIEW: The key concern in this section is contained within the capital letters in the last line of the above paragraph. The process to carry out and achieve the objective written above should be **managed and led** *by a professional mental health counsellor experienced in the use of Cognitive Behavioural Therapy, ideally arranged by your GP.*

For your interest and understanding, here are a few ideas that could be part of your counsellor's regime. They would apply actions and plans in a particular order and way appropriate to **their view of your situation and their individual preferences.** It is essential that, before you carry out any actions, you discuss with your counsellor all aspects of their planned activities. It is vitally important you work closely together through everything. You need to develop a mutually trusting and respectful relationship to achieve the best possible outcome for the improvement and management of your future emotional health.

I believe that the **functional cause** for most patients suffering a serious degree of mental illness is they are experiencing an **elevated Ongoing Tower level of Emotional Stress** for an extensive period of time. This has resulted in many bad habits being perpetuated without much awareness in multiple aspects of their life, therefore requiring an awful lot of improvements to assist the patient in very gradually recovering from their mental illness.

Hopefully, the patient will buy into this philosophy, thus entering into the following treatment process with solid belief and commitment. Therefore, they will also fully engage their placebo effect, benefiting from this additional and extremely powerful healing agent. The patient stands the best chance of a successful treatment outcome by:

Action a) Identifying and generating a list of the **underlying causes** or situations in your life that create an individual block of anxiety and stress in your ongoing Tower of Emotional Stress.

Action b) Thoroughly analysing each of these situations or **underlying causes** of these blocks of stress and identifying what action/s you need to take to:

1) Make a decision to finalise as many aspects as possible.
2) Take as many resolving actions as possible.
3) If achievable, eliminate or ignore some situations.
4) If not possible, minimise those as appropriate.
5) Pass any of your difficulties or issues over to someone else who wishes to and can take it off you completely and permanently if possible.
6) Get some more information about some situations or difficulties, hopefully in order to resolve or at least minimise them.

Action c) Very importantly, in addition to the above, be open to investigating and modifying your view and/or reaction to at least some elements of these issues, situations or difficulties in your life. This will eliminate or at least reduce, the degree of stress you are experiencing from them.

Action d) On top of, and in conjunction with the above, investigate and understand why you are reacting so anxiously to these situations. This involves searching for the **underlying root causes** that generate your anxious reactions, which means considering the different elements your character comprises. Considering the qualities and personalities of your parents can be particularly helpful. Asking the opinions of your partner and close friends can also be useful, plus reviewing the history of the development of each situation can be enlightening. Think outside the box, consider the inconsiderable etc.

Action e) Also, you may be experiencing several of what I refer to as frequently repetitive, highly negative and extremely disturbing memories of some of your unpleasant past experiences. These keep forcing their presence into and circulating around your mind. They individually create their own block of stress, or collective blocks, referred to as **Post Traumatic Stress Disorder (P.T.S.D.).** They accumulate to a very significant amount of stress within your Ongoing Tower of Stress, during the day and probably at night in your dreams and other elements during your sleep.

It is absolutely essential that you tackle each of these in turn. Set out to banish them for good. Face up to them with courage and fortitude. Analyse them in detail. Answer how and why they occurred. Can you learn anything useful from them?

Refer to Subchapter 7.14, for more details about P.T.S.D.

Action f) Take a very large step backwards and openly and honestly review the whole of your lifestyle, activities and attitudes, both at work and outside work. Consider why you adversely react to some situations that make you anxious. Review your character, biases, and fixed attitudes and review whether you should attempt to modify or maybe even delete some of these to reduce your anxieties. Include your relationships with your family, relations and friends in this review. Examine whether any of these relationships contribute to your ongoing blocks of stress. If this is the case, conduct a review of what actions you should carry out to reduce or even eliminate these stress-creators.

Action g) With your counsellor, make a note of all of these actions you have agreed to carry out with approximate target completion dates. Decide which ones to action first, and agree on a date for your next review meeting.

Action h) Also, with your counsellor, regularly look back and evaluate how much progress you have made. Look ahead to see further targeted progress.

Action i) Continue this process until nominally, initially completed.

Action j) Crucially and importantly, at any time where you feel you are experiencing difficulties of any type or significance, don't leave it too long before contacting your counsellor to arrange a review. This could be during the initial process, at a later phase, or after the initial nominal completion of your first course. You mustn't fall into the self-creating trap of making this healing process for your mental illness become the cause of a huge block of Anxiety and Emotional Stress.

Refer to the **NB** relating to **physical health** in section ROLE E-1b) to see if regular exercise is something you need to include, increase or reintroduce into your life to help significantly reduce your ongoing Stress Levels.

ROLE F-8a) A much simplified and differently-presented version than in ROLE F-8 above. It covers the basic principles of the process for identifying and tackling the four layers of Causes of Anxiety and Ongoing High Tower Of Emotional Stress. This presentation may better suit some patients' different temperaments.

OVERVIEW: *One vitally important factor to achieve the maximum benefit from the course of treatment the patient is embarking on is that they understand the reasons and benefits for all elements of it. **They also believe in everything they will be doing and have total trust and confidence in their counsellor.** If all of these aspects prevail, the patient will engage, feel and benefit from the maximum potential of their placebo effect and should therefore make a full recovery back to excellent mental health.*

One other aspect that I believe can be a fundamentally important cornerstone of correct and effective treatment of people with mental illness problems is for them to have a simple picture of what is engulfing them, which they can understand and therefore relate to.

This picture can take the form of their difficulties being created and contained within an all-encompassing shell comprising of the following layers:

a) The outer layer, which is what I call the **SINGLE FUNCTIONAL CAUSE**, followed by:

b) The next layer, which I call the **MANY UNDERLYING CAUSES**, followed by:

c) The inner layer, which I call the **MANY UNDERLYING ROOT CAUSES,** and finally:

d) The core at the centre of the enclosed shell, which I call **THE MANAGEMENT CENTRE OF YOUR LIFE.**

The allied and extremely important points I wish to make are:

a) The patient is taken through each layer of causes, and the core, **in the order** I have detailed them above. This gives them an overall appreciation, understanding and a feel for what lies ahead for them in their journey back to good health. They also get a sense of the overall causes of their difficulties, so dispelling and slaying what may have been the causal monster existing within their mind.

b) Before any detailed work is commenced with each of these layers of causes, the patient must understand and accept the philosophy and future basic plans of actions with their counsellor. Therefore, they will totally commit to carrying out their agreed actions, etc., resulting in obtaining the maximum possible improvements in their mental health.

c) The outer layer is presented first and must be understood and accepted by the patient before moving on to the second layer. It is vitally important that the patient very clearly sees the foundational simplicity of what is causing their severe mental health difficulties and such disruption in their life.

d) Identifying and listing causes takes place in the second layer and, when appropriate, entering into the third layer is carried out as best decided by the counsellor.

e) Discussing the management centre of your life is best nominally left towards the end period of the patient's treatment and can be dipped into and out of as required. This is basically about asking the patient to describe how they manage their day-to-day activities and carry out any planning of them, etc.

The objective of this crucially important part of the patient's treatment is that they must buy into the fact that their counsellor can help them with advice etc. However, only they, the patient, can actually improve their ongoing life activities. They have to learn how to manage their life far better than they have to date. They must carry out many basic aspects regarding their actions and plans etc., in order to reduce their anxieties and difficulties as a major factor in minimising their stresses for the rest of their lives. The resultant obtained benefits are immense. No one else but the patient themselves can do this. They will get great satisfaction when they feel and see the benefits that this aspect of their life achieves, all of which will be further advanced and enjoyed by their placebo effect.

ROLE F-9 What is the process that makes anti-depressants, in many cases, effective in alleviating the symptoms of poor mental health, and is the placebo effect involved?

I believe that the effect of taking anti-depressant drugs is that they cause an ongoing <u>interactive emotional chain reaction</u> which is as follows:

177

a) In proportion to the strength, type and dosage of the drugs and, in combination with the <u>reaction you have as a unique individual</u>, they de-sensitise/reduce your emotional reaction to what you perceive as difficult situations in your life.

b) This diminished reaction <u>reduces your previous anxiety and the degree of emotional stress</u> you experienced regarding these numerous difficulties in your life that you have previously been struggling to deal with.

c) This process above is repeated with each of the other life situations that had previously caused you significant anxieties. Hopefully, now, you will react less stressfully and thus be able to resolve at least a good number of them permanently.

d) This then creates the collective net benefit that your overall degree of Ongoing Emotional Stress is gradually reduced over the period when you are hopefully successfully dealing with the prevailing difficulties in your life better.

NB In addition to the above, I believe that, for the vast majority of this category of patients, who have probably become so desperate to move into a better day-to-day world as soon as possible, the additional, significant benefits of **the placebo effect** will prevail.

This placebo effect is so beneficial, crucially because:

1) <u>The patient genuinely believes</u> that their anti-depressant drug will **help them** become emotionally less stressed about

the difficulties in their life. Part **a)** of this <u>emotionally uplifting beneficial reaction</u> occurs <u>immediately</u> when they are <u>told they</u> will soon **receive help** and be prescribed the medication. Part **b)** is due to the patient being promised instant, <u>additional help</u> to deal with their mental health illness, the topic of which will be of absolute major importance to them and their whole life.

2) When the patient actually receives their anti-depressant drug, and it has become fully effective, this will create part **c)** of their <u>emotionally uplifting beneficial reaction</u> by them becoming emotionally less stressed about each of the difficulties in their life.

3) The three anxiety-reducing benefits listed in **1)** and **2)** enable the patient to crucially get better quality sleep, which in turn will give them a part **d)** benefit of a <u>further, significant reduction</u> in their overall level of anxiety and stress concerning their previous difficulties in their life, including lack of sleep.

4) There is one final benefit following the creation of the placebo effect as above. Due to its existence, it engenders a focus, attitude and belief that every action that forms part of the work to repair your mental health is carried out with maximum confidence, focus and dedication. These attitudes achieve the best possible improvement in the patient's mental health, which will create a part **e)** of an emotionally uplifting beneficial reaction.

NB For the placebo effect to operate, i.e. for the anti-depressants to have an <u>additional</u> health benefit for the patient, it is imperative that the patient genuinely believes the drugs will work, not just <u>says</u> they will, which gives the patient much appreciated help.

I apologise for the repetition in the above section, but the placebo effect shows the immense power for beneficial effect that your brain's mind can offer you when you have an important need for help.

TO FINALISE: I feel that I must ADD TO THE ABOVE, a point that I feel extremely strongly about. The above medication process does not identify and address the patient's Underlying Causes and the Root Causes of their anxieties. Nor does it provide them with the tools of control to deal far better with each cause and their life generally. It is treating the symptoms of their difficulties and not the underlying reasons.

Despite these aspects, if the patient is severely emotionally ill and depressed, the above process creates a channel of connection and hope for the patient. It reduces the degree of emotional ill health they are suffering and can in so doing, assist them in turning the corner towards better emotional health. At this stage, and when they have become stable for a month or so, with their full understanding and support of what lies ahead, they can be supported to wean off their anti-depressants gradually. They can then begin the process of identifying the underlying causes of their high Ongoing Tower of Stress and their underlying root causes.

This sequence of collective help will hopefully lead to, <u>allow and eventually enable them</u> to manage their lives significantly better for eternity! This last statement of life management is the most important factor of very many. I believe it is the **key to unlocking their door** to a future life that can make the very best of what they are potentially capable of enjoying.

ROLE F-10 An overview of your brain's extreme complexity and interactive functionality, including, when you are suffering from poor mental health, the risks caused by some of the treatment regimens employed.

NB 1 I believe that your brain's interreactive, dynamic, complete breadth and range of functionality and capability is awesomely powerful, complex and fast. Currently, as I perceive it, <u>the understanding of your brain's functionality</u> in all of its facets, during every operating state, through each possible range of input data it is capable of receiving, across the spectrum of conditions that it is presented with, ostensibly, at the same time, <u>is worryingly incomplete</u>.

This is confirmed due to, as I understand it, the current situation, which is that no one is yet able to offer a detailed definition of what human consciousness is, the comprehensive process of how it is derived, how it functions and what its objectives are, or how and why your brain actually works.

Because of all of these factors, I believe that <u>manually interfering</u> with your brain's functionality is potentially

extremely dangerous and inherently risky to the patient's future functional capability and mental health.

In my opinion, this manual interference occurs when, for example, to cure/improve a patient who suffers from extremely debilitating and embarrassing seizures or dysfunctionalities, the surgeons, having identified a part of the patient's brain they believe causes this particular behaviour, cut it out. Due to the extremely high processing density of the brain, even a minute amount of brain volume contains and represents many thousands of processing circuits being removed.

NB Work of this nature, particularly in some areas, requires professional people who are blessed with significant courage, skill, capability, knowledge and the extremely strong wish to help others. Without them, many of us would be in real life-changing trouble.

I believe that each patient's brain is comprised of the same basic format of design and functionality for their mind, soul, and consciousness as everyone else's. However, the contents in the many departments and subdepartments in the brain of every human being are unique.

The consequences of all of these factors are that a medical regime that may be helpful to some patients may not be beneficial to others, even when they each appear to have a similar set of symptoms. The vast number of the three types of departments and their subdepartments that comprise your brain, plus the activities within your mind that are involved with the creation of your current consciousness, emotional mood or state and each consideration and action, are always dynamic. They are constantly in an active, changing state, condition or value. They respond to states or values in other departments for each prevailing decision and its related considerations, plus various input data with their ever changing meanings and values.

Additionally, what concerns me is where drugs only nominally change one or two parts or areas of the extremely complex and total set of conditions and functionalities that combine to constitute the total processes of your mind's operation. These few parts are altered, without any reference or connection to other parts of your mind's processing activities, as is the case in the normal operation of your healthy brain. Also, the drug-induced one part fixed dosage change, comprises ostensibly of a non-changing condition or value that will undoubtedly gradually reduce to zero effect as the drug dose dwindles or because it has a slow release activity.

These areas of functionality are very different to how a **healthy brain actually functions**. Manually applying a mind-altering drug of some type and strength, once per day, or at whatever frequency, even if it releases its dosage slowly, is at the worst end of the Control System spectrum, compared to how the brain actually functions. It is at the other end of the Control System spectrum, with the most complex and best possible benefits.

Because of the above aspects, I believe that the common practice of prescribing powerful, mind-altering drugs to alter the balance of the brain's existing functionality in patients **whose minds are already sick, unstable and therefore not**

functioning healthily is fraught with risk. There are possibilities of very serious risks to the patient's future health from:

a) **Some** severe side effects from a very long list of possibilities that <u>add</u> to their existing symptoms.

b) **Becoming** addicted to a particular drug, and being unable to be weaned off it due to serious adverse reactions from withdrawal.

c) **Having long term,** seriously negative consequences suffered by a certain percentage of patients.

d) **Under** the welter of a significant percentage of the above negatives, the patient feels overwhelmed by it all. Their hopes which had become an expectancy of being cured, sink with despair. The unhealthy height of their Tower Of Emotional Stress and Anxiety returns, and their degree of mental ill-health worsens significantly.

e) **They** lose faith in their medical helpers and the treatment regime, so the blackness of emotional despair and depression prevails. They return to the base of their mountain, which they must then climb again to the top of their good health condition.

Having said all of the above, due to the nature of mental illness treatment being fraught with the combined **extreme challenges** highlighted, I am fully aware of the need to use drugs when a patient experiences emotional ill-health to a significant and, in some cases, extreme degree. <u>In these instances, which may involve high risks of suicide and/or even further degradation of</u>

their ill health, to commence effective treatment at all, the use of drugs is the only available and viable option.

However, hopefully, after comforting and positive treatment is prevailing, there is always the intention with the patient's treatment regime, to crucially, with their full and detailed participation and knowledge, gradually and extremely carefully, wean them off their medication.

Even if, in the future, a full and complete understanding of the whole of the brain's functionality under all conditions, and variations of multiple conditions, etc., is finally achieved, for all of the reasons above, I take the view, that it is best not to use any medication to treat a patient with a mental health illness.

Instead, always, firstly attempt to strive to slowly expose, understand and make a detailed plan to resolve, each of the three layers of causes of anxiety as detailed below (plus correct the core of your life's poor management) that are combining to create their emotional ill-health. This should always be done with the knowledgeable consent of the patient and with careful use of counselling.

I most strongly believe that to achieve a successful outcome in recovering from mental ill-health, it is crucially important encourage the patient to practice self-help at every opportunity. Along with firmly believing that all planned actions will benefit them, each step of improvement will constitute their complete journey back to the life and health they strive for.

Encouraging this positive, confident attitude will engage the patient's placebo effect. In turn, this will emotionally uplift them and thus reduce their degree of prevailing anxiety which their M.C. will detect, further causing their brain to reduce the patient's anxiety level in response.

NB I strongly believe that the <u>functional cause</u> of most people's mental ill-health is excessive <u>ongoing Emotional Stress</u>. This is due to many <u>underlying causes,</u> including the situations in their life that cause them to have significant anxiety. For some people, they are unable to resolve them entirely or even reduce them very much at all. It is so important for the patient, with their counsellor, to evaluate each underlying cause extremely carefully and fully understand all aspects of them. They can then collaboratively draw up a plan of action, with the ultimate objective being to resolve each one completely.

Underneath these two layers will be their <u>underlying root causes</u> of why they react emotionally to these situations and why they are not resolving them. Some of these root causes will no doubt, to some extent, be interlinked, and they will each combine to a certain degree from the following list:

1) Their inherited genes
2) Their character
3) Their lives experiences
4) Their ambitions
5) Their physical and mental health
6) Their biases
7) Their lifestyle

In order to evaluate the patient's unhealthy lifestyle, without leaving any stone unturned, discussions should include reviewing their eating regime, weight and regular exercise regime, if they have one. Regular exercise is so effective in keeping their anxiety levels at a low healthy level. For more details, refer to ROLE E-1b) in the **NB** section on physical health.

It is important to obtain the patient's willingness to investigate how to reduce, as much as possible, all conditions and lifestyle activities that are contributing to their ongoing, total Emotional Stress Level, thus maximising the number of ways of reducing their mental ill-health issues.

In addition to this, it is advisable to only use medication, with as small an amount as is possible and with the lowest degree of strength and frequency of use, **as a last resort,** when the above process has failed to achieve a significant and sufficiently successful outcome or at least a fair degree of progress.

NB It is crucially important to note and become aware of, during the above process, whether the patient is taking or has taken drugs that have affected brain functionality or caused damage, thus creating additional extremely disruptive thoughts, attitudes, behaviour and actions. If this is, unfortunately, the case, then noting this aspect, with the patient's knowledge and approval is certainly another element to consider to improve the recovery of the future health of the patient.

ROLE F-11 A detailed example of how I believe your brain uses the conditions of pain, discomfort and

functional disabilities to assist in healing your migraine illness.

Please note that this is fundamentally the same as ROLE E-1b) except that it presents the solution in quite a different way which you hopefully will find useful.

OVERVIEW: _People suffering from migraine illness experience_ <u>_extremely debilitating headaches,_</u> _sometimes with additionally_ <u>_quite_</u> <u>_disturbing dysfunctional symptoms_</u>_. It affects a significant percentage of the population and, quite often, for some people, they are an ongoing feature in their lives,_ _REMOVE and can have a devastating impact upon them._

1.0) Here is a list of some of the different types of common headaches experienced:

a)   A tension headache
b)   A painkiller headache
c)   A sex headache
d)   A cluster headache
e)   A tooth grinding headache
f)   A monthly headache
g)   A coat hanger headache
h)   A migraine headache
i)   A poor eyesight headache
j)   A sinusitis headache

2.0) Some of the various types of common dysfunctionality symptoms experienced could be one or more of the following difficulties:

a) Your vision in a number of different details of conditions.

b) Your speech in a number of different conditions. **c)**

c) Your brain's ability to reason, think clearly, quickly, rationally and confidently, which is sometimes called brain fog.

d) Your body experiencing aches, pains, numbness, or tingling in a variety of parts of your body at different times.

e) Your body experiencing physical tiredness, stamina fatigue and joint problems.

NB The severity, frequency and location of these extremely debilitating headaches and the disturbing dysfunctional symptoms you will experience at times will depend, to a degree, upon several factors. These include your character profile, physiological and genetic makeup and will also relate to the extent of unhealthy Emotional Stress you are currently suffering from.

3.0) The reasons you are suffering from these headaches and dysfunctionalities are:

a) Your brain is subjecting you to all of these symptoms above because it has noticed that the degree of your daily/ongoing

Anxiety and Emotional Stress has become damagingly high for a period of time.

b) Your brain is desperately trying to slow you down and de-stress you. It is making you unable to continue doing all of the activities and expressing the attitudes that are contributing to your elevated level of ongoing Emotional Stress and therefore causing you significant mental ill-health.

4.0) Further key aspects that prevail with your migraine ill-health:

a) Your M.C. will recognise, from previous similar episodes, the cause of each of your symptoms. Therefore, it will commence to deal with and resolve, or at least minimise, the underlying causes and possibly some of the underlying root causes that raise your Tower to an unhealthy level of ongoing Anxiety and Emotional Stress.

b) Each of these underlying causes will no doubt mainly be contained within parts of your life generally and components of your unhealthy lifestyle. The way you strongly and adversely react to each of these **underlying causes** will be due to your many **underlying root causes.** One of these will be your character. If you are not consciously aware of its traits and/or are unable to accept that some of them are troublesome, it is extremely difficult to manage/minimise their negative effects.

c) You will probably have been far too active and busy in your life at work and at home, causing far too high a level of Anxiety and Emotional Stress and, among other difficulties, being unable to unwind effectively by relaxing.

d) As your M.C. sees that you are beginning to reduce and remove, where possible, these unhealthy factors from your daily life, the benefits of your placebo effect will be activated, resulting in a reduction in the degree of your symptoms. Also, the height of your Tower of Emotional Stress will again reduce, thus further lowering the degree of your headaches and/or dysfunctional symptoms.

e) As your Anxiety and Emotional Stress Levels reduce, your quality and quantity of sleep will improve which will inherently further reduce your stress levels.

f) I believe that the above monitoring and responses in your brain are automatically managed by the appropriate, dedicated Category 1A and 1B departments and, extremely importantly, under the supervision of your M.C.

g) To see if regular exercise is something you need to include or increase in your life to significantly lower your ongoing Stress Levels, refer to ROLE E-1b) and the **NB** section on physical health.

h) Also of major importance, if you **totally believe** in the process detailed above, you will fully engage your placebo effect, which will cause an additional reduction in the degree of your symptoms.

i) Additionally, be mindful of is whether you have been prescribed medication to help treat/minimise your migraine illness. This medication could be significantly contributing to your difficulties due to the side effects you may be experiencing.

In conclusion, a critical point to make at this stage is if, despite the above procedure being followed as described and in spite of your best efforts, your symptoms and their degree, plus the state of your mental health is not improving or getting worse, you must stop. Seek the help of your GP straight away, inform them of your situation and bring up the topic of your medication.

ROLE F-12 The immense potential healing power of you/ your M.C./your intelligence/your mind/your brain/your placebo effect and helping you achieve goals is very under-appreciated, misunderstood and therefore much under-utilised.

OVERVIEW: *Additionally, from my own experiences in many different situations, observations of many other people and after much thought over many years, you must have your mind working for your benefit. If not, it may, in reality, be working against you sometimes without you being aware of this.*

I believe that the placebo condition or effect is not solely associated with you taking medication or having an operation, both of which are to make you better. It is also a condition or effect created by what you are doing to help yourself achieve something, anything, in your life that you deem very important. In these cases, it is an **attitude of mind** that has been created from a lot of thought and consideration. You have developed a planned list of several activities, all of which, when eventually completed, combine to achieve your objective.

The uplifting, invigorating and confident attitude of mind that the combination of these activities creates is immense. It spurs you on to achieve even greater efforts of standard and achievement levels as your mind sees your objective gradually become closer to realisation. You are so incredibly consciously aware that everything you are doing is exactly what is necessary to achieve your goal, to the point that, at times, you almost feel you are being carried along on your journey by some unseen hand.

There are so many immensely effective, powerful, efficient and strongly achieving attitudes, methods, tools, revision plans, other plans, proven systems, practices, getting super fit, etc. They can be successfully employed, individually and collectively, to achieve so many different objectives throughout every single walk of life. All activities in life can be carried out under the probably unspoken banner of the collective effect and beneficial help of the placebo effect.

I will identify a few examples of these objectives which prevail in everyday life and will include quite a bit of detail to explain the background required to create success. Please note that I am not attempting to put them in order of ranking, benefit or importance.

1)   From a pre-selection game, you have been selected to attend a residential weekend training at an elite sports centre which

193

culminates in a trial for being selected to play in a team at the highest level in your favourite sport. You take this opportunity extremely seriously and decide to gradually raise your normal weekly physical training routine to a much higher level in the two months prior to this weekend. You want to ensure that your level of physical fitness and stamina is at an extremely high order so your body can perform at the level your brain demands of it without any physical limitations. You also decide to attend extra technique practice training sessions during this period.

As this time passed, your focus of effective effort at your fitness level and at the practice training sessions created an emotional intensity and buzz within your mind that you had not quite experienced before. As you prepared yourself, you had the total belief that your preparation plan was one hundred percent appropriate to achieve your objective.

When the day of the weekend arrived, and you got out of your car and walked towards the meeting location, your mind and body felt so alert, alive and focussed, with a physical, emotional and technical performance confidence that you had never felt to this degree before. All of the additional work you had put in to be prepared for this challenge had created the utter belief that your physical, emotional and technical capabilities were ready, tuned and sufficient to achieve your goal of selection for this elite team.

The plans you laid down and the dedicated and effective execution of them all were a consequence of your mind creating the placebo effect. It raised your attitude, confidence and physical performance to an even higher level and you successfully achieved your objective, even exceeding it because they selected you as team captain.

2) You have some very important exams coming up at the end of the financial year. You are totally focussed on achieving the top grades you need to obtain a place at a particular university. You have not achieved your required grades previously, so you sit down one evening at home with your father at the start of your final year and discuss what changes and activities you should make to finally achieve your requirements.

Your father asks you how serious you are about actually achieving these grades. He makes the point that unless you are totally committed to all of the actions you write down to do over the next six months, including the very detailed revision plan, you will not achieve your goal. You have to believe that all the actions you list must be carried out every day, every week and month, as detailed in your plan. You must trust that if you carry them all out throughout this period, with total commitment, effort, confidence and belief, plus design and follow a detailed exam practice set of rules as part of your plan, you will achieve your grades.

You entered into carrying out each of the actions you listed and found that the attitude of mind the plan created filled you with a fire and belief that you had never felt before. You found that you worked increasingly harder as each week passed. Your father regularly checked up on your activities and progress, and his increasingly complimentary praise spurred you on even more.

When the day of the first exam arrived, you had never before felt that level of quiet but powerful confidence you experienced then. It was a wonderful feeling with which you entered the examination room, and actually, you couldn't wait to attack the exam. All of the planning, preparation and actual execution of the revision, etc., had created an extremely strong belief of success. In itself, this had generated additional benefits due to the creation of a very powerful placebo effect within your mind, with which you tackled each of the exams. You achieved top grades in all your subjects and received a lovely hand-written letter of congratulations from the school headmistress. You will treasure this for the rest of your life, particularly because you knew that she never thought you could achieve such success.

3) You have been asked by the C.E.O. of your company to give a presentation lecture to the C.E.O. of the worldwide organisation your company is part of. You are very keen to get promoted onto the board of your company, and this lecture would be an excellent stepping stone to achieving this if it went very well.

Your great difficulty is you have a major fear of giving presentation lectures like this, particularly to high-level people you have never met before. You contact the local college asking for help. You undertake a course in how to give such a presentation and do several practice presentations in front of different people in the college.

You are provided with a list of various aspects of how and how not to present your information. You must put the work in to master, understand and remember all of the aspects of the information you wish to present. You are shown various methods of jogging your memory in case you have a bit of stage fright. You give a lot of presentations and gradually become more confident in carrying out this exercise.

With all of the practice and work you put into this exercise, your confidence grows and grows, and you achieve a level where you eventually feel you are prepared and ready to perform. This has been arrived at due to you having the courage to admit that you have quite a serious fear. However, you also have the guts to face up to it with experienced and knowledgeable help and advice. Through your extremely hard work and practice, you have been able to develop a placebo effect and a sufficient level of confidence. This enabled you to be able to stand up, deliver this presentation and do a job that was so good that shortly afterwards, you had a promotion on to your company's board.

There will be so many more important objectives to you in your life beyond the few examples above. Some will be even weightier and more important than those above, but so many others will be a lot less important, as considered by other people. However, they will be extremely important to you, which is what always matters. Therefore, each time, you must carry out the exercises as in the examples above. Consider, plan and execute the required actions to achieve your objectives, therefore, creating and engaging your placebo effect.

ROLE F-13 Two final examples of how the power of your mind, its placebo effect and the healing and management power of pain is utilised by your brain for managing chronic knee and back problems.

OVERVIEW: Many millions of people in our country suffer from significant chronic lower back and knee problems. The common treatment prescribed is taking painkillers, with some form of anti-inflammatory medication, initially coupled with rest, at least during the onset phase. The treatment may also include anti-depressants due to suffering a degree of depression and quite often, particularly for serious chronic knee problems, a steroid injection up to a maximum of three, each separated by a number of months.

If you suffer from a physical joint type of difficulty, you have a number of options:

a) You could immediately go to your doctor, put your hand out, ask for tablets, go home and just take the tablets. Maybe you will go back and say they are not working well enough in an attempt to be given stronger and/or different ones.

b) Alternatively, you could engage the power of your mind and activate your placebo effect. Carefully and meaningfully consider your current difficulty. Investigate what you could do to help yourself make your situation better, perhaps by not doing some things for a while that aggravate your condition. Search Google to look for useful information and ask other people who may have helpful knowledge.

If you fail to make acceptable progress, **then** go to your doctor and ask them about all of the things and exercises you can do to help yourself. Avoid taking painkillers as a primary objective. The pain is there to warn you when you are doing something that aggravates your condition, so you stop doing it. Medication may also give you troublesome side effects.

When your attitude is as described above and you truly believe in the regime you are adopting, you will fully engage the placebo effect within your mind. This will significantly assist your healing and recovery process and reduce the discomforts you had previously been experiencing.

c) You could apply a general treatment regime that I believe, based on personal experience, is very effective to try for the majority of cases and can be fine-tuned to best suit your particular set of conditions.

It is very important you understand that with the chronic physical ailments of bad backs and bad knees, complete recovery is not realistically achievable. The aim is to manage the condition and minimise symptoms, whilst living your life to the full, as much as is achievable. Ideally, this is done without worsening the condition and keeping what you were born with, as long as that is the expedient option.

To benefit from your potential placebo effect when dealing with your chronic conditions, it is of absolute importance that you engage in the regimes detailed in ROLE F 13-1 & 13-2 with a strong belief. You need commitment and confidence that, if you follow it as a daily way of life relating to your chronic problems and you genuinely enjoy carrying out the regime, you will gradually see the benefits that will emerge. The total degree of your benefits will be significantly greater if you have fully engaged your placebo effect.

NB It is strongly advisable that you maintain these daily regimes with chronic conditions because they are likely to rear their heads again with a vengeance if you don't.

My current situation:

I have suffered from a serious chronic lower back problem for thirty-one years, from playing an awful lot of sport. The surgeon studying my back scan said, "Any more bad collisions into your back from playing sport will cause you to be in a wheelchair for the rest of your life because we will not be able to operate on you. Your back is in a seriously bad state."

I also suffered from a chronic knee problem in my right knee for sixteen years. Another surgeon studying my scan said, "You will have to have a replacement knee. We can't do anything else for you."

Thirty-one years later, my left knee is worse than my right knee, but I can dance a whole range of different dance styles and swim the crawl to a very good standard. All this is done with sensible care, knowing my safe limits and listening to the help of my brain when it sees me overdoing some physical movement. I have managed to achieve this current status by following the exercise regimes detailed in ROLE F 13-1 and 13-2 every day.

These regimes have suited me with my particular chronic conditions, which I would judge are pretty common conditions. However, **everyone is unique in all of their details,** so if you have problems at all as a result of practising any of my regimes at any time, **please don't blame me**.

Please, please bear in mind all of the advice I have given you in this ROLE F-13 section if you are experiencing difficulties of any kind. You can hopefully solve them and if not, stop doing some and change for others, do things less vigorously, stop completely for a while or seek advice from a physiotherapist – take care of yourself.

My primary purpose in writing this book is to help as many other people as possible. I am doing this by sh3ring all of the knowledge that I have derived and developed from my beliefs about your consciousness, and the activities, rules and objectives your brain operates with and by. For this reason, I felt I had to share my regimes with you because back and knee problems can decimate people's day-to-day lives with strong medications etc. Some of the exercises are very standard, but I must stress that if you find any exercises that don't suit your chronic state of back and/or knees, stop them immediately. Try other ones and, if necessary, stop following them.

One final note, but an extremely important one, is that the combination of all of the exercises and the details of how to do them are obviously a significant part of achieving success. BUT, in addition, it is so, so important to adopt the correct psychological attitudes plus observe pain signals etc,. from your brain, as I have detailed. If you employ the correct attitudes of your mind, you will create and enjoy the full benefits of your placebo effect, which will be of major benefit to your cause.

I wish you the very best of luck.

ROLE F 13-1 A detailed regime for managing your chronic knee/s problems.

a) Keep using your knee/s as much as you can comfortably manage. In principle, the worst thing to do is to sit down, overprotect your knee/s and do as little movement and exercise, walking and using the stairs etc., as possible. Try and get in a brisk walk of at least 30 minutes per day and preferably two sessions of 30 minutes. Whenever you are effectively exercising, using the stairs etc., do it briskly and if your knees ache, this is ok. If they give you pain, ease off because you are overdoing it.

b) The main objective of **a)** is to create and maintain good blood flow around the chronic joint to promote healing and reduce inflammation, which decreases swellings within the joint and reduces pressures between the joint's components.

c)   The other objectives of **a)** are to promote your whole body's good all-round physical and muscular health. Good muscular strength around the knee and generally in the leg area assists in reducing the load stresses within your knee joints. The last but not least objective is to keep your mental health in excellent order. This is vitally important with the potentially emotionally lowering effect that chronic back and knee conditions normally create.

d)   Whenever exercising, maintain full, normal walking movements of your legs and knees etc., to sustain normal muscle strength and fitness. This preserves the control movement quality of your Developed Semi-Automatic Open-Loop Control Systems for all of your walking and other complex movement action requirements. If you stop using these skills within your brain for too long, they will begin to lose some of their very fine, complex control qualities, which will have to be recovered/re-learnt afterwards. Also, walking incorrectly will cause other joints, for example, your hips, to move poorly and ultimately cause them to develop problems.

e)   At all times, keep your knees warm, particularly when walking outside in the cold, etc. Do not allow them to become cold and continue using them because the blood flow will reduce. Their constituents will become cold and thus decrease in size minimally. They will then probably physically interact more with each other, creating additional wear and tear.

203

f) When exercising your knees, whilst walking or dancing – two excellent hobbies to keep your knees in good order – do not initially put too much effort and strain on your knee/s. Make sure you have gradually warmed up to your normal level of activity and therefore loosened the whole joint and its constituents.

Swimming in a pool with warm water is great, but never with the breaststroke. This puts enormous strain on the inside of your knees, particularly if you are swimming hard.

It is very good practice whilst working the knee joints fairly hard to wear a relatively snug-fitting knee bandage for reducing the strain on your knee and also keeping it warm. However, you must remove it after exercise to avoid losing muscle power around your knee area.

g) If your knee/s is in a somewhat poor state, which is a fairly subjective judgement, you should avoid any strenuous exercise, particularly running or even very slow jogging. This is especially relevant on roads and pavements, as they are more of a strain than exercising on dry grass.

If you have a good relationship with your brain, I would expect it to play a large part in this judgement. If you get this decision wrong, you will notice that your general base condition is significantly worse after you have carried out this activity, immediately or the following day. You may experience pain very soon after commencing the activity, in which case you should stop immediately. Revert to using your knees with care as they gradually recover and before returning to your daily hard exercises but most crucially, continue with a three times daily application of Ibuprofen gel as detailed in point **j)** below.

h) Don't do the following activities:

Don't stand still for too long.

Don't twist and turn wearing ordinary trainers and walking boots.

Don't jump up or down.

Don't put all of your weight on one toe and turn with some vigour (a dancing move).

Don't gain weight. Keep your body weight down to your ideal fitness weight.

Don't run up or down stairs too quickly.

Don't carry heavy weights, particularly only on your bad side. If you have to carry weights for a short time, try to separate them. Balance each side so that they are approximately the same and walk with a correct, upright stance.

If you experience any pain, stop immediately.

i) If you are overweight, it is very important to reduce it **gradually** to ideally your optimum weight. This helps reduce the loading stress on your knee in proportion to the percentage of how overweight you are. Hopefully, you will be firm and kind with yourself about this objective due to the benefits that your knee/s, heart and more will gain. So, go for it slowly.

j) At least twice a day, but ideally three times every day – before breakfast before your evening meal and again before

205

bed – carry out a fifteen minute exercise routine for your knees maintenance as described below.

NB Even if only one knee is a problem, it pays to treat the other knee to prevent/delay the possibility of it becoming an issue. It is a possibility that the other knee, whilst not as bad as the known one, is not 100%, so it will pay to work that one also.

1) To relax your knees and legs, carry out the following exercise for one cycle.

Lie flat on your back on a firm rug or carpet with your legs stretched out away from you. Stretch out your hands, flat on the floor behind you, to try and reach the wall behind. Hold this position and try hard to stretch out your whole body whilst slowly inhaling and exhaling for one minute. The objective of this is to stretch all of your joints along the whole length of your spine. This releases any tension anywhere and frees up any of its constituents that are locked or partially locked up. It will increase blood flow with all of the resultant benefits.

2) Sit on a carpet, with your legs straight, stretched out together in front of you and your knees completely relaxed with no tension in them. Your knees and all of their constituents are totally relaxed, so your massaging fingers and thumb can make good contact with your knee joint components.

Start off slowly and increase the effort to warm up the knee, promote very good blood flow and feel the comforting and healthy warmth.

With **both hands on one knee,** concentrate more on the areas where you experience pain. Rub and massage vigorously with the tips of your fingers and thumb over the top, sides and underneath of each knee for one minute. Then change on to the other knee and massage for one minute. (2 minutes in total)

Please note that when you are not using gel (point 4), I find it more effective to massage through a pair of tracksuit bottoms or similar.

3) To give a different massaging effect with **one hand on each knee at the same time** constantly move your hands around the whole of each knee for one minute. Change hands to the other knee to give a different massaging effect for one minute. (2 minutes in total)

4) Finish with exposing your knee/s and massaging into each bad knee until fully absorbed, an inch-long bead of Ibuprofen 10% strength gel. **Apply it to the area/s where you experience pain when you are overdoing exercise.** If only one knee is a problem, it is also worthwhile applying a half-an-inch-long bead of Ibuprofen gel to the other knee in the same area as your bad knee to help keep at bay any potential future problems with it.

NB The primary benefit of this gel is to tackle any inflammation in your knee. It also provides an excellent lubricant to be extremely effective in massaging your knee and promoting excellent blood flow. The other effect that Ibuprofen gel creates is taking the edge off any pain you may have, although I would prefer this feature was not part of its effect. It is excellent at tackling inflammation, and you are applying it directly to the location of the problem area, unlike anti-inflammatory tablets.

If you overdo some physical activity with your knee which causes a continuous or semi-continuous **ache condition** when using your knee, **increase** the regime in **j)** above. Start to do it three times per day and **reduce** your knee activity regime (walking, swimming, dancing etc.) a little until recovery.

If you suffer a continuous or semi-continuous **pain condition** when using your knee, increase the regime in **j)** above. Begin to do it three times per day and stop your high impact knee activity regime for a day or more until your knee recovers its previous base line state.

If it's taking time to recover, try **including** FlexiSEQ in your treatment regime once per day, which is focused only on lubricating your knee joints. It can be used successfully along with the Ibuprofen gel, but not at the same time. Use your Ibuprofen first, and after 5 hours or so, apply your FlexiSEQ. You may decide to continue on a regular basis with FlexiSEQ but always apply your daily Ibuprofen treatment three times per day as a foundational treatment.

During all of the above, if you are overdoing exercise or anything that is too much physical strain for your chronic knee to stand, you will therefore make its condition worse. In response to this, your brain will give you pain, which could be an extremely sharp pain, and it is to tell you to stop – your knee can't cope with it. If this occurs, you must immediately take the weight off your knee to remove the strain of what you are doing.

I most strongly believe that one of the reasons your brain uses pain is to tell you to stop; for example, your poor chronic-conditioned knee is not capable of doing something without making its condition worse. If you take painkillers, the stronger they are, the more they will inhibit your pain signal, the more you will put stress on your knee without being told, "Don't do that. Your knee is not capable of doing it without suffering possible degradation."

The consequences of this painkiller regime are that you will continue to damage your knee. The worse its ongoing baseline state will become, leading you to experience increasing pain etc. and possibly need a completely new knee.

So, **throw away the painkillers** (the knee killers), have trust in and work with your brain to help manage your chronic knee to the optimum achievable. If your brain sees you carrying out this regime to help manage your poorly knee, it will only give you knee pain when you are doing something wrong. This may seem alien and silly to you, but I believe it is how the partnership works.

If you carry out all of these practices, you will hopefully prevent your chronic condition from deteriorating whilst, at the same time, doing as much as you can within the whole of the rest of your life. Please don't forget to engage the immense healing power of your Placebo Effect (please see the section on ROLE F-9 for more information) and maintain the enjoyment of helping yourself!

ROLE F 13-2 A dedicated regime for managing your chronic back problems.

OVERVIEW: This treatment and condition management regime is basically for the very common problem of having a chronic lower back issue where you have a bulging disc/s, pressure on your nerves from the swollen disc/s and other swollen parts and/or inflammation of your nerve cases. These combine to cause interference with the brain's signals transmitted along your nerves to control your muscles below the damaged area in your lower back. The consequences of these problem conditions are that you experience some of the following symptoms: significant pain, numbness, loss of muscular power, swelling, numbness, aches, pins and needles, tingling, reduction of feeling and blood flow in parts of your body below your lower back, down to and including your feet.

Here is a basic general treatment regime that I believe is very effective for most cases. You can fine-tune it to best suit your particular set of conditions at the time.

a) Keep using your back as much as you can comfortably manage. In principle, the worst thing to do is to sit down, overprotect your back and do as little movement and exercise, walking and using the stairs etc., as possible. Try and get in a brisk walk of at least 30 minutes per day and preferably two sessions of 30 minutes. Whenever you are effectively exercising, using the stairs etc., do it briskly and if your back aches, this is ok. If it gives you pain, ease off because you are overdoing it.

b) The main objective of a) is to create and maintain good blood flow to promote healing and reduce inflammation, which decreases swellings and reduces pressure. It helps to improve all of the problem conditions and symptoms you may experience with lower back issues.

c) The other objectives of **a)** are to promote your whole body's good all-round physical and muscular health. Good muscular strength around the knee and generally in the leg area assists in reducing the load stresses within your knee joints and therefore takes the pressure off your back. The last but not least objective is to keep your mental health in excellent order. This is vitally important with the potentially emotionally lowering effect that chronic back and knee conditions normally create.

d) Whenever exercising, maintain full, normal walking movements of your legs, knees, back etc., to sustain normal muscle strength and fitness. This preserves the control movement quality of your Developed Semi-Automatic Open-Loop Control Systems for all of your walking and other complex movement action requirements. If you stop using these skills within your brain for too long, they will begin to lose some of their very fine, complex control qualities, which will have to be recovered/re-learnt afterwards. Also, walking incorrectly will cause other joints, for example, your hips, to move poorly and ultimately cause them to develop problems.

e) At all times, keep your back warm, particularly when walking outside in the cold, etc. Do not allow it to become

211

cold because the blood flow will reduce. Its constituent parts will become cold and thus decrease in size minimally. They will then probably physically interact more with each other, creating additional wear and tear.

f) When exercising whilst walking or dancing – two excellent hobbies to keep your back in good order – do not initially put too much effort and strain on it. Make sure you have gradually warmed up to your normal level of activity and therefore loosened your whole back and its constituents.

Swimming in a pool with warm water is great, but never with the breaststroke. This puts enormous strain on your back, particularly if you are swimming hard. Only the crawl or back-stroke are good when suffering from back problems, but never with swimming too strenuously. This can cause you a reaction that can take months to recover from if you are lucky.

Unless you have extreme back problems, it is far better **not** to wear a back support. It will encourage your surrounding muscles to become weak. It also reduces all of the constituents of your lower back problem area to having less movement whilst you are walking etc., and generally supporting your back. Therefore, it will significantly reduce your blood flow in that area which is a major negative.

g) If your back is in a somewhat poor state, which is a fairly subjective judgement, you should avoid any strenuous exercise, particularly running or even very slow jogging. This is especially relevant on roads and pavements, as they are more of a strain than exercising on dry grass.

If you have a good relationship with your brain, I would expect it to play a large part in this judgement. If you get this decision wrong, you will notice that your general base condition is significantly worse after you have carried out this activity, immediately or the following day. You may experience pain very soon after commencing the activity, in which case you should stop immediately. Revert to using your back with care as it gradually recovers and before returning to your daily hard exercises. Most crucially, continue with a three times daily application of Ibuprofen gel as detailed in point **j)** below.

h) Don't do the following activities:

Don't stand still for too long.

Don't twist and turn wearing ordinary trainers and walking boots.

Don't jump up or down.

Don't put all of your weight on one toe and turn with some vigour (a dancing move).

Don't gain weight. Keep your body weight down to your ideal fitness weight.

Don't run up or down stairs too quickly.

Don't carry heavy weights, particularly only on your bad side. If you have to carry weights for a short time, try to separate them. Balance each side so that they are approximately the same and walk with a correct, upright stance.

Always keep your back's lower/lumbar region concave, with your upper back vertical and your head/neck vertical.

213

This all helps to keep your disc/s away from pushing on to the nerves in your lower back which is of major benefit.

Don't sit for too long, and have a very good chair for correctly positioning your back.

Avoid heavy lifting and, if you have to lift, maintain the correct back posture, lifting with your legs.

Never bend over anything for longer than a second or two.

If you experience any pain, stop immediately.

i) If you are overweight, it is very important to reduce it **gradually** to ideally your optimum weight. This helps reduce the loading stress on your back in proportion to the percentage of how overweight you are. Hopefully, you will be firm and kind with yourself about this objective due to the benefits that your back, heart and more will gain. So, go for it slowly.

j) Each day, before breakfast and again before bed, carry out a fifteen-minute exercise routine for maintenance of your prevailing back condition as described below.

NB If you suffer from chronic back problems, your symptoms will normally be significantly worse with you standing and sitting during the day. This is due to all of the significant weight of your upper back and above, bearing down upon your lower back spine components, your discs particularly, which will probably be pushing onto your nerves, causing you pain and other symptoms.

After a good night's sleep, lying out flat instead of standing or sitting, the components of your spine with no weight on them, will have physically relaxed. This creates more gaps between the components, thus reducing or removing the physical pressure on to your nerves and reducing or removing symptoms of numbness, tingling etc. In this improved physical state of your spine, it is the best possible time to carry out all of your exercises, improve the movement of your lower back components and blood flow and reduce the inflammation in your chronic back area.

1) Lie flat out on your back on a firm rug or carpet with your legs stretched out away from you. Stretch out your hands, flat on the floor behind you, to try and reach the wall behind. Hold this position and try hard to stretch out your whole body whilst slowly inhaling and exhaling for one minute. Relax for 30 seconds and repeat this for three cycles. The objective is to stretch all of your joints along the whole length of your spine, release any tension and free up any of its constituents that are locked or partially locked up. This will increase blood flow with all of the resultant benefits.

2) Turnover and lie flat on your stomach with your legs flat on the rug. Place your hands flat on the rug just above your shoulders and, keeping your legs flat on the rug, push up slowly on your hands. Raise your upper body as far up as you comfortably are able to and hold for one second and lower down fully. Repeat this 30 times.

215

The exercise aims to push your bulging disc/s away from your nerves carefully and to free up and move your disc and nerves and the constituents of your chronic problem area to promote blood flow in and around them. This promotes healing and the reduction of inflammation and the swollen conditions of the items that are inflamed and the resultant contact pressure between them.

3) Sit on your rug with your legs crossed over and under each other and rest your hands on your knees. Sit like this for a few minutes whilst carrying out several neck stretching exercises for any neck area spine problems. This position also helps to improve the health of the spine in your lumber area.

Move your head/chin fully out and hold for 3 sec., then fully back and hold for 3 sec. Turn your head to the side, looking behind with your mouth fully open and hold for 3 sec. Do the same for the other side. Whilst looking ahead, with your left hand holding on to the top of your head, slowly bend your head to the left side and hold for 2sec. Repeat the same for the other side. Carry out each of the above exercises ten times in their pairs of movements.

Never try and rotate your head all of the way round in a circular motion. If you have a neck joint problem, it can lock up your neck joints and be a big problem.

4) Sit up on your rug, with your legs stretched out in front. Slowly move your right leg over the top of your left leg and, holding the ankle of your right leg, carefully slide your right leg along your left leg as far as it will comfortably go

and hold for two seconds. Bring down your right leg to the original position and repeat this exercise with your left leg. Build this exercise up from one cycle per leg to six per leg as you are comfortably able to.

5) Repeat 1) above.

6) Repeat 2) above and add on placing your hands onto the rug and carry out 10 more push-ups. At the end of each push-up, raise your feet and legs (one after the other) up in the air as far as possible and lower immediately to the floor again. As you carry out this raising and lowering of your legs and feet, when the joints of your back spine area become a lot freer, you should feel the joints in your spine making a click-type feel/sound. The purpose of this particular exercise is to increase the movement of your spine's joints to promote blood flow amongst each of them.

7) Rise up on to your toes, stand and complete 40 raising up of your knees to your waist to stretch your lower back.

8) Repeat 1) above.

NB If you overdo some physical activity that causes a strong **ache or a stab of pain** in your lower back area, or a degree of tingling or numbness in one or both legs, please:

a) Stop the activity or activities that you were doing.

b) Reduce the total amount of time each time you are sitting down and also how often you sit down. Look to improve the back protection qualities of the chair you are sitting on or replace it with a more suitable one.

c)   Also, decrease the length of time you are standing still to possibly only a few seconds.

d)   The best time to carry out your massaging routine is before you go to bed, after the last part (section **j**) of your regime for the day.

Each time, massage an inch long squeezed bead of Ibuprofen gel 10% strength onto the area of your lower back where the actual back spine problem exists. This is not something you can do effectively and correctly on your own. To make it 100% effective, you need to get your partner to carry out this massage, with you lying flat out on your stomach, relaxing your back with both arms down by your side and totally relaxing your body. Lying on a bed is the easiest way to achieve this position. This enables the massage to penetrate the troublesome area to create good blood flow, which promotes the healing and reduction of the inflammation in the area.

The troublesome area required to be massaged should be prominent by presenting itself as an area that feels knotted, lumpy or gritty when being massaged. Also, the patient will probably say it is painful when you begin to massage this area, but this pain should subside as you gradually and carefully massage it.

Check to see if the same area on the other side of the lower back is the same and if so, or even if not as bad, massage that as well.

Be careful not to massage too vigorously, starting off very gently, and as the area becomes a little less knotty, increase your massage effort a little. Continue massaging until all of the gel has been absorbed.

In addition to massaging as directed, also, very carefully and lightly, massage along the length of the spine in the lower back area. This is to free up any joints of your spine which may have become slightly stiff and troublesome.

e) Continue this total daily regime until your body is free of unpleasant symptoms and the knotted area/s of your back are clear. The period of time required to achieve this status depends upon a number of related factors and could vary from several weeks to months. **NB** If you suffer from a continuous or semi-continuous pain condition, probably brought upon by exposing your back to stresses beyond its capability, immediately switch into a very low key activity regime. Take care not to worsen the already delicate state of your back. If you are comfortably able to, carefully continue with your daily exercise routine (section **j)** and most crucially, as a minimum, continue with your daily application of Ibuprofen gel as detailed in section **d)** above.

Try and avoid taking painkillers, but if you find this hard, take as small a dose as possible and wean yourself off them as soon as possible. Follow all of the good things to do and don't do any of the bad things to do, as detailed earlier.

Don't stay in bed any longer than usual. Get up and move around as much as you can comfortably and listen to the symptom signals from your Brain. Gradually, as your back recovers and your symptoms reduce, increase your level of movement and return to your daily regime of exercises, lightly and carefully at the start.

NB During all of the above, if you are overdoing exercise or anything that is too much physical strain for your chronic back to be able to cope with without making its condition worse, your brain will tell you. It will give you a pain, which could be an extremely sharp pain, and is to say, "Stop that – your back can't cope with it." If this occurs, you must immediately take the weight off your back to remove the strain of what you are doing, and the pain should disappear. If the pain does not cease immediately and continues, stop doing all of this exercise regime until your back recovers. When you do resume, start with extreme care.

If you carry out all of these practices, you will hopefully prevent your chronic condition from deteriorating whilst, at the same time, doing as much as you are able to throughout the rest of your life.

ROLE G – Your <u>brain's seventh</u> fundamentally important role is to remember. It needs to retain and recall all of the required details from your experiences and data or information that comes in via your senses.

Your brain needs to remember all of the learned conclusions you have derived from your mind's internal thoughts and considerations related to all aspects of your past, present and future life at work, home and at leisure, throughout the whole of your life.

NB I may have placed this role as the last on my list of roles for your brain, but this is not because it is the least important. Far from it, for without your ability to remember, you could not partake in life at all. Each of these listed roles is important because you could not function normally in your life without the complete set of them.

OVERVIEW: I believe that you will need to keep some information for relatively short periods. Some for a few seconds, a few hours, or maybe a few days or perhaps weeks. However, some information requires retaining for a number of years, and some for the rest of your life.

*Without being able to remember information **at all**, even from a second ago, you would not be able to take part in any of the everyday activities that being alive involves. You would be incapable of communicating with anyone, and they would be incapable of communicating with you. You would be isolated from the world around you and also be isolated in detail from your own world, within your body and being. You would be the absolute epitome of Manuel, from Fawlty Towers, who knew absolutely nothing because, as Basil Fawlty said, "He's from Barcelona."*

Here are some questions I would like to consider with you:

Question 1 – In very basic terms, how does your brain remember or store information?

OVERVIEW: In relation to an item or sets of items of data coming into your brain via your senses, or within your brain, from your

B.H.S.M.S. and your internally recollected thoughts, I define what is classed or referred to as:

a)   An item of memory or experience

b)   An item of data or information

c)   A combination of a) and b)

These types of items of data and experience are used as a priority for updating your consciousness and also, where relevant and required, for storing or updating your memory.

Definition 1 – A memory is:

A remembrance of an experience that comprises a collection or set of activities, thoughts, observations, feelings and information, coming into or from within your brain, as described above. All of this data is stored as a collection/set in one of your Category 1B Memory Experience departments within your brain. It is labelled appropriately and available for you to recall, review and therefore remember whenever your M.C., assisted by your intelligence, requires.

Definition 2 – An item of data or information is:

Data or information coming into or from within your brain that fundamentally provides you with a piece of information about the situation you are currently in. It is used in the process to update your consciousness and is also utilised for knowledge about a topic or aspect in life that will be useful now and perhaps in the future.

I propose that these items will be stored in one of your appropriate Senses, Memory or Category 1B Knowledge Departments, with an appropriate label. For example, a collection of data from your vision would be stored in one of your Vision Memory Departments and a dataset of sound would be stored in one of your Sound Memory Departments etc. Alternatively, in many cases, as described later, your sighted vision of a dog would be stored in the same memory subdepartment as the sound of a dog barking.

The labelling and storage location for individual memories is decided upon by what will give the shortest time to be able to locate and recall each stored memory. This assists your brain to access and process data in the fastest time possible.

I propose, for consideration, that the data providing you with knowledge from your five senses, via seeing, smelling, touching, tasting and hearing, will be stored in the relevant brain departments, as you have a multitude of Memory, Category 1B Knowledge Departments and subdepartments.

Rather than all data being stored in one extremely large memory department, each will have a particular type or category, some with multiple categories and subcategories or sub-subcategories of knowledge. Your M.C., assisted by your intelligence, can request information from any of these departments when required.

This arrangement, I suggest, will enable far greater efficiency of recall of any required data. This will result in a much shorter retrieval time than a huge Memory Department arrangement with only one category of data stored in each Memory Subdepartment would create, compared to, in many cases, having multiple data categories in the same Memory Subdepartment.

I proffer, for consideration, that your memory of an experience, which, as previously defined, comprises a collection or set of activities, thoughts, observations, feelings, smells and information entering your brain via one or more of your senses etc., are all stored in the same place. This place is your Vision, Category 1B Memory Experience Department: the memory storage location for all of the data connected to this particular experience memory.

I propose this memory storage arrangement in order to:

a) Use one of the Category 1B Visual Departments, because the vast majority of the data with most group experience memories will pretty certainly be in <u>visual form.</u>

b) Make the localisation of a memory and therefore the recall of each separate set experience, containing all visual data and all other data memory categories as fast as possible. You only have to access one memory location, *the visionary one*, to obtain all the other different categories of data that contain the whole of this separate set of experience.

c) Make the complete process of *localisation, recall* and *use* of this data, as fast as is possible. Consequently, the recall and response time performance of all of your brain's activities, is as efficient and fast as is possible.

This is one of its vitally important priorities, as it studiously attempts to look after all your safety and all your other needs throughout your lifetime. It can only successfully satisfy these needs when a rapid response can be achieved under all conditions. This is particularly important relating to maintaining your safety when this objective, at times, over an extremely short period, requires the lightning processing speed of a huge quantity of data.

Question 2 – In very basic terms, how do you access or recall memory information stored in your brain?

Example 1 – Viewing a chimney.

Each time data enters your brain via one of your senses and you have previously learned what this particular item is and its purpose, for example, you see a *chimney* with your *vision*, the process is as follows:

Step 1 Your eyes have received visual data of a chimney.

Step 2 Your brain has received a set of Visual information representing this chimney into one of its Category 1A departments, which is an Incoming Data Coding Section. The data is coded in the form of electrical current signals in analogue format.

NB At this moment of time in the process, your brain has <u>no idea</u> what this information means, other than it is visual and in analogue format.

Step 3 I propose that the data is automatically re-coded into a DNA-type of Analogue Format.

Step 4 Your brain has to search your Vision Memory Departments to find a match for this set of visual analogue information, now re-coded into a DNA-type of Analogue Format.

Step 5 When your brain finds a match, which will be in the memory cell location labelled *Chimney*, it then knows its name and can find out, from the information stored inside this memory cell location, what the purpose of a chimney is, etc.

NB If you see something that you have *never seen before*, the above process takes place, but because you are seeing it for the first time, at the end of step 4, you will not have found a match. Your M.C. will conclude, I don't know what this is. Therefore, it will have to find out with the learning process and commit this vision with its description to your memory for future use when you have learnt the relevant information. Meanwhile, this memory of the chimney remains in its Coded DNA-Type of Analogue Format, waiting to be processed in the Category 1B department allocated to this dedicated role.

When attempting to recall any particular memory, I propose that it is obviously significantly easier and quicker for you, and you will remember more detail if you are <u>at the scene</u> where <u>the original</u> memory occurred. This includes some of the basic views being the same as they were at the time of the initial memory. If you are detached from the scene, you have to rely totally on your recall of stored memory data. However, I suggest that if you recall a memory whilst at the location of the original memory, there is an inherent risk that the original details may be overwritten/corrupted. Some details and perhaps relationships related to the initial memory have changed from the time of the original event and you will probably be unaware that these changes have occurred.

Question 3 – In very basic terms, what format does your brain store or remember information in and why?

I believe that your brain receives updates and stores information or data in the state in which it is delivered into your brain system. For each of your senses, this is Analogue Format. Your senses collect their data in Analogue Format because this is the format that the data exists in at its creation.

N.B. Converting data from Analogue to Digital form will always incur a loss of detail. This can be very significant, for example, when converting sound from its original state of creation into Digital Format. Data conversion into some other format, from your brain's data receipt to brain storage is also best not carried out due to the additional time period for the conversion activity and storage process. Therefore, maintaining the original format improves/reduces your brain's response time when it is using data items to perform any of its tasks.

Question 4 – In very simple terms, what form or coding does your brain store information in and why?

Due to the enormous quantity of data that your brain is required to and does store, plus the incredible processing speed it operates at, coupled with the rate of data and memory recall that it achieves, I propose the following. Fundamentally, the **form or coding** your brain stores data in is in the structure used for **genetic coding**. However, it is very much tailored to an Analogue Format, which suits the particular use of this form and data for two reasons:

a) The basic D.N.A. format already exists within your functionality, and therefore your brain already has the means of understanding, communicating and generally working with it.

b) It is extremely efficient at storing a very high density of data per unit of its volume, resulting in a DNA-type of Analogue Format.

Question 5 – Why doesn't your brain get clogged up and full and therefore can't store or remember any more information?

OVERVIEW: Whilst you are awake and with your eyes open, depending on what you are doing and where you are, out of the data your brain is processing, nominally:

a)   50% will be from your vision

b)   20% will be from your hearing

c)   25% will be from your thoughts and deliberations (processing your consciousness data)

d)   5% will be shared between your other three senses plus your B.H.S.M.S.

If you remembered or attempted to remember, every single piece of all of this information, including each fine detail in all of your fields of vision, every activity, every second throughout your life, **despite your brain's incredible capacity** and capability, I think its total data storage limit would be reached in your early years.

Long before then, your data recall efficiency, which would have gradually declined, would have become significantly impaired. Your brain would be unable to function fast enough to keep you safe. It would be unable to complete decision making and action taking effectively and productively, to keep you capably involved in your everyday work and life.

Therefore, I propose that the answer to Question 5 is the brain employs various strategies that collectively prevent this wholly unacceptable and dangerous situation from ever occurring to you. These include:

1) If my proposal that all of the data within your brain is stored in an Analogue DNA format turns out to be correct, then this one feature would, in itself, allow an enormous quantity of data to be stored there, even though your brain is really quite a small volume.

2) Each time data is placed in memory, I proffer that it is stored with the amount of storage energy proportionate to how important you feel this data is to you. The energy imprint in its memory location enables it to remain in existence and therefore be available for immediate recall when required.

Every time a memory needs to be retrieved, it will be available for use and, at the same time, will automatically have its storage energy refreshed again after use. If a memory has not been refreshed for a while, its storage energy gradually reduce, resulting in it noticeably taking longer to be recalled. Sometimes it may be a few minutes or much longer before it can be recalled. Meanwhile, your M.C. will probably have been working on other activities, in addition to your Data Search networks, continuing to find the required memory.

If a memory has not been recalled for a long time and therefore takes a lot longer to be remembered, your brain will make a judgement of its future importance. Your brain will decide whether it needs to be used again and, if so, what level of storage energy it should be refreshed with. This will be one of the items of work carried out by your brain whilst you are sleeping. When a memory has not been recalled for a significantly long time, it will eventually disappear. This automatically clears out data that is no longer required, vacating that part of your memory to be available for use.

3) I propose that each time basic data from your Vision, Sound, Taste, Smell and Touch is received, it is simply refreshed if it is found to be in memory already. However, if it is not in memory, its meaning is to be established and stored under an appropriate label for future use if it is decided to be kept during your next sleep review. As opposed to basic data, which will be processed immediately, quite complicated sets and therefore large quantities of data go into a short term Memory Department. They will have their meaning established and reviewed to be retained or deleted during your next sleep.

4) I also suggest that, when you receive any basic data from your senses or thoughts, after processing it to understand its relevance to you in that moment, your brain will decide whether it is required as part of your consciousness update or not. If required, your brain will use and then discard it or delete it immediately if it is not required.

5) I believe that, apart from on specific occasions, when you require greater detail, in order to save an extremely significant amount of data memory storage capacity, your vision memories, in particular, do not carry all of the vast numbers of visual details of the original vision. Instead,

they only maintain details of basic framework, outlines and colour. This is sufficient to remember rudimentary layouts and relative positions of the main features in relation to each other, so that you can recognise/remember these repeating visions in the future.

The recognition or recollection of each of these visual memories of people's faces or views etc., are significantly aided by the other items of related memory. These include, for example, what job the person did, their character or voice, the beautiful weather that day, other emotions stored, etc. The most appropriate of these details are attached to the basic visual memory, located on the appropriate **Category 1B Vision Department's Cell Door,** thus enabling the fastest possible memory location and recall of Memories to be achievable.

6) During your sleep, I believe your brain does the following:

a) Reviews your recent memories of that day, both in your short and long term memory departments and deletes any that are not required.

b) Retains seemingly relevant memories for longer, until no longer deemed useful.

c) Updates those as required.

d) Relocates, as appropriate, memories to their permanent Memory Category 1B Department.

e) Refreshes any, to support their continuing retention, located in their appropriately labelled Memory Category 1B Department Memory Cell.

NB Some of the above processes involve your M.C., aided by your intelligence having to be extremely selective. It has to decide what it stores to memory and with how much detail. To do this, your M.C. has to complete this ongoing process.

a) Absorb the meaning and relevance to you of all of the data, with its multitude of items of finely absorbed detail per second. This information comes from the moving pictures and changing conditions of data you are receiving via your senses etc., to observe and understand all of the activities of the world around you.

b) The purpose of these observations and activities is to update your consciousness and then attend to all the prevailing considerations, related decisions and actions it brings to your attention. Your M.C. needs to ensure your safety is maintained and that you attend to situations requiring your attention and resolution. By the time this has been completed, your brain will have already discarded and redundant items of data, and all other data items you don't require in memory will be discarded.

c) Another significant saving of memory storage capacity occurs when, the moment you receive a data set from any of your five senses, if you deem any of it purely transient and not worth storing it for any length of time, your brain will immediately delete/discard that element. This action most frequently applies to your Vision, followed by your Sound.

Question 6 – In some detail, how are your memories and information located and recalled so incredibly quickly when required?

OVERVIEW: *Please take a moment to consider the absolutely gargantuan range of different topics and for each one, its range of items and sub-ranges and sub-sub-ranges of related data and experiences that continually flood into your brain via your senses, particularly throughout your waking life. All of this previously experienced data, information and experiences that you decided to commit to memory, will be stored in your Category 1B Memory Departments within your brain. Despite the enormous quantity of stored data that this equates to, how on earth does your brain manage to locate and retrieve any item or set of information from these memories as quickly as it does each time?*

The faster your brain operates to retrieve data from your memories, the quicker you process and update your consciousness with that available data. Therefore, the quicker you can respond to any danger that it sees you facing and ultimately remain safe.

I propose that this outstanding performance of your brain is achieved by combining all of the relevant operational aspects that it employs, as detailed in this book up to this point. These are in addition to the following list of features.

1) My estimation of the fundamentally awe-inspiring operating speed at which your brain processes all data, considerations, activities and actions during its ongoing updating of your

consciousness whilst processing all of its additional ongoing workload is calculated in this way.

*Your brain's processing involves a **significant number of millions** of multi-step, sub-processing activities and self-operating capability activities, **EACH OF WHICH contains and processes** millions of points of data every second.*

Dependent upon what type of data and the data processing workload this equates to, I estimate it very approximately to be: **8 million x 50 million points of data being processed every second by your brain.**

For the development of this estimation refer to Subchapter 4.1, Subchapter B. B2) & B3).

To continue with the list of features:

2)   The efficiency of retrieval of information is due to the vast number of Memory Category 1B Departments residing in your brain and the division and subdivisions within each of these departments and subdepartments. It is also due to the highly efficient and fast Data Search Facilities available within your brain that coordinate with each Memory Category 1B Department's in-house, automatic memory location search capabilities, which includes having complete knowledge of its own contents.

3)   To achieve the shortest possible retrieval time due to:

a)   Each of your senses having a dedicated set or group of Memory Departments dedicated to them. For example, any incoming data from your Vision, will be stored and labelled in a **Vision Memory Category 1B Department.**

b) For every <u>single item of data,</u> for example, when you see a Horse, the memory would be stored in a Vision Category 1B Department Memory Cell labelled 'Horse.'

c) For each <u>Multi Set of Senses Experience Memory</u>, comprising data from most or all of your senses, all related experience data would be stored in a memory cell with a Vision label on it. For example, when you wish to store in memory an experience on a family holiday of sunbathing, boating, fishing etc., inside the memory cell called 'Polperro Cove' would be all of the details of your experience for you to read and recall.

4) Each Memory Category 1B Department has its own set of Neural Networks working with your M.C. for automatically deleting, storing, updating, locating and managing all of the data stored within its domain.

When an item of data or information must be located, the following points are considered:

a) If the item of data is an *external, incoming one,* say, from your Vision, it will automatically be presented to your Vision Memory, Central Locating Department. This will automatically *present this data item coded in a set of DNA-type of Analogue Format,* to be seen by all single-item data Vision Memory Departments. The department where it is located will automatically recognise it by comparison matching the two sufficiently identical set of Analogue signals and provide the details of what it is.

b) If the item of data or a request for information is an *internal one from within your brain*, e.g. a request from your M.C. to locate a data item, say a particular type of horse, which it requires information about, it will request the recall of the details. This request, which would be in the DNA-type of Analogue format, detailing the name "Horse" and its type – "Dray." for example, would be presented to your Central Locating Department. It will automatically submit this request to be seen by all of your Horse Memory Departments.

The department where it is located will automatically sufficiently match the request with the labelling coded data on the Memory Department Cell door. Opening up this Memory Cell will present the required information for review.

5) An extremely beneficial factor contributing to the overall operational speed of memory recall is called Parallel Processing functionality. This takes place when an item of data or a Memory Experience is being searched for. The time taken to locate it is significantly reduced due to all Memory Departments that may contain it searching their own contents simultaneously. Many other related processing activities will also happen at the same time that searching for the Memory Cell location is occurring.

6) Particularly whilst you are awake, your M.C. is continually updating your consciousness. It keeps you safe by dealing with all safety-related conditions it flags up, and it handles all non-safety related conditions by deciding what actions are required. Consequently, most of the memories and their related Memory Departments that you require to be open will primarily be in the same areas of any additional data that enters or is internally requested. Therefore it is likely it will take significantly less time to locate existing Memories for any extra data that is required.

7) Storing all data items comprising of each basic memory experience set of activities and emotions within the same memory experience location label and cell gives a much reduced data search time. It also saves a lot of search and processing time, recalling, collating and understanding another range of items of data from many other separate and individual memory locations.

For example, take the word 'sand.' You have a large number of different colours, textures and compositions of examples of sand, with a wide variety of locations related to your experiences, several uses, and knowledge of things that live in and travel on sand that you encompass during your life.

You could have all data relating to sand, including its different aspects, mentioned within your memory under a common label of 'Sand.' Within this label, you could have separate labels and sub-sub-labels for all of the different aspects and details mentioned. This would mean that you would have many hundreds of *individual* memories related to sand. This would not lead to quick recall and understanding when **recalling memories that included some aspects of sand.**

But, in addition to the arrangement above, I believe that in the example of sand, you will have one Memory label of **Sand/General**. All of the general data about sand would be stored here, and relevant information from this Memory Label would be recalled when required. Meanwhile, any particular details relating to sand within a General Set of experiences would be included within the Memory details of this General Set of experiences.

8) I propose that when you are searching out a high percentage of information from memory and are trying to recall some details, you don't remember specific points in *words format*. Instead, you search out the required detailed answer from studying the basic picture memory of the area or situation. Included in this picture memory cell, is other data from your senses, as they are part of that Memory Related Cell, to provide all of the required information.

With this system, compared to one where you stored all data from all of your senses in word format, grouped as appropriate, you would have to store a huge amount more sets of data covering your memories. For example:

You are searching out some information about a tennis court you played at on holiday 50 years ago. You are trying to remember where the hitting the tennis ball practice wall was in relation to the main entrance of the tennis clubhouse. You don't remember in specific details in words where it was, but you search out the required information from recalling and studying in your mind. To obtain the answer, you retrieve the basic picture location memory of the related area, and what was there in relation to each other.

NB All of the details above and below are my proposals. They are to convey some ideas of methods and possible structures for consideration by others – at the very least, it's a starter to build upon.

Proposal 1

For consideration, with more details than before, of how your brain may actually process the data that comes into it and, importantly, how it utilises labelling and the data layout construction within your Memory Cells to maximise the efficiency and, therefore, the resultant speed of this complete data processing cycle.

Example 2 – Your vision sees a horse. How does your brain process it?

For clarity of understanding, let's consider a single part of what would normally be a far greater amount of data involved with the process of Updating your Consciousness. We will focus on just a single item – the vision of a horse – coming into your brain as part of the next update of your consciousness.

How is this vision received by your brain and processed to full understanding, being included, or not, in that update of your consciousness?

OVERVIEW: I propose that, even for your brain, there is far too much processing, decoding and understanding of the extreme amount of micro-detailed data if all of this Vision Data is presented into only one of your Category 1B departments for all required processing. The consequentially awesome amount of processing necessary for you to understand sufficiently well, clearly and quickly enough all of the significant elements with sufficient detail of each picture your Vision is presenting to your brain makes it an impossible task.

A) Therefore, I propose that the different aspects and categories that comprise each picture are received and initially processed by the separate, specialist, dedicated Category 1B departments to suit the type and composition of the data they are processing. After a tremendous amount of processing by these different departments of your brain, the initial interpretation of the fine details of each electrochemical analogue format elements of the complete Visual Data set (the picture of the horse that enters your brain via your eyes, the following takes place:

A1) These fine details, still in analogue form, representing attributes about the colours, the shape, the movement and all other visual aspects about the horse, are collected and combined when they enter your brain's Incoming Category 1B Developed, Semi-Automatic Coding Department.

A2) I believe that this Coding Department is one of a set of seven departments in a particular area of your M.C. that comprise your consciousness creation process. At this stage, the picture of the horse is in a form and detail condensed from the incredible amount of very fine detail presented initially into your brain as above. Consequently, the picture bears an

241

excellent likeness to how the horse appears in real life (to other people) within the limits of it being seen by your brain, which has worked with the eyes of the beholder, i.e. you. **NB** The most important factor to be understood at this stage of the process is that you do not have <u>any idea</u> AT ALL, what you are looking at.

A3) I propose that a set of all of this incoming data is converted into a type of DNA Analogue Format, reproducing the colours, shape, movement and all of the other details of the horse as you actually saw it in the first place.

NB All data is stored within its particular Memory Cell, which has a door allowing access to various data related to what is stated on the Memory Cell Access front door. On the front door of our example, we have the following:

- A label of the "<u>vision</u> of a basic horse," coded in DNA Analogue Format.
- A label of the <u>written</u> word "Horse" is coded <u>visually</u> in DNA Analogue Format.
- A label of the <u>spoken</u> word "Horse" coded as <u>spoken audibly</u>, in DNA Analogue Format.

Details of horse-related data are contained within the cell inside different subdepartments for each category of information.

This cell would be split up into subdepartments, of all of the different types of horses that exist. Each subdepartment would be labelled with a vision of a particular kind of horse and would contain knowledge about that breed, detailing their different roles in life, where they originate from, etc. So, the access route into this wide range of knowledge could be a basic picture of a horse, the written word "Horse" or the spoken word "Horse."

All the data within the cell is stored in <u>the written word</u>, coded visually in DNA Analogue Format. When you wish to find data on the horse, you use your Developed Category 1B Semi-Automatic Reading Skill to read the data within the cell subdepartment. This then encodes the words back to their normal human written form and then presents them to your M.C. to read with your Developed Category 1B Department Semi-Automatic Reading Skill within your mind.

A4) Your *automatic Memory Data Search Department*, which works with all of your Memory Category 1B Departments' in-house automatic neural networks, will be instructed by your M.C. In this instance, it will be told to search for and locate a Memory Cell door with a Vision Label of a horse on it, which at least approximately matches the basic vision of the horse that you have seen.

NB Your Memory Data Search Department will be satisfied if it initially finds an approximate match with your vision. If this is insufficient for your prevailing knowledge requirements, it will search through the other horse breeds within this horse Memory Cell Department's subdepartments for an acceptably comparable match with the horse you have actually seen.

A5) If it can't find one, it will select this type of horse to be added to this Memory Cell during your next sleep and try, by then, to find out some information to add to this kind of horse.

A6) At this point in the process, you can at least recognise what you are looking at and have basic knowledge about its role in life. This Vision Data is copied into the vision department of your seven department consciousness process.

A7) At this stage, your vision of the horse, along with the data and knowledge about it, is made available for your M.C. to study as part of its updating process of your consciousness. After study, your M.C., with your intelligence, will decide if this data creates any unsafe condition or situation for your safety. If it does, this data will be included in that update of your consciousness. If it does not compromise your safety, but it presents a situation that merits your attention, it will be included in the prevailing update of your consciousness. If it offers neither, your M.C. will immediately delete/discard it.

Example 3 – You have an internally created thought/ wish to recall a holiday with your grandchildren. How does your brain process it?

OVERVIEW: *Your internally generated thought was created by yourself because you day-dreamed when you had a period of available introspection whilst alone. You wished to recall the wonderful memories you and your wife have about your holidays of years gone by with your grandchildren.*

A1) For clarity of understanding, let's just consider this single part of the process of updating your consciousness using *one internally created thought/wish*, to recall one of your Multi-Sense Experience Memories, which are already within your brain. **As**

part of the next update of your consciousness, your brain will view and recall internally stored visions, smells, tastes, touches and sounds from your memory. How are all of these aspects of your Experience Memories recalled and reviewed by your brain, processed to full understanding and included, or not, in the prevailing update of your consciousness?

A2) Your internal thoughts are automatically directed into the Category 1B department for Internal Thoughts of your brain's consciousness, which comprises seven departments. *Your thoughts wish to recollect the many memories of great holidays you and your wife have experienced.*

NB The <u>most important fact</u> to understand <u>at this point in the process</u> is that you know you will eventually recall some holiday experiences, because that is what you wish to recollect. However, you do not have <u>any idea</u> AT ALL, what particular holiday/s and their detailed memories you will resurrect out of your memories.

The actual memory which you require to be searched for is on Caister Beach with three of your grandchildren. This detail is only able to come to your mind whilst you are searching through all of your holiday memories.

A3) Your Automatic Memory Data Search Department, which works with all of your Memory Category 1B Departments in-house automatic neural networks, will be engaged by your M.C. to search for and locate, in this instance, a Memory Cell door with a **written word** label on it, saying **Holidays.**

A4) When the required Holiday Memory Cell has been found, your brain will read search the list of contents using one of your dedicated Category 1B departments to find a holiday memory that you wish to recall.

A5) At this point in the process, your chosen holiday memory, which is of a particular time on Caister Beach, is copied into the vision Category 1B Department of your seven department consciousness. It is made available for your M.C. when it requires, to study it as part of its updating process of your consciousness. After investigating it, your M.C. assisted, by your intelligence, will decide if this data presents any condition or situation affecting your safety. If it does not compromise your safety but it offers a situation that merits your attention, it will be included in the prevailing update of your consciousness. If it presents a danger, your M.C. will immediately delete/discard it.

The most likely outcome of this situation is that you decide that your wish to recall and reminisce about this particular holiday will not jeopardise your safety. You then decide to deal with maybe one safety issue and a few other actions, for example, adjusting your seat position whilst intermittently thinking about your Caister Beach experiences. This same internal thought is constantly re-entered, 250 times per second, into the continuing process cycle, commencing with A1) above.

This means the previous scenario with these thoughts would be repeated, with other items of probably changing input data, over a ten-minute period, giving you the impression, at times, that you are experiencing these Caister Beach reminisces continuously. This feeling of experiencing a continuous experience is simply due to the awe-inspiring processing speed of your brain.

Question 7 – What thought language is used for two-way internal communication between your M.C. and other departments within your brain?

I propose that you **hear** the words **produced** by your mind when it ponders various thoughts about something you are considering or requests information from another department. This internally spoken word is spoken silently within your mind, but nevertheless, you can hear it as if it is real. It creates a set of electrical activities identical to the spoken word and will, therefore, generate an identical Audio-Coded copy in a type of DNA Analogue Format.

I believe this is the communication format or language when thoughts are used, for communication, between your M.C. and other departments, plus vice versa, within your brain.

This communication arrangement is also compatible, with the system for locating Data in your Memory Departments. Therefore, it leads to a high efficiency of functionality and extremely fast brain processing speed. All of these facets are necessary to stand the best chance of keeping you safe at all times and also process all of your other considerations highlighted by your Consciousness, suitably fast enough.

***ROLE G-1** Another example, so you have an appreciation of just how ferociously busy the recall from your memories is, at times, of so much that you have learnt.*

This covers such a vast range of topics and situations about life on knowledge, data, information, and making ferociously fast, accurate and complex judgements.

Also consider your many different thoughts, the number of life-threatening decisions, EXTREMELY DIFFICULT and, at times, conflicting conditions of requirements your brain is called upon to make at a frightfully fast processing speed, because of the number of situations that require resolving quickly.

OVERVIEW: To appreciate how incredibly busy your brain is sometimes forced to be in order to update your consciousness, keep you and other people safe and carry out all of your required considerations, decisions and actions during a very short timescale, please consider the following conditions.

Example 4 – Exploring how ferociously active your brain is when you drive your car in an extremely busy, unfamiliar high street.

You could be faced with having to be aware of and deal with many major challenges, including:

a) Pavements full of pedestrians, hectic traffic conditions, a dog off the lead, people only looking at their mobile phones, deplorable weather conditions, and all of this happening within an extremely noisy, distracting and unsettling environment.

In addition to each of these factors, you may also have to be aware of and deal with the position, distance, approaching speed and any other safety aspects in relation to your car, of a combination of some of the following:

b) A car close behind you.

c) A car in front of you.

d) A car travelling in the other direction to you, on the other side of the road.

e) A wobbling cyclist, in front of the car, in front of you.

f) A car, on screeching tyres, skidding up to a side road junction to your right, 10 metres along the road to you. Your brain has computed that this other car will not be able to stop at the junction, resulting in it hitting the offside side of your car where your daughter is at significant speed.

g) Your five-year-old daughter has started to scream in the back of your car not to hit the lady with a baby in a pushchair. You have already noted is panicking and compute that she could step into the path of your car within two seconds.

The data above conveys the details related to each person, car and all other moving items and changeable conditions created by the consequences of the above situations listed, from **a)** to **g)**. Some of these variables are:

1) Active at the same time.

2) Occurring one after the other.

3) Overlapping others.

4) Experiencing changing dynamics of speed, direction and positions relative to each other.

5) Removing themselves out of the zone of your immediate location and, therefore, your concern.

6) Being joined by new sets of situations and conditions which are within your zone of immediate potential danger.

7) Forcing you to keep reconsidering the actions that you are required to take to keep you and others safe within your zone of activity.

Data related to the above situations is flooding in, mainly from your senses, into your brain to be processed. This completes each cycle of the continuously updating and responding to the requirements of your consciousness, which is done 250 times per second.

During periods of this furore of activity, your memories supply you with a huge amount of information concerning the ever-changing situation you are immersed within. To fully understand the relevance of each data item or condition listed and to understand the inter-related and interreactive meaning of the conditions detailed, which are changing due to their individual dynamics, keeping you, your passengers and other cars, their occupants and all other people listed above hopefully safe, all of the activities your brain has to process in their very basic form are:

a) For <u>each item of data</u> coming into your brain via your senses, B.H.S.M.S. and any internal thoughts, your brain has to search in your Memories Cells, to locate a data set match for each item.

b) It then *decodes* what each item is; for example, this view is a car, a bicycle, a lady, a pushchair, a baby; this sound is of screeching tyres; these are the words of my daughter, she is extremely frightened etc.

c) It must *decide*, for each collection of inter-related items of data, for example, the lady, pram and baby are connected as a unit, what their particular relevance is to your car:

d) It then *discards* all data items that you have decided are not important regarding safety or other aspects in the moment. Your brain updates your consciousness with all relevant items of data, thus enabling you to know what decisions and actions you require to make to keep you safe.

e) For each car and everyone else involved with this situation, your brain, utilising your Computational Learned Automatic Skills (from several enlisted Category 1B departments), predicts the distance and the approaching time to you, plus notes any other safety aspects concerning them and your car.

f) Your brain views and considers each of the cars and people involved in the items listed in relation to each other to decide what options you have in each moment, in terms of the ideal objective, which is keeping everyone safe.

g) If at any time you decide that this objective is not achievable, you then have to decide what is the next best viable goal and what actions you as the driver of your car should take to achieve it.

h) You have to continually monitor the actual sets of conditions which are continually changing because the other cars and people involved are moving and changing their positions relative to you and each other.

i) Also changing by the second, which needs monitoring, is the degree of danger, from when each situation or combinations of situations commenced, through to their conclusions.

Your M.C. is attempting to repeat each of the above process activity steps and considerations fully, from **a)** to **i)**, whilst updating your consciousness at a rate of 250 times per second.

NB I believe that, despite the extreme complexity and difficulty of the conditions detailed above, which don't occur every time you go driving, but certainly can and do sometimes occur, the brain of an experienced car driver doesn't panic and manages to cope very well. This is due to a number of factors, including:

a) The crucial roles that your Category 1B departments play in having the Neural Networks with their automatic abilities, including the required speed of searching, locating and understanding the prevailing relevance of each item of data.

b) The speed at which your consciousness can be updated, thus providing the required, latest actions necessary to keep you safe.

c) The computational speed and accuracy of each one of your Learned Automatic Skills, Category 1B Departments you utilise for the computations required to estimate the approaching times to your car for each moving unit.

d) The speed, accuracy and correct decision-making of your M.C., ably assisted by your intelligence, working with all of its car driving, Developed, Category 1B Department, Semi-Automatic skills utilised for steering and manoeuvring your car in such challenging conditions.

e) All of the different departments your brain has utilised in the above process were continually very busy, carrying out their dedicated functionalities.

f) The crucially important role and incredible operational efficiency, speed, decision-making and management quality that your M.C. achieved by effectively utilising all of the data received from each of the departments involved with the complete process. This includes the ones containing the total, vast amount of knowledge and experience for safely driving a car you have gained from many years of driving.

NB Extremely challenging conditions, similar to those described above, also occur in several sports.

a) Footballers and field hockey players, attempting to dribble, weave and pass their way through a goalmouth area packed with moving opposition defenders. All of the players are constantly in motion, trying to score, prevent scoring, not break any rules, keep on their feet etc.

b) Rugby players are similar to football players, and many typical scenarios frequently occur within rugby matches.

c) In ice hockey matches, particularly in the area around the defenders' goal mouth.

CHAPTER 3.0 – HOW YOUR FIVE SENSES, M.C., B.H.S.M.S, THOUGHTS AND ALL OF YOUR BRAIN'S OTHER DEPARTMENTS CONTRIBUTE TO YOUR ONGOING DECISION MAKING AND ACTIONS EVERY SECOND OF EVERY DAY THROUGHOUT YOUR LIFE.

*OVERVIEW: In order for it to carry out its vital role within your brain, I believe that your Master Conductor is active at all times, through all states of your consciousness and your subconsciousness – **yes, your subconsciousness** – whilst you are **awake** and **asleep.** It will be at different levels of activity during sleep, dependent upon how much work it has to carry out in each moment.*

Your M.C. works tirelessly and incessantly within your mind in your brain, enabling you to carry out and satisfy all of your required Intellectual Objectives and Physical Functionalities to live the life you require and aspire to. It is functioning every second throughout the whole of particularly your waking lifetime. Whilst you are asleep, it plays a key role in re-ordering your brain's memories and status and also dealing with the prevailing emotionally stress-related difficulties and problems you have. Dreams play vitally important roles in helping you to de-stress and work towards resolving any issues.

I believe that your brain works tirelessly, throughout your life, trying to keep your physical, chemical and emotional health in the best of order. Its awesome functionality, effectiveness, accuracy and balanced control of all of its achievements are primarily due to its ongoing foundational functionality from which most of its other activities originate or relate. This is despite the frightening complexity it deals with and the vast number of activities occurring at the same time.

SUBCHAPTER 3.1: More details of the interaction between your M.C., five senses, B.H.S.M.S, thoughts and all of your brain's other departments concerning the ongoing creation of your consciousness and dealing with the information it presents to you.

The working relationship between your M.C., each of your five Senses, your Body's Health Status Monitoring System, your internally created thoughts and all of your brain's other departments, is **absolutely key** to how good or otherwise your life is. It needs to be ordered, enjoyable and satisfying, in terms of being kept safe and the degree to which you can approach achieving your maximum potential, and live your life to the full, within sensible and realistically achievable goals.

I believe that each of your brain's numerous, separate and independent departments are dedicated to their particular tasks. Some operate Fully Automatically under their own dedicated

Control System, and some operate Semi-Automatically in conjunction with your M.C. They all carry out their ongoing detailed second-by-second processing activities as their roles require. Some also respond to your M.C., which requests and receives their outputted processed data and seeks answers and guidance as appropriate to their dedicated and specific roles.

Under the management of your M.C. and the operation of their dedicated Control Systems, many departments have the ability, when they have the relevant data, to automatically adjust their process control functionality. Therefore, they can enhance their capability by learning from their experiences and improve their effectiveness at carrying out their dedicated role in looking after your ongoing needs.

Your Body's Health Status Monitoring System (B.H.S.M.S.) automatically detects whenever one or more of your organs, limbs, etc., has received an injury or developed an unhealthy condition that requires an appropriate corrective and/or protective response which it will immediately arrange. Your M.C. will instantly detect and recognise these conditions and their required and supporting responses from its knowledge derived from Learned Experiences, working them in with other prevailing considerations it may have to deal with.

I also believe that the other primary role that your B.H.S.M.S. carries out is to note whether your body develops any areas of infection, inflammation or diseases due to many causes. If this is the case, it sets out to tackle these states to eradicate them as soon as possible. Part of this eradication process may be that your M.C. notices the symptoms of the inflammation or disease and activates various actions to help effect a cure. This may involve arranging the basic measure of a visit to your doctor.

The other fundamental role for your B.H.S.M.S. is to note whether you are suffering from any mental illness condition and, if so, instigate the appropriate responses to deal with it.

SUBCHAPTER 3.1.1: The detailed, sequential functionality of the processing of your five senses, B.H.S.M.S. and your internal thoughts, when creating and updating your consciousness.

Please note that this section is vastly different from that described in subchapter 3.1 as it contains many more details. It describes the overall picture of how your consciousness is created and fits in generally with many other considerations.

Your five senses (sight, sound, smell, taste and touch) are independently receiving and immediately sending data into your brain continuously, throughout your life, whilst awake and asleep. During sleep, the frequency of data changing and conditions will normally be extremely minimal compared to whilst awake. Throughout your life, any data sent out from your B.H.S.M.S. and any existing internally generated thoughts will immediately be passed from within your brain, where they already exist, into one of the seven departments comprising your consciousness.

At this stage of this process, no understanding exists of what any of this data actually is and what it means to you.

A) *The first phase of this ongoing cycle of creating and updating your consciousness.*

a) Each data item from each source goes into a different and dedicated Category 1B Department as part of the analysis process which includes utilising your vast array of knowledge to commence understanding what they are and mean to you.

Each of these **separate processes of analysis** per item of data comprises a series of steps:

1) For each of your senses, there are **six separate process steps**. The first of which is to re-format the data into what I propose is a DNA-type of Analogue Format.

2) As your B.H.S.M.S. and existing thoughts are already stored within your brain, they are already in a DNA-type of Analogue Format, so they only pass through a **five separate step process,** the first of which is entering into their dedicated Category 1B department.

I proffer that this DNA-type of Analogue Format is the standard format that all data within your Brain is formatted in and remains in for all future processing.

3) The remaining process steps, when completed, culminate in you having established what they are and their meaning to you for each item of data.

B) The second phase of this cycle.

a) Each data item, its information, together with its meaning, is available for view and study by your M.C. in the appropriate dedicated Category 1B department.

b) Your M.C. studies the data with its innate and developed intelligence and can decide what data or datasets *in the context of your prevailing situation* present danger to you or, if not dangerous, require your consideration and resultant actions. All of this necessary data is sent to your Data Review Scanning System. It is identified in the category of 'danger' or 'requires attending to.'

   All other remaining data is deemed unimportant and is deleted by your M.C.

c) Thus far, you have established your updated consciousness, which is all of the data that requires processing and responding to nominally immediately, that has been sent to your Data Review Scanning System for review. This crucially enables these seven Category 1B Departments to be able to receive new incoming data.

C) The third and final phase of this cycle.

a) Your M.C. once again uses its inherent and developed intelligence to create the required and appropriate Thoughts of Consideration. It uses these to review anything in your Data Review Scanning System that indicates danger to you. In order of priority of importance, you can then consider what actions are necessary to deal with them individually or collectively, as appropriate.

b) Your M.C. then instigates each of the required actions to prevent or dispel each of the dangers. This could be, for example, by it sending instructions in software format to several of your Category 1B Developed, Semi-Automatic Skills Departments to operate walking, speaking, reading or fighting, or perhaps carrying out some more thinking and very many other possibilities.

c) Additionally, your M.C. will engage its inherent and developed Intelligence to address each of your Non Safety related issues and requirements, nonetheless important ones, whenever it has the time, in between keeping you safe mentally and physically. It will manage these by giving each one the appropriate Thoughts of Consideration it has created and issuing the fitting instructions to the relevant departments in your brain to achieve the related action/s it has decided are required.

NB Your five senses, B.H.S.M.S, internal thoughts, Data Review Scanning System, **is** continuously scanning around the complete set of analysed data that hasn't been processed yet, in the same order, one after the other every 1/1000 sec. Most crucially, immediately after an item of data has been successfully processed, it is deleted from the Data Review Scanning System, thus making more room/time for processing new data.

Via your Data Review Scanning System, your M.C. studies each of your items of analysed data. Its study time for each item of data which I call Dwell Time, is variable, over each 1/1000 second cycle from nominally 1% to 100% of the 1/000 sec. The Dwell Time is continually set to the requirements of your M.C. by a dedicated Category 1B Department. The time your M.C. spends reviewing each sense's data is depends on what importance your M.C. places upon that particular data and in proportion to the amount of other data that may require critical review in that **particular moment**.

Due to what I believe is your brain's first priority – to keep you safe at all times – even when you are asleep, your consciousness is still active and is constantly being updated with data from your Senses, your B.H.S.M.S. and your thoughts. This is simply to ensure that whilst asleep, any data you receive _at any time_, which may pose a danger to you internally or externally, is received by your brain as fast as possible to deal with as quickly as possible. The difference during sleep is that your vision will be zero and, during dreaming, your physical movement will be disabled to prevent you physically acting out your dreams and causing harm to yourself and your sleeping partner.

Whilst asleep, even with zero vision data, and far less changing data from all of your other senses, what data is being detected from them, your B.H.S.M.S. and any thoughts you have still go through the same processing system as A), B) & C) above, but take much less time to process than whilst awake.

I believe that, due to the extraordinary high speed of your responses and actions, they all occur below your conscious awareness, i.e. they are your **subconscious processing thoughts.** But nevertheless, your M.C. is involved with **managing the**

process to ensure you maintain an overall, balanced, controlled and safe status in absolutely the fastest possible time your brain and bodily functions are capable of achieving. Part of this process is to engage your Developed Semi-Automatic Skills and Actions as much as is appropriately possible. Another condition that helps achieve your brain's fastest possible processing speed is that four of your five senses' data input positions are located extremely close to your brain, thus the length of the data input transmitting circuits are extremely short. This reduces the transmission time for this data to begin to be processed by your brain to be the shortest possible. Your Touch Data is the one sense this doesn't apply to, except for the data transmission from your head and inside your mouth. This is of great potential benefit because you will respond extremely quickly to any threat to the safety of your brain.

Due to your extremely high Scan Rate per second, it **appears** that you are continually and consciously monitoring each of these items of data from your 5 Senses, B.H.S.M.S. and thoughts **at the same time**. However, I do not believe this to be the case, but rather that you are scanning around them one at a time, as I have detailed above. This method allows you to concentrate exclusively on each one as required.

Additionally, when you wish to focus intently upon only one item of data from **one** of these sets of data, I believe your M.C. can alter your prevailing senses/B.H.S.M.S./internal thoughts scanning dwell time. It stops this normal scanning routine and focuses primarily continuously, for nominally as long as it wishes, only upon the data that it has selected.

263

Crucially importantly though, in the interests of maintaining your safety, whilst your M.C. is continually focusing on one particular item of data, all of your other Category 1B Departments are continuing as normal, to study their sense's completed Analysed Data as B) b) above.

From their Memory Cells, if they note any conditions that pose a risk to your safety, they will immediately notify your M.C. It will instantly observe and assess the situation in conjunction with the other data it was currently focused on to decide which to prioritise. It may well choose to deal with each condition on a progressively alternating basis. Your M.C. has to consider any limitations within the <u>possible time boundaries imposed</u> by the initial prevailing conditions, their objectives and the <u>finite limiting</u> response and completion times of your different intended actions, which your M.C. has to accept, relate to and operate with.

I believe that these are some of the reasons why at these times, when your M.C. has to respond to your consciousness, the conditions of which are changing at a rapid rate and presenting it with partially conflicting objectives requiring extremely complex solutions or forced pragmatic solutions, you bump into something in front of you. For example, you might collide into a lamppost (but it could be anything physical) whilst walking along a very busy pavement. This is because you have been intently focused on another object which related to a particular prevailing priority objective for you, <u>within your field of view that also contained the lamppost.</u>

The operating reality of how your M.C. will actually manage all of your activities you are surrounded and affected by, hopefully achieving the expedient balancing of needs and priorities is, at times, highly complex and forever changing, the busier your activities, conditions and situations are. At times of significant complexity, your M.C. engages your Intelligence for assistance.

Above all else, your inbred priority is always keeping you safe. If you have completed all safety issues, have moved on to a non-safety issue, and your M.C. has noted a new safety issue has occurred, it will immediately stop attending to the non-safety issue and focus on the safety one.

Also, if you have dealt with half of **a)** issues and a new safety issue appears, which is of more consequence than those to be dealt with, you will prioritise processing the new one.

In reality, dependent upon what you are actually doing, you may prioritise stopping a goal being scored in a football match, despite having noted that in doing so, you are presenting a serious safety risk to yourself of perhaps a severe head injury.

Also, the usual sequence of events will be that, as your consciousness is updated with safety issues of major or minor importance, and with more or less important data, situations, or decisions to be made, your M.C. is attempting to conduct a masterful orchestration of the ever-changing conditions with which you are surrounded. It prioritises moving some actions along, then goes back to a previous activity and moves that along, balancing and sometimes cajoling extremely challenging and complex situations. Again, your M.C. will enlist the help of your (its) intelligence when required.

I believe that the potential confliction of priorities occasions relating to critical situations or significant danger to you, such as described above, is one of the times where *your perception of real-time appears to slow down.* In proportion to the importance to you of the prevailing conditions, I propose that the reason for this phenomenon is to give your M.C. significantly more time to review all of these prevailing **conditions** to make the best possible decisions and actions in response to each of them.

At times such as these, decisions of expediency and compromise may have to prevail. I have experienced conditions similar to these on many occasions whilst playing sport and participating in an extremely important competition, where you go into what is commonly called "the zone." You feel as if you have entered into another dimension when time appears to have significantly slowed down. It is an incredibly empowering, effective and out-of-body-type experience, during which time it enables you to totally focus and be emotionally detached from all around you. You feel you have more real/actual time to analyse the situation and make decisions whilst being completely aware of all that's around you. You feel confident and totally in control of it all, allowing you to achieve an unbelievable degree of physical and emotional sporting performance beyond what is normal to you.

I have spent a lot of time considering, testing and evaluating this extremely fundamental aspect of your data management functionality of external data from your senses and data from your internal sources, as detailed above. I was struggling to obtain strong confidence in finalising my thoughts until, one morning, I was casually looking out over the side of our docked Fred Olsen Cruise Ship at one of the mooring posts it was docked to. The usual, continuous, fairly loud exhaust sound of one of its diesel-powered electrical generator engines could be heard, continually imposing itself on my conscious senses. Suddenly, I found myself *focused extremely intently* upon a particular unusual detail on this mooring post. At the end of this very short period of time, around three or four seconds, I realised, with great clarity of realisation, understanding and confidence, that **I had not heard/ been aware of this engine's noise at all**.

Understanding the significance to me of this experience, I instinctively shouted out, "That's it! I have got it" to the puzzlement of my wife and all others in the vicinity.

It was the classic "eureka moment," to me anyway.

I have since had this type of experience repeated with different situations whilst driving a car with passengers.

Since this **unplanned experience** and many others, I have found that if you **deliberately** carry out this experiment/ simulation, you **don't quite** experience and can't quite grasp this very fleeting condition quite as clearly and definably as when it has **occurred naturally.** As in my case, you also need to be primed to review what you have just experienced to notice, appreciate and understand what has just happened. This topic and experiences takes us nicely into the next subchapter.

SUBCHAPTER 3.1.2: More details about the operation and functionality of your Data Review Scanning System from which your M.C. reviews each of your data items as part of the process of creating, updating and acting upon the requirements of your consciousness.

OVERVIEW: Because this process is one of the most foundationally important operational features throughout the whole of your brain's functionality, I felt at this stage, it warranted an overview to add to the information already presented. Hopefully, this will provide complete clarity of understanding of how and why it all functions as I believe it does. The principles of which are:

SUBCHAPTER EXTRA 3.1.2 a), b), c), d) & NB

a) I believe that your Data Review Scanning System, which allows your M.C. to study each item of data coming into your brain from outside it and also data already within your brain, operates continuously throughout your lifetime.

b) It operates extremely fast, completing one scan cycle around all of your different items of data **every 1ms, thus completing 1000 scan cycles every second**. This means that during the **total cycle time of 4ms,** in which the complete Cycle of the Creation, Updating and acting upon the requirements of your consciousness has occurred, your Data Review Scanning System will have carried out four complete cycles.

c) I believe that each different item of data will each have its own nominal value of Data Review Time required by your M.C. during each <u>unique</u> Data Review Scanning Cycle. These are as indicated in the examples below and are expressed as a percentage of the 1ms scan cycle time.

d) <u>The hugely beneficial aspect of this arrangement of functionality is that</u> the completion of the processing of any particular item of data may take longer than, let's say one Scan Cycle, i.e. 1ms, or say 15ms or even more, due to any number of reasons. For example, you are struggling to find a match-up of an incoming data's information profile to any stored anywhere in your memories, so you are unable at this stage to recognise it and therefore understand its meaning. This hopefully does not matter! Your M.C. would then move on to reviewing the next item of data.

If the delay is connected to data dealing with your safety, the resolution of which is to be as soon as possible, then any time delay could matter and your M.C. would perhaps have to make a judgement of expediency.

NB If any one or more of your senses' dedicated Category 1B Departments, which carry out a **separate process of analysis** of each set of data to understand its meaning, detect any danger to yourself, they will instantly notify your M.C of the threat. It will, as a priority, immediately take the appropriate actions to keep you safe.

SUBCHAPTER A) *How I arrived at estimating the speed of operation of your Brain's Data Review Scanning System.*

OVERVIEW: *The more I have thought about the processing speed of operation of your brain, in terms of its outputs, i.e. what it achieves over an incredibly short time, the more I stand in absolute awe of how fast its processing speeds actually are. Playing all of the sports that I have done really gives me a pretty accurate feel and judgement of how fast it actually has to be for your mind to achieve all of its decision-making and your body to accomplish all of its movements in the extremely short period it does.*

With these prior thoughts in mind, please read the following account of a related experience I had, and I hope you don't think I am some sort of "quack."

During some Reiki exercises, which I once tried for a period when at home with some serious eye problems, I lay on my back with *my eyes closed.* I attempted to acquire a mental and physical state of total physical relaxation and to <u>approach</u> an emotional state of no conscious thoughts.

After a while and approaching the boundary of achieving this state, I noticed that my brain did not **feel** in a less active state than normal, despite nominally having very few conscious thoughts over 20 minutes. This is very difficult to describe, but my brain felt very much alive, in a vibrational, very high frequency, constant and steady functioning state. It had an extremely low, almost inaudible sound level, having a frequency compared to the C note on our piano, 3 octaves higher than middle C, which puts the frequency of this sound at 1000Hz., i.e. cycling one thousand times per second.

I reflected upon this experience, which was the first time I have ever been aware of this phenomenon and which I had not heard of before. I have since found it is a permanent state for me whenever I sense for it with my eyes closed with no/minimal thoughts.

I propose that it could be the sound caused by my brain's Data Scanning System as it permanently scans around each of my five senses, my B.H.S.M.S. and my internal thoughts, one at a time, for my M.C. to view and consider the data they are each receiving.

It will be very interesting to see what responses these thoughts have from readers of my book and those studying the functionality of your brain system.

Even if it is not concluded to be the sound I propose and is just your background environment noise, it does not change my other proposals about the functionality of your Data, B.H.S.M.S. and Internal Thoughts Scanning System and their processing speeds being in the order of cycling every 1/1000 of a sec. This is simply because of the sheer amount of data processing work that your brain carries out. This starts from the moment it receives all of this input data, through analysing it all, to considering and concluding decisions to it all and instigating and achieving all of your related actions in such an incredibly short time later.

In addition to all of this activity, there are all of the other incredible data processing workloads it also manages constantly. Having 1000 processing cycles every second is the required

271

order of performance for most other operating processes within your brain simply to be able to achieve all that I think it most certainly does achieve.

NB The possible reasons for this "sound of functionality"

Since I first wrote the passages above, I came to re-read, review and update my entire book from start to finish a few months before it was completed. During this latest review I sat and thought for a few minutes – how on earth and why on earth would the *processing functionality of your brain* **create a sound**? I had a flash train of hopefully correct or at least worthwhile considering, inspirational thoughts, which were:

a) Your brain, with its unquestionable mind-numbing functionality and processing performance, would not create something without a useful purpose.

b) I firmly believe that your ongoing consciousness is the foundation upon which all of your deliberations and related actions emanate from.

c) I think that each of your brain's different processing activities will operate at nominally the same processing speed so that there prevails an inherent natural efficiency of communication. The product of the fastest speed of communication between each of these processes results in the vitally important aspect of achieving the quickest completion of all considerations and each resultant action, keeping you safe at all times and also making the best decisions and actions for you.

d) This vibrational sound condition may be the foundational, underlying processing base or timing clock upon which each of your brain's different processing systems function. This will inherently impose an overall control, balance and symmetry throughout the whole of your brain's immense processing activities during every second of your lifetime. It will impose a reference point for all processing functionality, continuously. It will naturally, simply and easily impose order and status of functional calm over what could easily be, at times, a degree of chaos over your brain's immense processing workload. This is particularly the case when many different departments are busy processing their duties at the same time, combined with a high level of intercommunications prevailing.

e) This condition of very low energy, high frequency with a very small amount of movement, may well have additional benefits of creating a cleansing of your brain's physical structures. It also encourages and allows your brain tissues to keep in a physically and functionally healthy state whilst enjoying a long life in order to satisfy your life spans' requirements.

SUBCHAPTER B) *The extreme importance of your sense of vision.*

Your vision is by far the most detailed, data-devouring data item compared to the others. This is due to all of the colours, their vast number of shades and the extensive amount of other high-density details that can be contained within what your eyes can see. But, I believe that your brain optimises the required quantity of vision data that goes into your brain by controlling how much detail your eyes are actually seeing. You decide, <u>in the moment,</u> what is important to you and, therefore, how much detail you allow to pass into your brain. If you feel there is no need for any Vision data *for a particular period of time,* **you will close your eyes,** for example, whilst processing a thought. <u>During this time, you will have zero vision data entering your brain and have a Vision Review Time set at nominally 1%.</u> This will free up a lot more review time per scan for other data.

As in most times, **when you have your eyes open,** and you decide that you have no prevailing need to look out for some particular vision data, you will be slowly scanning around with your eyes and idly taking in a minimal density of vision data detail. <u>During this time, you will have a low quantity of vision data entering your brain and have a Vision Review Time set at nominally 5%.</u> Again, this will make a lot more review time per scan available for other data deemed more important.

In most cases, **when you have your eyes open,** if **you** have a specific need to look out for some particular person, thing or situation within your vicinity, you will be intently studying every little visionary detail in a relatively small area of view, as your eyes slowly scan around, devouring everything in sight. <u>During this time, you will have an extremely high density/ high quantity of vision data entering your brain and have a Vision Review Time set at nominally around as high as 60%.</u>

However, this depends upon the environment you were in and the consequential importance of other data entering your brain during this time, as always with particular reference to the priority of keeping you safe.

This range of different situations, reasons and the required density, amount of data required and variability of the settings of your Data Review Time described above for your vision, at all times, applies for each of your senses, your B.H.S.M.S and your internal thoughts.

The **time settings** of your **Data Review Time** are extremely flexible and are always liable to change from moment to moment. They could change from a large percentage down to a much smaller percentage of time value, or vice versa. These changes are always driven by your M.C. to suit its Data Information knowledge requirements in each moment. This is always in relation to fully satisfying the prevailing requirements of your consciousness in terms of your M.C. having sufficient time to evaluate each item of data and then having adequate time to consider the required actions to keep you safe. It then attends to the other important decisions and actions you should take as driven by your prevailing consciousness.

NB I propose that, during times of absolute <u>maximum Emotional and Data assessing frequency and intensity</u>, when the data coming into your brain *is at the highest speed possible, with immense and immediate danger to yourself, your Dwell Time arrangements will be fundamentally altered, but only for the period described.* During these times, each scan cycle will not scan all categories of data but will focus on the categories of the highest worth concerning the prevailing extreme situation.

Real-world examples of how you <u>utilise, review and act upon</u> the incoming data from your senses and the data from within your brain in the most optimum, efficient and effective manner in relation to your surroundings and prevailing objectives.

Example 1 – Shopping in a very busy high street.

The scene: Whilst walking along the *pavement* of an extremely *busy and unfamiliar high street shopping area,* you have the usual shoppers, pedestrians, children, dogs, cars, lorries, buses and bicycles etc., to be aware of and take the appropriate actions in respect to all of the activities within your vicinity of passage. In addition to your shopping requirements, your additional prevailing objectives are, at all times, **to proceed with sufficient safety and care for yourself and for all others you encounter within your zone of activity.**

The data from your senses, B.H.S.M.S. and any internally generated thoughts you may have are all being scanned by each Data Review Scanning Cycle, taking 1ms to complete. During this time, your M.C. is reviewing all the data.

In order to deal with and satisfy the above conditions and objectives, I believe that your M.C. arranges for:

Your sight to occupy approx. 60% of your M.C.'s review time per Data Scanning Cycle.

Your sound to occupy approx. 30% of your M.C.'s review time per Data Scanning Cycle.

Your internally generated thoughts (which will normally be a small number and at times zero) to occupy approx. 5% of your M.C.'s review time per Data Scanning Cycle.

The remaining data from your B.H.S.M.S, smell, taste & touch senses share equally over the period of approx. 5% of your M.C's review time per Data Scanning Cycle.

This equates per scan, per set of your data with your:

Sight being reviewed <u>continuously</u> for 0.6ms during each scan cycle.

Sound being reviewed <u>continuously</u> for 0.3ms during each scan cycle.

Internally generated thoughts being processed <u>continuously</u> for 0.05ms during each scan cycle.

The remaining Data from your B.H.S.M.S., smell, taste & touch share equally and over the period of approx. 0.05ms during each scan cycle.

NB The times spent observing the data flooding into your brain from each category of data are proportionate to the **quantity** and **importance** of the type of data relating to the conditions and your prevailing objectives. Therefore, the Dwell Time figures above are very nominal. They will change when your M.C. requires longer, Focused Intent dwelling on some of your senses requiring different dwell times from those indicated above. This will be to study with a particular focus what is the key data you

277

require at that moment about what is happening around you, within your zone of activity which affects your safety.

Hopefully, you will not miss any important data coming in and will carry out sufficient data assessment consideration time to make the correct related thoughts and decisions in every moment such that you will satisfy all of your objectives at all times, whilst in this general shopping environment.

NB For those who are not used to "feeling" or being aware of how long one millisecond (1ms) is, the time it takes to blink your eyes from open to close to open is approximately 300ms. In other words, I believe that the **set of review actions** detailed above are taking place incredibly fast at 1000 times every second.

This means that during the time it takes to complete one blink of your eye, all the data coming in from your senses and from within your brain will have been scanned 300 times.

This mind-blowing speed of just one part of your brain's functionality is why so much of your brain's activity, with which your M.C. is involved, occurs well below the awareness of your conscious mind. You just experience it and accept it without really being aware of it. It also gives an appreciation of the spell-binding speed of the functionality that your brain processes information, considers information, arrives at decisions and instigates resultant actions. Whilst this process is taking place, many, many other parts of your brain are in true parallel operation also carrying out their own processing activities simultaneously.

Example 2 – Participating in a very busy meeting

How you utilise, review <u>and act upon</u> the incoming data from your senses and the data from within your brain in the most optimum, efficient and effective manner concerning the discussions and presentation of data taking place within your surroundings whilst at work and about your objectives during a meeting in the real world.

The scene: You are the Chairman of a very important meeting at work, in which 25 people are present in the same room. Some have come from other companies, and all of them have various interests in the meeting's agenda, which all attendees have been provided with an advanced copy of. In addition to your ensuring that the agenda is adhered to throughout the meeting, with a little pragmatic tolerance, your additional prevailing objectives, are to clearly see, hear and understand all information that each person is providing through speech, visual and audio means. This is all achieved by the data from each of your senses, your B.H.S.M.S. and any internally generated thoughts being scanned by each Data Scanning Cycle, taking 1ms to complete. During this time, your M.C. is reviewing all the data.

It is vitally important to understand that your M.C. uses its inherent intelligence to **create the Thoughts of Consideration** to review all *remaining data that has completed its analysis process*, solve any safety issues and also process any non-safety requirements. It carries out this work during the second phase of updating your consciousness. The time required for this is not required as part of your Data Review Scanning cycle.

279

In order to deal with and satisfy the above conditions and objectives, I believe that your M.C. arranges for:

Your Sight to occupy approx. 45% of your M.C.'s review time per Data Review Scanning Cycle.

Your Sound to occupy approx. 45% of your M.C.'s review time per Data Review Scanning Cycle.

Your internally generated thoughts (which will normally be a small number and at times zero) to occupy approx. 5% of your M.C.'s review time per Data Review Scanning Cycle and:

The remaining data from your B.H.S.M.S., Smell, Taste & Touch shares equally approx. 5% of your M.C.'s review time per Data Review Scanning Cycle.

This equates per scan, per set of your data with your:

Sight being reviewed <u>continuously</u> for 0.45ms during each scanning cycle.

Sound being reviewed <u>continuously</u> for 0.45ms during each scanning cycle.

Thoughts being reviewed <u>continuously</u> for 0.05ms during each scanning cycle

Smell, Taste, Touch and B.H.S.M.S. <u>each</u> being reviewed <u>continuously</u> and equally over the period of 0.05ms during each scan cycle.

These times spent observing the data flooding into your brain from each of your senses are proportionate to the **quantity** and **importance** of data of each sense concerning the prevailing conditions and your prevailing and longer-term objectives.

Hopefully, you will not miss any important data coming in and will carry out sufficient data assessment consideration time to make the correct related decisions in every moment to satisfy all of your objectives whilst in this meeting scenario.

These figures are very nominal and will change because, at times, your M.C. will dwell longer and with Focused Intent on some of your senses, requiring different dwell times from those indicated above. This will be to study with a particular focus the key data you require at that moment. This relates to who is speaking, what they are saying, their body and facial language, the importance of the topic they are talking about, the current and future observations and decisions you wish to develop, and the objectives you want to achieve in this meeting.

SUBCHAPTER 3.1.3: General aspects and relationships of your M.C., with your five senses, internal thoughts, B.H.S.M.S. and all of your brain's other different and fundamentally independent departments carrying out their designated roles.

Real-life examples of some of the interactions and operations taking place between your mind, body and senses, your B.H.S.M.S and some of your brain's other departments.

Example 1 – You are playing in a very important football match.

Your side is drawing, with five minutes left to play, and you are in the process of preparing to kick the football into the goal.

The ball is coming towards you in the air at shoulder height in a curving and dipping trajectory. It is also spinning during its flight, whilst you are struggling to maintain your balance and footing due to a slippery pitch and dealing with a strong gusty wind.

As you adjust your balance, your brain gives your left knee an extremely sharp stabbing pain, warning you to take some weight off your chronic injury. You do this immediately as an involuntary health safety response and make other compensating movements to re-establish your balance.

The combinational effect of all of these prevailing conditions, from when the ball was passed towards you to when the situation ended, required you to:

- Make continual adjustments to the whole of your body, arms, legs, your balance, your feet and toes, plus much more.
- Deal with the additional physical challenges and distractions of defenders trying to prevent you from kicking the ball hard, cleanly and effectively.

But despite the combination of all of these conditions and challenges you encountered, you scored a match-winning goal.

The very many reasons why you successfully overcame this extremely challenging situation was the result of you:

a) Having practised the extremely complex set of skills required to execute the above activity successfully, many thousands of times over many years. Therefore, you had developed the required physical fitness and physical capability, confidence and the resultant set of very many Developed, Semi-Automatic Skills required to succeed as above.

b) The resultant success was only made possible because your M.C. continually observed all of the data coming into your brain with information from your senses. It made you aware of the **unique details of the prevailing conditions** in which these skill sets were being applied and completed the **necessary fine-tuning and adjustments** to deal with the wind, slippery conditions, curving dipping ball, bright, dazzling sunshine, etc.

Despite the fact that you were engaging a lot of your vast library of Developed Semi-Automatic Skills, each time that you utilise a skill, during which your Brain is operating at an incredible speed of estimating the ball speed, trajectory, the closing time to arrive at a point where your feet need to be etc. Your M.C. is noting the actual prevailing conditions around, relating to and affecting the basic functionality of your Developed Semi-Automatic Skills. It continually makes fine adjustments to most of your body parts and balance in order to compensate for all of the prevailing, objective offsetting factors.

c) You brain's internal thoughts and objectives of being on guard from the knowledge you have about the opposition's centre back who will dangerously foul you just outside the penalty box if you are threatening to score a goal. Also, your internal thought about not attempting to score with your left foot is that your left Achilles tendon is very sore and is threatening to tear.

Also, just as you were about to kick the ball into the net just inside the near post, the goalkeeper moved to his right, leaning towards his near post and had nearly all of his weight leaning on his right foot. This forced your M.C., within the last half-second before shooting at goal, to change its goal mouth scoring target. This necessitated an awful lot of changes to your body positions with each of your limbs, waist, feet, toes, knee joints. Your M.C. issued probably hundreds of different instructions or adjustments to 100 of your Developed Semi-Automatic Skills to operate with directional targets, speed targets, power targets, turning, twisting, stretching and weight adjustment targets as you successfully executed your shot at goal.

NB During such an activity described above, the incredible speed and amount of calculations, assessments, decisions and actions triggered by your Developed Semi-Automatic Skills, overall managed and fine-tuned/adjusted by your M.C. is utterly astounding. All of these activities culminate with your basic body, many of your body parts and the related messages flying around a vast number of departments of your whole brain. The coordination and control of a phenomenal number of your muscles, plus the lightning speed of the processing functionality of your Developed Semi-Automatic Skills, managed and fine-tuned by your M.C., ably assisted by your intelligence's crucial contribution in updating your consciousness, are all taking place continually in each part of the blink of an eye.

All of these activities occur so fast you are not consciously aware of around 96% of them, so you feel that they all occur outside your control and are solely due to your Developed Semi-Automatic Skills. **I very firmly believe that this is not the case, as described in detail previously in the book.**

Every time the above basic skill or routine occurs in a football match, played by the same footballer, their highly practised and perfected routines are engaged and utilised. If they executed the above skills a total of 1000 times, each time, all of the many prevailing conditions that affect the ball's trajectory, the footballer's balance, the exact details of the defenders' positions and movements etc., would all combine dynamically to create a set of totally unique conditions.

I think it is worthwhile encapsulating the above in a slightly different way:

It is only due to the combined skills, knowledge and capabilities of your M.C. and intelligence that all the data coming into and from within your brain is scanned and responded to 250 times per second. Couple this with the complex achievements of very many of your different Departments, all functioning in parallel operation, and it results in a successful outcome being achieved, despite the extremely challenging conditions and required objective.

Example 2 – You have been carrying out a regular activity or process of car driving when you suddenly realise that you have not been consciously aware of the process conditions for a significant period of time.

You have been driving along a route that you know really well and have been heavily engrossed in deep thoughts about something that had been bothering you. Suddenly, before you were consciously fully aware of it, a car travelling at speed shot out of a side road in front of you. This forced you to execute emergency braking whilst executing evasive manoeuvring to avoid a child on a bicycle and an on-coming car, all of which you carry out successfully.

You realise that all of these aversion activities appear to have occurred in an extremely short period of time, apparently without your consciousness being involved. You also recognise that you have travelled some miles but can't recall any details on the route and feel a very strong sense of relief and luck that you have not had an accident. You then think, how have I managed to achieve all of this?

Driving like this is certainly not to be advised, but you will have handled the situation driving hopefully safely, on **autopilot,** by managing the traffic and all road safety-related occurrences and conditions around you. You will have noted the relevant incoming data presented to your M.C. by your senses which will have been used to update your consciousness continually. Your M.C. will then have responded, making the appropriate decisions and taking the related actions to keep you and other road users safe.

Your M.C will have also been employing many of your Developed Semi-Automatic car manoeuvring and decision-making skills developed and fine-tuned from all of your car driving experiences to date.

Prior to the potentially dangerous incident occurring, you will have dealt with fairly stable, orderly and comfortably predictable road conditions. Then, one or more of your senses, in this case your sight, plus possibly your hearing, will have detected a danger to yourself. Automatically, in their fastest possible response time, they will have alerted your M.C. of the threat. It will have triggered the range of appropriate Developed Semi-Automatic Skills, all executed in the shortest possible time and all appearing to be, but not actually being the case, without your M.C.'s involvement. Your M.C. will have taken other additional and related supportive actions as required.

NB The phrase used for driving your car, on "autopilot," is in no way the same or the equivalent facility, quality or capability as the increasingly frequently touted man-made autopiloted self-driving systems for driving cars and other vehicles.

CHAPTER 4.0 – WHAT DOES YOUR BRAIN ACTUALLY DO, SECOND-BY-SECOND, HOUR-BY-HOUR, DAY-BY-DAY, WHEN YOU ARE AWAKE AND ASLEEP, WHILST YOU ARE CARRYING OUT A HUGE VARIETY OF POSSIBLE ACTIVITIES?

Illustrations of how busy you and your brain could be cover an *extensive* range of possible activities, across a *vast spectrum* of busyness.

Example 1 – You are fully awake whilst alone sitting in your favourite chair, mulling over your life to date.

The scene: You are sitting in your favourite chair in your favourite room at home, alone, with absolute peace and quiet. You have your eyes closed most of the time, just letting your mind wander around the many years of the wonders of your life to date, from early childhood to today, your 65th birthday.

In this situation, the data coming in and the change of data coming in from:

a)   Each of your senses would be absolutely minimal.

b)   Your B.H.S.M.S. would probably be minimal to zero.

c) Your internally-instigated daydreaming thoughts would be relatively very busy.

You would probably have no safety concerns to attend to and maybe some very occasional remaining issues to decide on and take related actions.

Your ongoing consciousness creation, the ongoing updating and instigating actions from the data status of your consciousness would be updated with the same overall processing cycle time of 4ms, meaning it will repeat 250 times every second.

There is a significant reduction in the quantity of data that:

d) Requires evaluating

e) Requires deleting

f) Requires processing

g) Requires thought consideration

h) Requires any instigating actions.

Due to the change of details in **a)** to **h)**, with each of them lacking relative difficulty, complexity or urgency, the consequences are that your brain would be operating in **the lowest range of its overall Data Processing busyness.** This covers Quantity, Density, Speed, Urgency, Resultant Safety, Complexity, Difficulty and Range of Actions.

Example 2 – Playing mixed doubles badminton.

The scene: You are playing at, say, county-level standard in an extremely hard-fought, evenly matched game, which both pairs of players are extremely keen to win. The four players' ongoing consciousnesses are being updated at breakneck speed. Their senses are flooding into their brains, near their limit of its perception at times, as the shuttlecock is hit at breakneck speed around the court with cross-court shots, smashes, full-length shots and very slow, delicate net drop shots. At all times, each pair of players are making lightning-fast decisions based on their internal thoughts about if they should make their next return shot or whether it is better for their partner to play it.

Sometimes, this decision is aided by one or other of the partnership saying 'yours' or 'mine' and occasionally from what appears to be a telepathic link between them. I don't believe that telepathy is prevailing. Instead, this is due to their experience as players, particularly as partners. They are responding to situations very similar to what they have experienced many times previously. They are repeating the same decision, which probably is partly due to the bodyweight position, balance and indicators of who will play the shot.

Their vision, hearing and touch senses are all working in overdrive as they each track the speeding shuttle. They are estimating where it will go, plus where to hit it so their opponents will struggle to return it, and thus they begin to get control of that rally. They also continually note where their opponents are and predict where they will be in the next second, therefore knowing where best to hit the shuttle, so hopefully their opponents can't return it and they win that point.

This is an extremely challenging, almost non-stop, high-speed, high adrenalin sporting situation. A crucially important part of every player's decision-making logic includes the strengths and weaknesses of their partner and opponents relating to the prevailing situation at each moment. This crucially important data is processed by their internally generated thoughts. There is very little time between the completion of each point played for and the start of the next, culminating in the players having to perform at an incredibly fast physical and mental pace with almost no time to have a breather between points.

Each pair of players employs very intricate, interwoven and complex sets of thoughts, from which are created decisions and related actions and movements. In response to each player's prevailing consciousness and its many requirements, the total number of thoughts created and concluded, resultant decisions and actions, allied to the frighteningly complex type and number of physical movements processed nearly every second, is extraordinarily high.

Despite all these quite extreme challenges, most of the time, they can avoid physically clashing with their partner. They are able to reach the shuttle with good control and return it over the net with interest, hoping to win that rally. All these strategies are achieved 99% of the time by each couple without physically impeding their partner to any significant degree.

In order to achieve the <u>physical</u>, <u>athletic</u> and <u>mental</u> level of skill and <u>emotional performance</u> displayed by these sportspersons, they have to be:

a)   Superbly physically strong, fit and have plenty of physical stamina.

b) Superbly mentally and emotionally fit and determined, with plenty of emotional stamina and intent focus.

c) They also have to have practised for thousands of hours to develop their range of Category 1B departments, highly-developed Semi-Automatic skills which they employ to hit a large range of different types of shots. A part of these skills includes the intricate all-embracing body positions they have to adopt to play these shots.

d) They have to employ many of their Category 1B department's highly-developed Semi-Automatic skills for carrying out the mental calculations and predictions, plus the physical movements and decision-making as detailed above.

e) Their brain has to process the phenomenal amount of changing data continually flooding into it, primarily via their vision, hearing and touch (of their hands and feet). Their M.C. controls this, ably supported by their intelligence, masterminding and responding to the constant updating of their consciousness.

In addition to responding to their consciousness is their attention to their own ongoing safety. This is necessary to avoid dangerous collisions with their partner, prevent being blinded by the shuttle or being seriously injured by being hit by their partner's racket head.

f) Under extreme game pressures and despite tiredness at times, they have to keep a clear mind and maintain a game strategy with the confidence of believing they can eventually win, thus creating the all-powerful benefit of their placebo effect.

The consequences of all of the details and activities described above of each player's physical and mental activities would be that their brains would be operating at the **highest level of its overall Data Processing busyness**. This covers Quantity, Density, Speed, Urgency, Resultant Safety, Complexity, Difficulty and Range of Activities.

Example 3 – When the extreme importance of the ultra-rapid processing of your consciousness and your resultant actions are of life-threatening consequences whilst on patrol in enemy territory.

This is an extreme example of when, in response to all of the data entering and already within your brain, and the ultra-rapid processing of it, necessary to update your consciousness from which your decision-making and resultant actions are produced, the importance of accurate receipt literally has *life-threatening consequences*.

OVERVIEW: *You are a soldier, travelling on foot, on the frontline in a country where you and your squad of colleagues are outside the safety of your barracks. You are amongst the natural terrain of your camouflaged and hidden enemies, who are out to kill you, at any second, with concealed explosives, live rounds from all types of weaponry and small bomb-dropping drones.*

294

You are extremely hot and uncomfortable having been out continuously on active patrol for 6 hours with the occasional 5-minute rest, in temperatures of 45°C.

Your consciousness is being updated by your brain at the absolute maximum limit possible of its processing speed and response to incoming conditions. It is working at its absolute, 100% focussed maximum effectiveness within your mind, primarily to keep you safe and alive and, in the process, to attempt to capture, if possible, as many of your enemies that you encounter.

During all of this time, your senses will be straining and stretched to their absolute limit to collect all of the relevant data available to keep you safe. Your M.C. will be striving to process and understand it all by dealing with each of your prevailing thoughts with as much accuracy of reception, understanding and speed as possible.

This is all to update your consciousness immediately with any *new or changing incoming data*, supporting the objectives of your mind and, at all times, to end up making the correct decisions based on the meaning of all the data you are presented with from your updated consciousness.

Also relevant to your situation is that this group of enemies are believed to be holed up in a village and its outlying ditches and ravines. They are believed to be responsible for killing a squad of your comrades the previous month.

Because of the nature of your surroundings, the vast majority of the data coming into your brain will be immediately related or potentially related to your safety. Despite this fact, your

Observations, Thoughts, Decisions and Actions will primarily be unchanged and repeated. This is because the ***rate of change*** of this *safety-related data* coming in from your senses and being processed and understood by your M.C. is extremely slow 95% of the time.

In other words, this data <u>ostensibly remains unchanged</u>. Your vision sees the same detailed views of the landscape, including your immediate locality, down to the soldiers around you, and your hearing hears the same noises – or lack of them. You experience the same smells; your touch experiences the same occasional wisps of breeze and the constant weight of your high-powered rapid-firing submachine gun. Your touch sense notes each footstep as you carefully feel your way along the ground to avoid losing your balance or footing and creating unwanted noises.

Despite this period of slow change of incoming data, your senses will be strained to their utmost to detect any item of information that it is imperative they do not miss. These could be numerous:

The flash of part of a person moving ahead of them, the glint of sunlight from the muzzle of a gun.

The sudden, short sound of a flutter of alighting birds as they are disturbed by a potential enemy who could be your enemy.

The very short-lived smell of the strong spices from the favourite food that your enemies have eaten, born on the wind travelling down to you.

The fleetingly short-lived, muffled voice of a potential enemy – anything that gives you as much warning as possible to be pre-

prepared to take the required actions to fulfil your objectives, the moment in time when you have to take immediate and vitally appropriate actions.

Due to the extremes of the situation and the prevailing environment, your thoughts will be processing all relevant information presented by your consciousness. You will also be desperately trying to **predict** anything that may happen suddenly **before** it happens, which presents a danger to your life. This will enable you to take action to protect your life a few milliseconds sooner and hopefully keep you alive.

BUT – what your M.C. is waiting and waiting and waiting for is to observe a CHANGE of safety-related data or new safety-related data. This change could be gradual, like an enemy slowly coming into view and is almost within range of your fire. You respond very slowly, signalling to your comrades what you have seen. You all gradually make the appropriate changes to prepare for shooting at your enemy, or taking cover from being shot at, etc.

Or – your incoming data suddenly *changes in an instant.* Six of your enemy unexpectedly appear from behind a wall ahead of you, firing a maelstrom of bullets at you all, with three of your comrades falling immediately around you.

Your consciousness, mind and M.C. instantly burst into a frenzy of instinctive, practised and self-preservation **actions from your many Semi-Automatic Category 1B departments.** They are desperately attempting to take the most appropriate thoughts, decisions and actions, as soon as possible, to save your life and that of your comrades.

The number of decisions and actions taken during this period of time will be of the utmost possibly achievable by your M.C. and your mind. Nearly all of these decisions and actions will be deeply below your conscious awareness, due to the speed they are made at. Despite all of this, your M.C. will be organising and approving all of them so that they are safely and effectively coordinated, dynamically compatible, and, hopefully, none of them will compromise your safety or the safety of others.

NB As normal, the actual percentage of Data Scan time for your M.C. to dwell on and assess your senses and thoughts will depend on what data your M.C. currently requires and what level of priority of importance prevails for each of them.

During times of _minimum_ Emotional and Data assessing intensity, when the data coming into your brain **is very slow changing with no immediate danger attached,** I believe the following applies:

a)   The percentage of Data Scan Time for your Vision will be nominally 30%.

b)   The percentage of Data Scan Time for your Hearing will be nominally 25%.

c)   The percentage of Data Scan Time for your Smell will be nominally 20%.

d)   The percentage of Data Scan Time for your Touch will be nominally 20%.

e) The percentage of Data Scan Time for your Taste, internal thoughts, and B.H.S.M.S. will be nominally 5% shared equally amongst each of them.

During times of _maximum_ Emotional and Data assessing frequency and intensity, i.e. when the data entering your brain **is changing at the highest speed possible, with immense and immediate danger perceived via your Vision and Hearing,** *I propose the changed Dwell Time arrangement is:*

a) For the ***First Data Scan time***, the percentage of Scan Time for your Vision will be 80%.

b) For the ***First Data Scan time***, the percentage of Scan Time for your Touch will be 20%.

c) For the ***Second Data Scan time***, the percentage of Scan Time for your Hearing will be 80%.

d) For the ***Second Data Scan time***, the percentage of Scan Time for your Touch will be 20%.

e) For the ***Third Data Scan time***, it will be a repeat of **a)** and **b)** above.

f) For the ***Fourth Data Scan time***, it will be a repeat of **c)** and **d)** above.

NB During this modification of your percentage of Data Scan time, the Incoming Data entering the relevant Category 1B Consciousness Department set will recognise any incoming data from your Taste, Smell, B.H.S.M.S. and internal thoughts that represents a danger to you. That department will immediately inform your M.C. of this, so it will access the data and take the appropriate actions. This routine will continue until this level of danger has been dealt with or subsided.

As you make your way along this track, you will be scanning ahead and around you, including behind, as best as you can. With the utmost focused assessment, you take note of everything you can see in a *general state of detail,* seeking and searching for any visual information which critically relates to your safety and situation. You are desperately attempting to spot some potentially dangerous aspect a split second *before* it becomes a danger so that you can eliminate or at least reduce the level of threat and gain the upper hand upon the proceedings.

If your M.C. suddenly spots a visionary aspect that requires more detail, it will immediately home in on that particular part of the general view it previously assessed to garner more detailed information. It will then make a judgement of whether you need to take some action towards, for example, what you think is a sniper's telescopic sight targeting you or your partner to your side.

Whilst you are carefully making your way, you hear with the same intensity as you see. Both senses are placed on the highest of alerts, hearing and assessing all of the different sounds coming from everything around you, including behind, as best as you can achieve this. Again, as with your vision, if you judge that one particular sound from a specific area requires more understanding, you will focus on this to gather more detail. Then you can make a more detailed and hopefully better-informed judgement about it from which to decide what, if anything, to do.

The consequences would be different for both periods of time:

a) <u>Before</u> the sudden burst of enemy action:

Your brain would be operating in the <u>lowest Range level</u> of its overall Data Processing for Quantity, Density, Speed, Urgency, Resultant Safety, Complexity, Difficulty and Activity.

b) <u>During</u> the <u>burst of enemy action:</u>

Your brain would be operating at the <u>highest Range level</u> of its overall Data Processing of Quantity, Density, Speed, Urgency, Resultant Safety, Complexity, Difficulty and Activity.

SUBCHAPTER 4.1: Your brain's fundamental activities whilst awake and asleep

This section covers a complete, normal, basic list of what I believe are all of your brain's fundamental, ongoing activities whilst you are awake and asleep. They are of absolute major importance to your safe, healthy and productive continuing existence on this planet of ours, i.e. what your brain's total ongoing workload actually is. As well as the crucial managing role that your M.C. carries out, with its all-powerful use of its intelligence when required, what else helps your brain operate throughout your life without making even one mistake?

SUBCHAPTER A) What is your brain's total ongoing workload?

A1) Here are my thoughts about what is a significant part of your brain's workload. It is the process of your brain's ongoing activity of creating and taking action upon your consciousness, described in a step-by-step manner below.

Firstly, here is an explanation of each of the abbreviations used:

- **M.C.** denotes that your <u>Master Conductor</u> has an involvement with the activity listed, which always includes being ably assisted by its intelligence when required.

- **C.A.** denotes an ongoing <u>continuous activity</u>, irrespective of what you are currently engaged in and whether you are awake or asleep. Some activities will be more active at times, dependent upon what you are doing.

- **W.R.** denotes an activity that is only active <u>when required</u>, awake or asleep.

- **D.I.** denotes the <u>department itself</u> automatically conducts its own improvement refinements.

- <u>Creating your Consciousness</u> and taking actions indicated from its creation is a significant part of the ongoing workload of your Brain.

- **Category p)** are dedicated sets of Category 1B departments that use their selected automated <u>Sequential Processing</u> to decode and understand the meaning of all data entering your brain. They are crucially assisted by your M.C. and provide it with information from your memories.

- **Category q)** are dedicated Category 1B Departments that use their selected, particular quality of <u>self-operating capabilities,</u> managed and assisted by your M.C. when necessary, to carry out all of their required actions as indicated by your updated consciousness.
- Each main, separate activity is designated with its own reference letter, commencing with **a)**.

This is the description of the process **a)** to **f)**, to update and take actions upon your updated consciousness:

a)   <u>**M.C.** & **Category p)** & **C.A.**</u>The objective of **a)** is to analyse all of the data entering your brain via your senses, B.H.S.M.S., and your internal thoughts, which are already within your brain. This is to fully understand their meaning and relevance to you as part of the required process of creating/updating your consciousness.

b)   <u>**M.C.** & **Category p)** & **C.A.**</u>The objective of **b)** is for your M.C. to study all of the data that has completed its analysis process. With the help of its intelligence, it creates thoughts to review and decide whether any items of data can pose a danger to you in the context of your prevailing situation. Your M.C. also considers whether each item of non-safety-related data on its own is important to process. If not, it will immediately delete each of them.

c) **M.C. & Category p) & C.A.** The objective of **c)** is for your M.C., with its intelligence, to create thoughts to review and consider what actions are required to resolve each safety-related issue, identified within this latest update of your consciousness.

d) **M.C. & Category q) & C.A.** The objective of **d)** is for your M.C. to instigate the required actions specified in **c)** above.

e) **M.C. & Category p) & C.A.** The objective of **e)** is for your M.C., with its intelligence, to create thoughts to review and consider what actions are required to satisfy each non-safety-related requirement, identified within this latest update of your Consciousness and **then:**

f) **M.C. & Category q) & C.A.** The objective of **f)** is for your M.C. to instigate the required actions specified in **e)** above.

Activities **a)** to and including **f)** *continue ad infinitum* in the sequence detailed above.

A2) In addition to the activities listed in A1) above, the following activities listed below complete your brain's total ongoing workload:

NB Many of the activities listed below will be involved with the ongoing processing of the typical/normal incoming data, combined with the activities and objectives of **a)** to and including **f)** as described. The remaining ones will be active as required.

Category p) and/or **Category q)** will each contribute to your brain's ongoing total workload where Category 1B Departments are utilised, which will be in the majority of the activities detailed in **the following A2) list:**

g) <u>**C.A.**</u> All of your **Category 1 Department's** activities.

h) <u>**M.C. & C.A.**</u> All of your **Category 1A Department's** activities.

i) <u>**M.C. & Category p)** and/or **Category q) & W.R.**</u> All of your **Category 1B Department's** activities including, for example: Reading, Writing, Speaking, Remembering, Hearing, Seeing, Tasting, Touching, Smelling, Problem Solving, Planning, Processing, all of the vast number of different activities of your body's physical movements, your subconscious thoughts, your conscious thoughts from external data, your conscious thoughts generated internally within your brain, your instinctive thoughts, your involuntary actions and many, many more activities.

j) <u>**M.C. & C.A.**</u> All of your **M.C.'s Department's** activities, most of which are extremely busy night and day.

k) k) <u>**M.C. & C.A.**</u> The ongoing adjustments of your **Data Dwell Time facility** to study each item of Data to suit the prevailing needs of your M.C.

l) <u>**M.C. & W.R.**</u> All of the many vitally important activities your brain conducts whilst you are sleeping, the majority of which are only active whilst asleep.

m) <u>**M.C. & W.R.**</u> Whilst awake and asleep, the continued learning and memory storage of new knowledge, the development and updating of existing knowledge and the deletion of redundant knowledge.

n) **D.I. & W.R.** The refinement of your Category 1 Department's Fully-Automatic Control Systems.

o) **M.C. & D.I. & W.R.** The refinement of your Category 1A Department's Semi-Automatic Control Systems.

p) **M.C. & D.I. & W.R.** the refinement of your Category 1B Department's Developed Semi-Automatic Skills and a number of other Category 1B Department's skills.

In conclusion: What a list of an immense, gargantuan workload for your brain. What a BRAIN to be able to process it all with no mistakes, with the immaculate help of your Master Conductor!

SUBCHAPTER B) As well as the crucially important managing role that your M.C. carries out, with its all-powerful use of its intelligence when required, what else helps your brain operate throughout your life without making even one mistake?

B1) As I consider this question to be of immense importance, I will take the opportunity to remind you of part of the basic process of how your brain creates/updates your consciousness:

Your brain externally receives incoming data from your five senses plus data from inside your brain, from your internally created thoughts and your B.H.S.M.S.

Each set of data, for example, from your vision, is received by your brain as a complete set or package of data that represents the whole or complete vision you are seeing. I propose that this complete data package is then reformatted into a DNA-type of Analogue Format.

It is then passed into the standard facility in your brain to be processed by your **Category p) processing facility** (see Subchapter 4.1, A1). There it will be analysed by the multi-step, sub-processing activities carried out within your brain to understand exactly what all of this vision is and what it means to you.

a)   Your sense of vision (followed by your sound) will contain by far the most **separate points of data** compared to the other senses to accurately represent all of the visionary details. It will be in the order of many millions when all the required data points from all the other senses are processed in total, both in **A1)** & **A2)** where appropriate.

B2) I spent quite some time studying each of the separate items of your brain's required processing work, listed in A1), to be able to assess the related workload that each one required. I did this by evaluating the number of blocks or groups of processing activities carried out within your brain per second to enable each of the process activities and objectives to be fully satisfied. I chose to call them multi-step, sub-processing activities.

a)   I arrived at a ballpark figure of **a significant number of millions** of multi-step, sub-processing activities and self-operating capability activities carried out per second for **A1)** only.

b) I then proceeded to do the same exercise for the workload on list **A2)**. I arrived at an approximate figure of **a significant number of millions** of multi-step, sub-processing activities and self-operating capability activities per second.

c) I then considered how many data points were contained within each set or group of incoming data as detailed in **B1-a)** above in relation to **A1)** & **A2)** where appropriate. As a ballpark figure, the outcome was a **substantial number of millions** per second.

B3) In summary, your brain's processing workload is of a significant number of millions of multi-step, sub-processing activities and self-operating capability activities, EACH OF WHICH contains and processes a substantial number of millions of points of data every second.

Depending on the type of data and the data processing workload, I estimate that this equates to, approximately **8 million x 50 million points of data being processed every second by your brain.**

This is an OVERWHELMINGLY awesomely immense feat of processing, when you consider the following:

a) Your brain operates in this manner, albeit with a significant reduction in total workload whilst you are asleep throughout the whole of your life.

b) You make the occasional decision making mistake of logic, from too much emotion, etc., but your brain itself performs faultlessly, providing you take care of it and don't in any way abuse it.

c)   Your brain occupies its position inside your skull for the whole of your life. Despite the sum total of the indescribable workload and the amount of data processing per second it quietly deals with, it makes no fuss. It just does it all, every second, minute, hour, day, month and year throughout your life.

B4) The date of the question posed in Subchapter B) heading was 24th September 2021, which I will never ever forget!

This is because, on this day, my brain finally opened the window to me, giving total clarity of exactly **HOW** our brain is able to process its never-ending gargantuan processing workload, at the speed it operates throughout our lifetime, never making **even one mistake**.

These comments above may be confusing to you, but please read on for my simple, but, I believe, extremely powerful set of explanations of **HOW it is achieved!**

a)   The processing performance figures per second and ongoing workload obviously include elements of my beliefs, proposals and approximations. However, I am fairly comfortable with them at this stage, because they feel they are in the right ballpark. They relate to the observable performance of how fast your processing brain can respond to extremely fast-changing data input conditions, plus how rapidly it responds with its related actions/output activities as required by your updated consciousness.

How does it achieve all that it most certainly does achieve – the almost unachievable?

In my opinion, three simple words explain it all.

Can you guess what they are? They have 10, 11 and 9 letters: **simplicity, flexibility and constancy!**

b)   Yes, your brain has all of its required strengths, capabilities and more. Yes, it processes a mammoth workload updating your consciousness, which all of your decisions and resultant actions every second of the whole of your life come from. It is also processing all of your activities detailed and listed in **A1)** and **A2)** above. However, despite this utterly immense, permanent workload, it continues quietly with no fuss, no complaints, no change in its status in any way, whilst satisfying all of your requirements.

c)   Its workload is utterly immense. Its speed of operation is completely mind-blowing. The secret of its unquestioning success is the **simple** and inherently **flexible** operational process, as described in my book, of the permanent and ongoing **constancy** of the creation of your consciousness and how you take appropriate, straightforward actions to satisfy what your consciousness is requesting.

During the **constancy** of this process, you **always** apply the **simple rules** and **objectives** of each of these following steps:

a) Your first **simple objective** is to _establish the meaning_ to you of each different set of data presented to your brain.

b) Your next **simple objective** is to **identify** any sets of data that _present a danger to you._

c) Your next **simple objective** is to **identify** all _remaining_ data that requires _action._

d) Your next **simple action** is to _discard/delete_ all _remaining_ sets of data.

e) Your next **simple action** is, if there is more than one, to identify the _highest danger_ risk to you and **take action** to deal with it, then deal with the next one if there is one.

f) Your next **simple activity** is to _take action_ upon all remaining **conditions that require your action**, in the priority required.

Each cycle of the **constancy** of the process above takes 4ms. You **simply** follow each cycle of steps as above, with significant help from your Data Review Scanning System through the flexible and efficient way it operates, plus from your M.C. with its intelligence and organisational skills.

The process above, **simply** and **repeatedly** at the same speed and frequency without change, continues with the constant existence and flow of your life until your very end of life. Only then does it stop forever.

If your brain runs out of time, for example, to complete step **a)** for one data set, your M.C., with **flexibility,** will automatically **simply** ignore this situation during this cycle. Also, **extremely importantly** with **flexibility,** your **Category**

p) Sequential Processing Department will continue searching for the meaning of this data which will be processed during your next consciousness update cycle. If it takes three update cycles for the meaning to be found, this data will then **simply** be processed in the next cycle that comes along.

Also, if your brain has insufficient time, for example, to complete step **e)** for one set of data, because your **Category q) 1B Departments**, using their **self-operating capabilities** (with the aid of your M.C), have not completed their thinking process of how to eliminate this danger, they will, with **flexibility, simply** continue searching for a solution. When the solution is available and the next cycle comes along, this danger will be dealt with <u>as part of that cycle</u>.

The overall **capability, constancy, flexibility** and **simplicity** of this system supports your brain to allow more time to process parts of your consciousness update. It also facilitates this when dealing with danger if a very fast response is unnecessary. If absolute and immediate life-threatening danger has to be dealt with immediately or you are dead, this can also be accommodated by your brain with **flexibility** and **simplicity** due to its mind-blowing speed of response when required.

One crucially important factor that I must remind you of that plays a major role in the stability and success of your brain's processing work is your **Master Conductor's** involvement. Its invaluable input is mentioned in all of your activities (with almost the total exception of the operation of your Category 1 departments.) Its role is to be involved with all of your brain's ongoing processing activities; see **Subchapter 4.1, A1)** and **A2)** lists.

Your M.C.'s input is the final polishing influence that keeps the whole of your Brain's operating state in perfect order and balance.

B5) To answer the question posed in the Subchapter B) heading: *As well as the crucial managing role and the application of its intelligence when required, that your M.C. carries out, what else helps your brain operate all of your life without making even one mistake?* The answer is three things! Your brain operates within a system that operates at all times, in all situations with **Simplicity, Flexibility** and **Constancy.** *These are the three other reasons.*

I have spent some time presenting the above situations to highlight how **simple** the set of rules and objectives are. In addition, I have shown how extremely **flexible,** with **constancy,** the process of updating your consciousness is and **crucially, most importantly, must be.**

During your life, if the whole of your brain's processing activities didn't follow all of the factors and aspects detailed above, the **worst-case scenario risk is** that some functional brain faults would occur. These could cause the immediate and **earth-shattering consequences of you going instantly and utterly out of control.** This would be due to the juggernaut of your brain's workload coupled with the momentum from its sheer speed of operation, causing it to run off the rails of your consciousness. Can there be a more frightening thought?

CHAPTER 5.0 – WHAT INFORMATION AND CAPABILITIES ARE YOU BORN WITH, AND HOW DOES YOUR BRAIN DEVELOP AND ADD TO THEM DURING YOUR LIFE?

OVERVIEW: The way your vast array of skills, knowledge, capabilities and incredible flexibility are developed is just awesome. Some exist before birth, with continued development afterwards, and others are encouraged or produced after birth, also with ongoing, continuous evolution. Each develops to a level of outstanding reliability, flexibility, lightning speed of functionality and the capability to be instantly applied, individually or collectively.

When you add to the above attributes that they are each capable of automatic, continual, self-learning and improvement, I keep running out of different suitable descriptions that do justice to the amazing living partnership of your human body and brain. So-called robots or bots, auto-pilot cars and artificial intelligence systems – eat your heart out. However, that is impossible because they don't possess one (an intelligence) and never can. More importantly, they also don't have human consciousness and many other human attributes and never will be able to, for some fundamental and absolute reasons. The word 'Artificial' in their name is a big clue.

Where human intelligence is not required, these AI facilities with one dedicated function can perform their task quicker and perhaps better than humans in particular applications. But when you consider the immense depth and range of skills and capabilities that the average human being possesses, these AI-driven machines bear no comparison.

They will never be able to match the immense number of different skills that an average human being has and can select from to deal with whatever unexpected scenario they meet whilst coming around any corner, anywhere on the planet, at any time. The awesome depth and breadth of your human consciousness is the cornerstone on which all human beings keep safe, make multiple decisions and take their related actions, 240 times every second, throughout their individual and unique lives.

It is the platform upon which they drive cars, play all sports, react to an ever-changing, interreactive and inter-dynamic one hundred and one people situations, ebbing and flowing all around them. They are able to cope admirably with any situation they are presented with, even if they haven't met all of the detailed conditions before in the context that prevails. This is due to the capabilities described above plus, their ability to apply their intelligence, intuition and vast expansive range of knowledge.

Question 1 – What information, knowledge, facilities and capabilities were you born with?

OVERVIEW: Providing you are not born with any brain damage or disabilities, I believe you are born with your brain having certain information installed. You have some facilities with a basic level of capability and a significant number of other facilities that are <u>actually fully functioning before your birth</u>. This range of capabilities and facilities commence with the **three different categories of Automatic Control Systems.** *Each one resides within its own department, of which vast numbers are located within your brain.*

Refer to Subchapter 2.2.3 for more information on the above, if required.

a) Your Fully-Automatic, P.I.D. Closed-Loop Measurement and Control Systems
(A Category 1 department facility)

These are the many Control Systems that maintain your brain and body's vital services, organs, conditions and facilities active and functioning correctly and, therefore, keep you alive and healthy. They are for controlling your heart, blood sugar level, chemical health, body temperature and many, many more elements.

I believe that these Control Systems are innate and are potentially there at your conception. They fully develop in the womb <u>prior to birth, as required. Thereafter</u>, each of them automatically develops and fine-tunes the operation of their neural networks to improve the effectiveness of their control and operation of what they are controlling for you.

b) Your Semi-Automatic, Open-Loop Measurement and Control Systems
(A Category 1A department facility)

These are the many Control Systems that keep your brain and body's core states and conditions in good order. This preserves a robust state of health regarding your Emotional Health and Stress, keeping you hydrated and controlling your food intake and many, many more factors.

I also think that these Control Systems are innate, potentially from conception, developing in your mother's womb before birth, with some fully developed by the time you are born. After birth, they will each fully develop where required. All of them will automatically fine-tune the operation of their neural networks to improve the effectiveness of the control and operation of what they are controlling for you.

c) Your Semi-Automatic, Open-Loop Control Systems
(A Category 1B department facility)

These are the vast multitude of Control Systems that provide the Primary Processes, Functionalities and Skills required to enable your mind and body to achieve each of their ongoing objectives and related actions during the whole of your life. They provide your reading and writing skills, walking, running and general moving skills, management skills and multitudes of so many more.

Again, I consider these Control Systems to be innate and potentially there at your conception. I believe they are passed on in your genes from your parents and their forefathers. Some develop in the womb prior to birth, with some more developed than others by the time you are born and with some fully functioning as required before birth.

To improve the effectiveness of the control and operation of their dedicated role, they each automatically, develop and fine tune the operation of their neural networks. This occurs naturally in some, from your life's experiences, and with deliberate practice in others, where the will prevails, continuing to improve throughout your lifetime.

d) Your genes

I believe that at birth, the genes that you were born with, passed on from your parents and, to a lesser extent, their parents etc., will be resident and functional where they can. This will be in all the departments of your brain and elsewhere in your body, when and where their influence is required.

e) The ability to receive information

I propose that you are crucially and importantly born with the abilities to start to learn to receive information. This comes to you as data via your five senses, that they all sense in every moment through their data input receivers – your eyes, ears, tongue, nose and tips of your fingers, etc. Their exclusive data format converters change the data into a format that can be ultimately recognised/understood by your brain. Therefore it is processed and stored in the appropriate departments for future use.

Each of these departments is dedicated to managing solely your vision, sound or smell data etc., so that all incoming data can be successfully received, processed and utilised by your brain, commencing from birth to a very minimal extent. You need many neural networks, within a large number of Category 1B departments, each of which has the required functionality to automatically carry out all of the detailed data processing and provide your M.C. with the data necessary to fulfil its objectives.

f) Your M.C. and the Category 1B Departments it comprises at your birth.

The department housing your character and soul, plus all of the other departments which comprise and operate as part of your M.C., working with your Category 1A and 1B Departments, form part of your extremely limited amount of knowledge at birth. However, most crucially and importantly, they are all able to **start practising**, developing and employing the vitally important abilities of:

- Assessing your surroundings.
- Creating your consciousness.
- Keeping yourself safe.
- Carrying out your decision and action making skills.

I believe that these conditions and facilities will gradually and automatically develop and improve as you, your Character,

Soul, M.C., and all of your Category departments store more and more data, plus evolve and mature their characteristics and processing capabilities as required.

g) A basic, foundational framework of abilities

At birth, I propose you are born with the very basic, foundational framework of abilities that, when appropriate to each prevailing skill to be ready to be developed, begin to be able to commence very early. These help you learn to:

- Talk
- Read
- Write
- Walk
- Think
- Remember
- Hear
- See
- Taste
- Touch
- Smell
- Problem-solve
- Many, many more skills.

h) Other early-onset skills

Also, at your birth, or soon afterwards, you begin to develop the ability to be able to:

1) Speak with a range of sounds.
2) Independently move all of the very large numbers of parts of your limbs and all of your body.
3) Feed from your mother's breasts.
4) Indicate when you are hungry, unhappy, happy, tired, excited, and able to respond to various stimuli.
5) Pass urine, defecate and many more bodily functions.

Question 2 – How does your brain acquire and develop all of its incredible breadth and depth of knowledge and capabilities?

OVERVIEW: I believe that you are born as detailed above, with a significant amount of functional and learning capabilities. The sum of these abilities, if measured in numbers of available and active neural networks and brain cells, plus overall available and active capability, is incredibly high, compared to the total capability of say, a standard laptop. However, if measured as a percentage of your entire brain's total available potential capacity and capability, it is incredibly low – only about 0.15%. This is an assessment from considering all different types of each of your Category 1B departments and their capability at birth.

An extremely pertinent point is also that, at your birth, the capability of your Category 1 and 1A departments will be at around 90% of their designed maximum potential. However, the capability of each of your Category 1B departments, which are by far more numerous within your brain, will range between 5% to 10% of their designed maximum potential. This is due to this category of department in your brain being entirely empty of acquired knowledge and capabilities derived and developed from your experiences. At birth, they only contain their neural software processing systems ready to grow to full capability with gradual use, and receive, process and carry out their pre-dedicated roles when capable.

This feels to be an almost unreal and frightening situation. But crucially importantly, the capabilities that you are born with are safely and reliably sufficient to keep your body and brain healthy, alive and functioning correctly, coupled with the range of help and support from your mother and family. They also enable you to begin the earliest of your learning stages with the tiniest glimmer of understanding to commence practising:

1) Assessing your surroundings, which enables you to:
2) Begin practising creating your consciousness, which lets you:
3) Begin practising keeping yourself safe and also stimulates you to:
4) Begin practising carrying out your decision-making and related actions processes.

Also, you are born with the capabilities that, crucially and importantly, allow you to immediately begin the lifelong (if you wish) process of learning and developing an awesomely wide and deep range of topics that this wonderful world has waiting for you to experience.

a) At birth, I believe that your brain is <u>virtually empty</u> of any knowledge and capabilities derived from your experiences.

You will only have acquired a very small exposure to some data before birth. This is because the stupendously vast majority of information and capabilities you have gained when you are 60 years old, for example, will have been accumulated and stored in your brain, resulting from the incredible amount and range of data and experiences that you have been exposed to from birth.

b) Every waking second of your life, particularly initially, is a learning process for your brain.

This is due to every data item and collection of data of which each experience comprises being new to you. All of the data pouring into your brain from your senses has to be received, viewed, considered, studied and understood in the following way, where possible – what it is, what it is called and what relevance to you it has.

It then has to be stored in the relevant Memory Department in your brain for future use in updating your consciousness, keeping you safe and assisting in making decisions, taking actions and basically living and hopefully enjoying your life most of the time.

c) Just stop and consider for a second how much of a learning process it has been for your brain to immediately recognise many thousands of different noises.

1) All the *sounds you hear* throughout all of the varying situations in your life.

2) The different *words you hear* during everyday life.

3) The *voices* of all of the people you know.

4) The *sounds* of different animals, working activities, the weather, the birds in the countryside, walking in a busy city centre – the list goes on and on.

For each sound, your brain has to learn to recognise and differentiate it from the others. This means knowing its name, what causes it, what aspects of life it occurs in and its meaning to you and others. Does it represent a danger to you, and do you have to take any decision and related action to it in that moment?

d) Think about your vision sense.

Consider all of the big pictures of information you can see if you are travelling around cities, the countryside, coastal areas, driving a car 600 miles through a whole range of sceneries, visiting a huge museum, etc. The list can be endless.

Every different item you see in each image and view of your world, your brain eventually has to learn to instantly recognise it from all others. It has to know its name, its role, how many different types exist, and what aspects of life it relates to and affects. Additionally, your brain has to learn how all of the individual items within each picture connect and relate to each other immediately, to manage, as necessary, all that you see and sense around you fast enough to keep you safe.

e) Consider the formal schooling system that you pass through.
This is the foundational learning process from which you learn so much about the world and all its facets to prepare you to move on to further education and then into the world of work. Alternatively, you may bypass further education after senior school and move into work, ideally combined with further education whilst on the job. However, this could be a block release arrangement or whatever suits your working ambitions, academic skills, practical skills and prevailing financial situation.

It is so important that this formal learning process includes not only academic learning and experience of the other facets that lead to a balanced healthy life, including sporting activities, chess clubs, or any other available pastimes. From all of these enjoyable learning experiences, you continue to develop interpersonal skills and your own character, obtain satisfaction from achievements, self-confidence and self-esteem. All of these provide you with the tools to healthily and successfully steer your path through life's challenges whenever they materialise.

f) What you can expect as you grow and develop, providing you remain healthy and retain your zest and energy for life.

1) You will continue to accumulate new experiences, data and knowledge in your life. This adds to the range and depth of your general knowledge of so many topics that this magically fascinating life comprises. When acquired, all of this new data, experiences and knowledge becomes stored within your Memory Cells for future use.

2) Your list of Developed, Semi-Automatic Skills will continue to grow. By exposing yourself to new experiences and *gradually practising* and improving, your existing Semi-Automatic skills required for all things increase. These skills include: crawling, walking, running, talking, playing sports and dancing, interpersonal skills, logical reasoning, planning, communicating with others, forward-thinking and a vast multitude of others.

3) Your depth and range of character, soul and intelligence will continue to develop, mature and change at times. This is a consequence of battling with extremely challenging situations and by increasingly achieving more and more goals and different targets in your life at school, work and in your home life and within hobbies, pastimes and holidays. Each achievement you obtain builds your self-esteem and self-confidence from within, plus hopefully from people around you expressing their congratulations and admiration of your accomplishments and prowess, in many different ways. A crucially important and valuable end product acquired from each of your achievements is a feeling of satisfaction for a job well done – even more so when you had to overcome some extremely challenging hurdles on the way. The units of well-earned satisfaction are worth so much more than money.

4) Your advancement of years and continuance of learning brings an increased ability of your M.C. to be able to efficiently utilise all of its departments and all of your brain's other departments to construct your ongoing consciousness.

This is the foundation upon which you keep safe and oversee, manage and coordinate each of your prevailing thoughts, considerations, decisions and resultant actions. It also allows you to manage the whole of your life on a day-to-day basis, in a more balanced, controlled, satisfying and enjoyable manner.

5) Your ongoing process of learning, and your increasing number of experiences in all of the vast range of facets of life have crucial benefits. All of your brain's departments gradually store more and more knowledge and information and/or acquire increased capabilities appropriate to the Category of Department they are in and the related dedicated role they each carry out within your Brain. Providing you remain physically and mentally healthy, coupled with the retention of a zest for life and a need to learn, the increasing accumulation of your knowledge and capability enables you to make faster, better quality decisions and actions than any time previously in your life.

Question 3 – Imagine if you were born with all of your faculties, capabilities and senses in pristine health apart from one – the key sense of your vision.

You would have been unable to see at all from birth!

Then one day, when you reached 40 years of age, you wake up and find, to your total astonishment, that you can see perfectly.

1) How would you feel emotionally?

2) How would you cope with this sudden, vast amount of data pouring into your brain?

3) What would you do immediately?

4) Would the sudden explosion of this extensive amount of new data to you be good for you?

5) Would it improve the quality of your life?

6) After a few weeks of acquiring this sense, would you prefer to lose it again?

I believe that each person, being a unique individual, would react differently, but some of the realities of such a situation would include:

a) You would certainly have had numerous people describing everyday things throughout your life, so you will have had some description in your mind's thoughts, of what they look like. But, your brain will not have any visionary data of anything at all that you are now seeing, so it will not have any images in any of its visual Memory Departments, each of which will be entirely empty of data. Also, it is likely that some of these departments will have been used for other memory storage and processing roles. If this is the case, this could compromise your brain's capability of having sufficient, maximum storage capacity as your total vision memory storage grows in the future. Additionally, your brain's many departments that would have been used and developed from birth to execute the vast amount of highly complex super-fast additional processing of your Visionary Data, even if still available, they will not have evolved as normal and will seriously struggle to cope and develop 40 years later.

b) Emotionally, I propose that, particularly if you were on your own, you would feel swamped, confused, uncomfortable and emotionally unbalanced by this vast amount of data exploding into your mind. Your brain would not be able to recognise any of it, simply because it had not seen it before. Therefore, it could not compare it with data in its visionary memory cells because they were all empty.

c) I have my doubts, but let's consider if my concerns detailed in a) above are not as close to the extreme as I have painted. Suppose you have sufficient capacity and capability within your brain to at least be able to commence your visionary learning process to acquire a reasonable visionary capability. In this case, to protect your emotional health, I believe your brain would make you immediately close your eyes, shut out all of this unrecognisable data and call out to someone for help. Hopefully, you will be able to engage the help of a knowledgeable person. They would probably suggest you start to, very gradually, at a comfortable learning pace, expose your brain to short periods of different visionary experiences, and, before each visionary view, a sighted person explains what you are about to see and what it all means.

In this way, you will gradually enable your brain to go through the extremely long road of learning. Eventually, you will have developed your visionary knowledge and included visual memories in your life experiences from this new period, in addition to the audio and other of your senses' memories. Hopefully, out of this process, you will be glad that your vision came to you and that the quality of your life eventually was enhanced significantly and permanently.

However, going through the above process would require an awful lot of determination and tenacity to continue the learning process. You would need the help of the correct type of committed person and require perhaps some years of significant learning. You would also need significantly more sleep than before, to assist your mind with processing, understanding and storing this vast amount of new knowledge and experiences.

CHAPTER 6.0 – RESPONSES TO MANY ONGOING TOPICAL QUESTIONS IN THE MEDIA ABOUT US, OUR BRAINS AND THEIR FUNCTIONALITY AND CAPABILITY IN RELATION TO EVERYDAY LIFE.

OVERVIEW: Up to this juncture, my book has focused fundamentally upon what your brain comprises in terms of functionality, its roles and priorities, Its objectives and how and why the whole of your brain actually functions. I have given many examples along the way as a means of demonstration and hopefully with a good degree of improved understanding. This section focuses on topical questions related to your brain, each with my detailed related answer. I hope that this process will further cement at least some areas of your existing understanding of our brain and its relation to our everyday lives, about all that you and it does and why.

Before you read on, please refer again to AN EXTREMELY IMPORTANT POINTER in Subchapter 1.1.

And also, before you continue, please <u>read the following point</u> that I would like to make, covering, in particular, Chapters 6.0 and 7.0, but also covering the whole of my book, which is:

Throughout my book, my comments are my honest, genuinely held and personal beliefs always without exception.

They are intended to be constructively helpful to those who take the interest, time and effort to read my book. These comments are always entirely my opinions, to which others may quite rightly, acceptably and properly hold different views to mine. At no time whatsoever are my comments intended to be critical of anyone, professional person or not, practising work I have passed my opinions upon, suggesting that they consider other aspects in addition to their current ones. Any work, of any type, connected with the functionality of the brain is, by its fundamental nature extremely complex and challenging. It can negatively affect one's mental and physical health and, at times, be life-threatening.

In some areas, in particular, work of this nature requires professional people who are blessed with significant courage, skill, capability, knowledge and the extremely strong wish **to** help others. **Without them, many of us would be in real life-changing trouble.** Please read on.

SUBCHAPTER 6.1: Your human consciousness, mind, soul and you. What are they? What are their precise roles? What do they comprise of? How do they function, and how do they interact with each other?

Due to the ever-increasing interest in brain functionality, partly caused by the increasing use and, more importantly, the increasingly 'projected use' of robots, autopiloted vehicles and automated systems in general, there is an increased frequency of using this vocabulary and related questions. People have concerns about what automation may mean to the future of their jobs and to that continuity, even of the human race itself, added to the ever rising concern about people's poor emotional health leading to significant mental illness.

Despite worldwide lifetime studies done over centuries by countless numbers of highly trained, committed, extraordinarily clever and academically-gifted people, as I understand it, no one has yet proposed, with any degree of confidence nor significant depth of detail, the definitions of what could be described as a deep understanding of your consciousness, mind and soul.

This open situation was the catalyst for me to finally commence writing this book. Also, because – and I genuinely hope this statement is not seen as me being a ridiculously cocky upstart – I felt I could usefully propose definitions of these facilities and energies that we each have, which I believe are fundamentally at the core of us human beings, our existence and functionality.

To ask some absolute and fundamental questions:

a) Do you have any of them, or are they all an illusion?
b) If you have any of them, what is the basic definition of each of them?
c) Where are they located, and what are they comprised of?
d) Why do you have them, and how do they function?
e) Who and what is You?
f) How does your consciousness, mind, soul, and You co-exist, interreact and functionally operate?

OVERVIEW: *I believe that the creation, composition, functionality, potential capability and utilisation of your consciousness is at the core of all of your brain's functionalities, ably supported by your mind, your M.C. and soul. Your brain can achieve and create the incredible control and outputs that it produces in such an overall balanced, stable, efficient and effective manner, due to the collective contribution and capability of your consciousness, mind, soul, and M.C., supported by your multitudes of Category 1A and 1B departments.*

Your brain operates at an incredibly fast rate, producing an awesome number of processing activities and resultant actions per millisecond, throughout the whole of your life, whilst awake and continuing, albeit with a much reduced workload, whilst you are asleep. Despite the mind-numbing processing performance of your brain, coupled with the incredible range and number of all of the resultant actions carried out by your body, for example, over a two-hour virtually continuous period of highly intense and extremely complex movements, **your brain and body produce a faultless performance.**

NB If the person is carrying out this performance during a sporting activity and they make a faulty decision-making mistake by giving their opponent an easy winning return shot, forgetting that was their opponent's forte, I don't define this as a mistake by their brain. I define it as a human error category mistake!

I have noticed, more so since writing my book, that apart from a very small percentage of people, I guess everyone else, when witnessing such performances, just takes what they have witnessed for granted. Understandably so, if asked, they say, it's all due to the hard practice they put in – and muscle memory, of course.

The more I have pondered the workings of your brain, the more I stand in absolute and utter awe of its stunning, majestic power, immense flexibility and wondrously awesome range and depth of capabilities, the most important of which is genuine intelligence.

It is this awesome power with which your brain is able to not just receive information coming in from your senses, B.H.S.M.S and your internal thoughts. Additionally, it crucially selects the relevant details from all of this information, enabling it to understand the meaning and, therefore, the contextual relevance to you in that moment of your time and how to deal with and process it.

This intelligence is the primary factor that allows you, as a member of the human race, to be able to stand intellectually head and shoulders above so called Artificial (i.e. non) Intelligence-controlled machines. You can produce, when required, **<u>original</u> <u>thoughts</u>, which I believe are beyond the capability of machines now and will always remain so**. Artificial Intelligence must surely be the most miss-named title for anything in the history of mankind – the intelligent part.

SUBCHAPTER 6.1.1: Your consciousness

Question 1 – Do you have a consciousness, or is it an illusion?

I do not believe that consciousness is an illusion. I propose that it exists as an intellectual product of understanding, awareness, knowledge and intelligence. It is derived from the results of information collected, processed and understood as a result of the coordinated work carried out by many departments of your brain, each of which has an organic, physical existence.

Definition 1 – My Basic Definition of Consciousness.

Consciousness is the permanent and ongoing updated, intellectual product based on the receipt of the raw data entering your brain via your senses, Body's Health Status Monitoring System and your internal thoughts, its conversion, analysis and full understanding and particular relevance to you, in each moment of your life.

Question 2 – What faculties do you require to be able to create your consciousness?

Your full consciousness can be created by your brain, from your senses, B.H.S.M.S., and internal thoughts. Your vast storage of knowledge and memories, your mind and its M.C., all being in good operational health, also enables the accurate, detailed evaluations, conclusions and resultant updating and creation of your prevailing consciousness.

The most crucially important component of this process is the power, **utilisation and application of your intelligence**. This is what intellectually separates you as a human being now, and always, I believe, from man-made robots and all other such machines, none of which is capable and never will be capable of **original thought** as humans are.

Question 3 – What is the detailed process that your brain utilises to create your consciousness?

NB Please refer to the two other descriptions of how your consciousness is created. Each is presented differently, particularly concerning other activities happening around and within your consciousness – Subchapter 3.1.1 and Subchapter 4.1.

A) A basic description of the first phase of this ongoing cycle of the creation and updating of your consciousness.

i) Data inputs from your five senses automatically pass into their own dedicated Category 1B Department in your brain, as part of the analysis process. This includes utilising your vast array of knowledge in order to commence understanding what each data item is and means to you.

ii) Any <u>data inputs</u> from your <u>B.H.S.M.S.</u>, which are already within your brain, will automatically pass into another Category 1B Department, as part of the analysis process. This includes **utilising your vast array of knowledge** to begin the analysis, to comprehend what they **each are and mean to you.**

iii) <u>Data inputs</u> from each of your <u>active thoughts</u> you may have, already within your mind, automatically pass into another Category 1B Department in your brain as part of the analysis process. This includes **utilising your vast array of knowledge** to start the analysis, to understand what they **each are and mean to you.**

The prevailing processing status for each data item for all activities in **A)** above will nominally have been reviewed after 1ms by the end of the first scan cycle.

NB On some occasions, <u>not</u> all items of data will have completed their analysis process within this 1ms, simply because they comprise of data that requires <u>more processing time than 1ms to understand them fully.</u>

When these items of data are finally analysed, they will be entered into the system to be processed during a subsequent consciousness creation cycle.

B) The second phase of this cycle.

i) Your M.C. studies all of the data that has completed its analysis process. With the help of its innate and developed intelligence, it decides what data or sets of data in the context of your prevailing situation, indicate danger to you. Alternatively, they imply no danger but still require your consideration and resultant actions to deal with.

ii) All other remaining data which has no importance to you at that moment in time will therefore be deleted by your M.C. This deletion assessment activity is of prime importance to minimise the risk/difficulty you would otherwise occasionally encounter of being overloaded with too much data to analyse and process correctly.

iii) Thus far, you have established your updated consciousness, which is all of the data that requires processing and responding to nominally immediately, that has been sent to your Data Review Scanning System for review.

*The total time for all of these activities in **B)** above will be over a second Scan Cycle of 1ms.*

C) The third and last phase of this cycle.

i) Once again, your M.C. uses its inherent and developed intelligence to create the required and appropriate

Thoughts of Consideration. These thoughts review all of the remaining data that has completed its analysis process to consider any data that indicates danger to you in order of priority of importance. Your Thoughts of Consideration subsequently decide what actions you are required to take to deal with each of them individually or collectively as appropriate.

ii) Your M.C. instigates each of the required actions to prevent or dispel the dangers. This could be for example, sending instructions in software format to a number of your Category 1B Developed, Semi-Automatic Skills Departments to operate your activities of walking, speaking, reading or fighting, or perhaps thinking and very many other possibilities.

iii) Once again, your M.C. will engage its inherent and developed intelligence by addressing your Non-Safety related issues and requirements but nonetheless important ones, whenever it has the time, in between keeping you safe. It will address these by giving each one their appropriate Thoughts of Consideration it has created and instigating the fitting instructions required to achieve the related action/s it has decided are necessary.

*The total time for all of these activities in **C)** above to be completed within 2 Scan Cycles = 2ms.*

NB-X The total time from each of your Category 1B Developed, Semi-Automatic Skills receiving instructions to them actually being carried out physically and operationally will vary greatly due to a number of factors. For example, how long will it take for each particular instruction to be completed, which could vary from looking at a particular person's face near you, shouting a warning to someone, walking towards the end of a wall to read a notice, etc.

The total time for all of these activities in NB.X to be completed nominally from 2ms up to a possible wide range of a number of seconds.

D) The next cycle commences with its first phase exactly as A) above.

i)   It is for analysing the incoming data which may include **NB-X** and one or two of the results and consequences of some of the instigated Actions in **C-ii)** above.

ii) To note and address all other data inputs as **A-i)**, **ii)** and **iii)** above where, in each case, some data inputs have not yet completed their required processing.

iii) To continue to deal with every data item that has completed its process of analysis in order to understand what they are and mean, moving them along through this ongoing process of updating your Consciousness and dealing with all of its requirements.

And so your brain's complete processing cycle of the creation, the ongoing updating and instigating actions from the data status of your consciousness continues. Your reactions to its requirements continue, ad infinitum, as described in each cycle, detailed in **A)** to **C)** above, repeating itself throughout your life every 4ms. *This means it will have been repeated 250 times every second, ad infinitum.*

Question 4 – What are the criteria by which your brain decides what conditions or situations to prioritise taking action upon?

Above all else, your brain's inbred priority is always keeping you safe. You will always deal first with any safety issue that presents the biggest threat to your safety and proceed on this basis. If you have completed all safety issues and have moved on to activities **C)** but your M.C. has noted a new safety issue has occurred, it will immediately stop attending to activities **C)** and return to **A)**. Also, if you have dealt with half of **A)** issues and a new safety issue appears, which is of more importance and consequence than those being dealt with or those pending, you will prioritise the new one.

In reality, dependent upon what you are actually doing, you may consciously decide to prioritise something that goes against your inbred objective of keeping you safe at all times. An example is stopping a goal being scored in a football match, despite noting that in doing so, you are presenting a serious safety risk to yourself of perhaps incurring a very severe head injury.

Also, the usual sequence of events will be that, as your consciousness is updated with safety issues of major or minor importance, and with more or less important data, situations, or decisions to be made, your M.C. is attempting to conduct a masterful orchestration of the increasingly and rapidly, ever-changing conditions with which you are surrounded. It prioritises moving some actions along, then goes back to a previous activity and moves that along, balancing and sometimes cajoling extremely challenging, interactive, non-static and complex situations.

Question 5 – How important is the activity of filtering/ignoring some data carried out within the creation of your consciousness?

I firmly believe that the action of your M.C. in filtering out/ignoring unimportant incoming data in the context of your current situations is absolutely crucial for updating and creating of the most valid, worthwhile and useful state of your consciousness. It means that you stay safe and only process the conditions and situations that are important to you in that moment. On some occasions, you may filter out as much as 90% of all incoming data.

Frequently, this filtering will crucially prevent your brain from becoming totally overwhelmed with too much incoming data, the consequences of which could be, at worst, raw, emotional fear, confusion and possibly a life-threatening situation and, at best, leave you in a state of significant confusion.

Question 6 – Is some form of awareness (people commonly say self-awareness) part of your consciousness?

I believe the answer to this question is most certainly yes. Your updated consciousness provides you with and makes you aware of all information that you are surrounded by, which relates directly to you and your prevailing circumstances in that moment. Also, particularly at times, a vitally important part of the detailed makeup that your consciousness should include is awareness of your emotional state and the emotional climate existing around you. This emotional climate relates to and connects with your prevailing situation and circumstances and is generally created by one or more individuals who are also involved.

This produces, on occasion, quite a complex set of interreactive emotional conditions due to the emotional complexity of the situation combined with the complexity of the characters of the people who are involved with you. We humans, some more than others, are highly complex creatures and require immediate and careful understanding and dealing with.

Part of the human decision-making process always includes the element of our prevailing Emotional State, which can be overpowering if left uncontrolled. Therefore, it is of great importance to be aware of both your and other people's Emotional State whilst your and their consciousness are being processed. This awareness will potentially produce far better quality and appropriate decision-making conclusions and their resultant actions for all concerned.

Question 7 – Where does reality fit with your consciousness?

I think that your consciousness can also be referred to as your reality. This is because it's exclusively related *to you* with your unique personal perspective, individual view, exclusive sense and understanding of the world you are in and surrounded by in each moment of your time on this earth.

I believe that it is essential to know and therefore be aware that someone standing next to you at any time will ostensibly be experiencing the same sights and information coming into their brain from their senses as you. However, despite the aforementioned, they will not have developed *exactly the same consciousness* or describe the same set of reality relating to their senses.

In the same moment, if your consciousnesses could be compared in detail, they would be found to have some significant differences, particularly in some categories of incoming data and also in what incoming data was to be acted upon.

*You could say that each person's **unique** reality is **uniquely** processed within their **unique** brain – what a powerful statement of the resultant combination of three uniques!*

Question 8 – To what extent does each person's level or degree of intelligence affect the development, breadth and depth of perception of the creation of their

consciousness and, therefore, its resultant worth and value to them?

OVERVIEW: I believe that fundamentally, your overall level of intelligence is created from the interactive combination of all of your prevailing characteristics, capabilities, skills and knowledge. All of these qualities comprise of many factors, and each factor has a certain level of quality or contribution to the resultant level of your intelligence.

These qualities reside within your Master Conductor's departments. Whenever your intelligence is required, your M.C. brings it to bear, to assist in processing the situation, which, in this case, is the creation/updating of your consciousness.

Your intelligence plays a key role in the detailed process of the creation of your consciousness, not only but specifically with its ability to create your original thoughts.

Question 9 - Where is your consciousness?

I believe that your consciousness permanently resides in its current updated state, within your brain and your mind, It is located inside a department in Section 1.0. in a group of departments within the extensive set of departments that I collectively call your Master Conductor. (See Subchapter 2.2.1, Question H for more information about Section 1.0.)

Question 10 – Why do you have your consciousness and how is it utilised?

I believe that the two primeval, fundamental reasons for the creation of your consciousness are:

a)   To meet the <u>priority</u> objective of constantly keeping you physically safe, having a healthy body and an emotionally healthy mind throughout your lifetime.

b)   To provide <u>the foundational part of the process</u>, enabling you to make the <u>most appropriate decisions and actions</u> to achieve your optimum intellectual and functional objectives during each moment within your world and throughout your lifetime.

I believe that your consciousness is the *absolute foundation* upon which you as a unique individual functionally stand and can so successfully operate, with and within this incredibly complex, fascinating, ever-changing and challenging world, for fourscore years or more.

Your brain performs faultlessly, and your M.C. functions with a small percentage of mistakes, dependent upon the prevailing state of your Emotional Health combined with your personality and with any ongoing self-created difficulties.

I believe that your consciousness is also utilised by making you fully aware of everything around you and what it all means to you. It makes you aware of all details **relevant to you** as a unique individual in the moment on this earth, including your own bodily state, thoughts and all of the states and conditions in your immediate vicinity and beyond. All of this culminates in giving you a sense of self. You are consciously, fully aware of yourself – who you are and how you are as a person, plus how you relate to other people and the detailed world of your surroundings and beyond in each moment of your time.

Whilst you are awake, I think your consciousness exists on an ongoing and continually updated, constant and complete basis and continues to exist at a very much reduced state of awareness whilst you are asleep. This is mainly because your visionary senses are shut down and because the rate of change of the data sensed by your other senses is significantly reduced during this time.

During sleep, the primary purpose of your consciousness is to attempt to ensure the safety of you, your wife, children and or others who you care for, who may also be in your vicinity. As you sleep, the source of incoming data from which your consciousness is derived is primarily your hearing, B.H.S.M.S. and your internal thoughts. With some degree of sensing ability, a small element of data comes from your taste, smell and touch, but zero from your vision.

SUBCHAPTER 6.1.2: Your mind

Question 1 – Do you have a mind, or is it an illusion? If not a myth, what is it fundamentally?

I believe that your mind is not an illusion. It exists as an incredibly powerful intellectual facility – the product of a vast number of all of your different Category 1B departments within your brain, each having a biologically physical existence and clearly defined role within your brain's ongoing functionality.

Question 2 – What are your mind's fundamental roles?

I believe that, in order for your mind to carry out its numerous and vital roles for you, it is active at all times, whilst you are awake and whilst you are asleep. It operates across an extensive range of levels and types of activity, dependent upon the type and quantity of work it has to carry out in each moment.

You mind works with your M.C., continuously and tirelessly, with the objectives of keeping you safe physically, functionally and mentally. At the same time, it attends to your prevailing needs, enabling you to execute and satisfy all of your required Intellectual Objectives and Physical Functionalities to live the life you wish, every second throughout your lifetime.

Question 3 – What is your mind comprised of?

Within the boundary of your total and complete mind, which is the only one you have, I believe the following two major collections of departments of your brain exist:

Collection 1 – Many multiples of groups, the majority of which are your vast number of Category 1B departments.

Collection 2 – Your M.C.'s family of numerous departments, comprising the remainder of your Category 1B departments that are located within your mind.

Your M.C. is comprised of sections 1.0 to 11.0.

Section **1.0** is where your updated consciousness is housed in your Data Review Scanning System.

Sections **6.0** and **8.0** are where a large part of the creation of your intelligence is sourced.

Section **7.0** is where your soul resides.

(See Subchapter 2.2.1, Question H for more information.)

I believe that your mind does not contain or have any actual control of any of your brain's other two departments (Category 1 and 1A), as they are located within the core of your brain.

Question 4 – Where is your mind located?

I believe that the Category 1B departments that comprise your M.C. are located inside a shell formation, around the outside of the central core of your brain. This position offers the vitally important conductor of your mind and brain's functionality excellent protection from physical harm and attack from serious infection. The remaining vast number of Category 1B Departments are located within a thick casing which completely encompasses the shell formation containing your M.C. departments.

Your Category 1 and 1A departments are located in the central core of your brain. Collections of these vitally important departments for your brain and body's continued healthy functionalities are located on both halves of the core. This arrangement offers these collections maximum protection from physical damage and attack from any serious infections.

This positioning achieves the overall shortest length and time for data transmission and receipt for these departments' most important communications. This enables your brain's processing time to be the fastest possible, providing you with maximum possible safety and your body's functionality to ensure safety and many other benefits rapidly.

Question 5 – Where does your mind originate, how does it develop, and what are its responsibilities?

Potentially, I believe that your mind exists at conception, with its vast number of departments growing, developing and improving, many before your birth and most beyond. Some will continue to improve to the end of your life, providing you remain in good emotional and physical health, retain your zest and energy for life and continue to learn.

Your mind is responsible for every consideration, objective, thought and related action you take throughout your life. The only exceptions to this are the processing of the considerations and their resultant actions of each of your:

a) Fully-Automatic Control Systems, housed in your Category 1 Departments which control, for example, your heart and blood sugar level.

b) Semi-Automatic Control Systems, housed in your Category 1A Departments for bowel control, passing water, etc.

Question 6 – What is the relationship between your mind and your Master Conductor (M.C.)?

I believe that your Master Conductor exists at the core of and is the hub of your mind. It is You_In terms of managing, influencing, overseeing and effecting most of your brain's activities. In my opinion, your M.C.'s role within your mind is absolutely the most important and critical one of all of the collection of activities throughout the whole of your brain.

Under the management and control of your M.C., it and your mind work together. They are continually presented with ever-changing, ongoing, incoming situations, varying conditions and questions that you, as a person, are challenged with, have to consider and deal with at every waking moment.

Your mind and M.C., with its crucially important intelligence, make considerations, decisions and take actions, based upon all the data which your prevailing consciousness comprises.

Question 7 – How does your brain keep you safe at all times?

I have often referred in the book to your brain's first priority, which is to keep you safe at all times. To look more closely at this, we can split it into two questions:

a) **Where in your brain is this rule located?**
b) **How in detail is this objective actually achieved?**

Answer to a)

This priority and instinctive drive is located in Section 7.0, inside one of the departments of your Master Conductor, where your **soul resides**. This department likely originates before birth and grows in content when accompanied by other extremely important priorities and rules that you experience, learn from and adopt as you continually develop as a person.

Answer to b)

To achieve keeping you safe, all the numerous departments containing many different skills and knowledge under the key roles of your soul and, most notably, under your M.C., all exist within your brain. Their collective knowledge and capability required encapsulated by your intelligence, when called upon, are brought to bear to satisfy each unique prevailing objective fully. This means you can react and respond rapidly and appropriately to any danger or threat, maintaining your physical, emotional and mental safety.

SUBCHAPTER 6.1.3: Your soul

Question 1 – Do you have a soul, or is it an illusion? If it does exist, what is it?

I believe that the soul is not an illusion. It exists, not as a physical presence, but as a set of information and descriptions that collectively represent all of your behavioural characteristics, attitudes, priorities and potentially related actions. It also includes very important rules, objectives and limits. All of these conditions are wrapped up in such a manner that when other people meet you, what they see and emotionally feel about you relates to what your soul is projecting outwardly towards them. This mainly comes from your external facial expressions and body language. However, it can also be seen from within by some people, through your eyes or as an aura around your head.

Question 2 – What is the basic definition of your soul?

In my opinion, your soul is defined as the very essence of what you are like as a person and human being. It comprises your codes and rules of conduct, intellect, emotional and physical energy, your spirit, emotion, humour (or lack of), plus your degree of detailed awareness and empathy towards other human and living entities, especially when you sense they are in trouble.

To emphasise this, if you were to look at the face of a robot, I believe you would never see or feel any of the elements stated in the definition above, even with the best possible quality of manufacture, care and attention put into its creation. It is primarily for these reasons why I think some people feel a degree of emotional discomfort when interacting with robots compared with interacting with humans.

Question 3 – Are there different types of souls?

Yes, there are many kinds of souls. Here is a list of some of the different types and variations. Your soul is likely to comprise a combination of a number of them:
- A hardy soul - A kindly soul
- A troubled soul- A tortured soul
- A happy soul- A brave soul
- A godly soul- A fatherly soul
- A motherly soul- An artistic soul
- A creative soul- An enlightened soul
- A conscientious soul- An angry soul
- A lazy soul- A hardworking soul
- A frightened soul

Question 4 – Can you see someone's soul?

I believe you feel that you are looking at a person's soul whilst studying someone's facial expressions. If someone allows you to do it, you can look **into** a person's soul whilst peering intently into their eyes. This is when you can emotionally connect incredibly closely. You can also see, smell and feel their fear (or other emotional states, if present) displayed in their eyes and on their face. I also think you can see it in someone's eyes if they are quite seriously ill, particularly emotionally.

Question 5 – Where is your soul?

I think your soul resides inside your mind, within your brain, in one of a group of departments in Section 7.0. They are within the extensive set of Departments that I collectively call your Master Conductor.

Question 6 – Why do you have your soul, and how is it utilised?

I believe your soul is a significant part of the decision-making process that your M.C. utilises when deciding on its objectives and what actions to take in response to every situation you have to deal with. It imparts a human element of consideration into every decision you make so that they are not based entirely upon cold, hard facts and logic. This would be the case if a man-made decision-making machine, for example, a robot, was employed, unless the human designer, for some particular reason, decided to include some emotional elements in the machine's decision-making process.

It is of the utmost importance that, for you to make the necessary and best quality decisions, to benefit yourself, at the time of decision-making, you are always consciously aware of:

a) Your emotional state.

b) The emotional climate around the decisions you are deliberating upon.

This will enable you to be aware, when your emotional reactions to certain situations are likely to play a dominant, if not overriding, role in your final decision. Therefore, you can control or moderate these emotional urges, enabling your final decision to be a good or, at least, a better one.

I believe your soul gives you a sense of identity, of how you feel about yourself. You have a sense of uniqueness that other discerning and observant people detect and connect with, hopefully to your mutual benefit. Your soul also enables you to give love to others and receive love from them.

In my opinion, your soul enables you to be emotionally receptive and sense emotional conditions from others, even when they are sometimes extremely subtle, having minimal substance and state. Therefore, it is a key player in enabling those who can to have gut instinct or feelings about other people and in many situations in life.

For example, during work interviews, I was able to feel, 'something is not quite right here.' I looked out for any particular category of question, which created a definite change and an air of unease from the interviewee. If and when I found this reaction, I would delve into this area of concern to unearth whatever was at the root of what I had sensed. I could then take the appropriate decisions and actions resulting from my findings.

SUBCHAPTER 6.1.4: Who and what is 'You'?

OVERVIEW: *I believe that this often used, very basic three-letter word, despite its relative simplicity, conveys a wide range of meanings and references to You and to every other living human being. It also embraces the very essence of how every living human, animal and living entity, having been born, functions, survives, grows up and lives its life.*

a) *You* are your brain, and your brain is *You*.

b) *You* is the sum total of YOU.

c) *You* are encompassed by the whole of your name.

d) *You* comprise all of your hardware and all of your software.

e) *You* comprise the whole of your body, including your entire brain.

f) *You* comprise the whole of your character and all of your soul.

g) *You* are a unique human being, compared with anyone who has ever lived, who is alive today and is yet to be born.

This statement is astounding and mentally tingling, but nonetheless, I believe it to be true.

h) _You_ comprise the trillions and trillions of detailed items and points of data and information encompassing all your experiences from the day you were born to NOW. This data is all stored in your many multitudes of billions of memory cells. Together with your character and soul, providing you have a fairly typical and healthy life, this data and these experiences combine to create your responses to the myriad of decisions you have to make and their related actions, multiples of millions of times every day.

i) If you took off all of your clothes and adornments, stepped inside a box and closed its lid, the box would contain all of _you_ – nothing more, nothing less. If someone opened the box and looked all around you, they would still only see the superficial you. They would have to learn about all of the contents and data within every department in your brain to know and understand the realities of what _you_ as a person are comprised of._

j) Last, but certainly not least, and the most important reference or meaning of You is that _You_ are your Master Conductor. This is the key part of _You_ that works with and within your mind, organising, planning, coordinating and utilising all your activities.

SUBCHAPTER 6.1.5: How do your consciousness, mind, character, soul, You, and your M.C. coexist and functionally interreact?

I believe that your Master Conductor is driven by your character, soul and its intelligence to manage and conduct its own departments, which collectively utilise your other Category 1B departments, all of which are housed within the boundaries of your mind.

Your Category 1A departments are not within your mind, but your M.C. is aware of their objectives and assists them when required. The combined results of the incredible power and capability of all of these departments, including your intelligence, consciousness and mind, with its all-powerful M.C., keep you healthy and safe. It also means you create all of your decisions and actions during every part of every waking second and at a reduced level of awareness whilst you are asleep for the whole of your life.

SUBCHAPTER 6.2: Why has your consciousness and its creation been so particularly hard for people to understand fully?

I think that there are a number of reasons for this difficulty that people have of understanding your consciousness. Here is a list of the ones that immediately come to mind:

1.0) A failure to see that your consciousness is involved with every consideration and the resultant action that you take.

2.0) A failure to see that your whole brain's functionality is always based upon the simplest possible way of carrying out everything it is doing. Looking for complex explanations of its functionality will never unearth its operating mysteries simply because they do not exist.

3.0) Your brain lives inside your body, and I believe that the fundamental _you_ lives inside your brain. However, because _initially,_ you see, feel and sense the world from _outside_ your brain through your eyes and other senses, it seems that you are looking into your brain from an external position. Therefore you feel, or some people feel that they somehow exist outside their brain. I propose that this feeling/perception significantly adds to the other difficulties listed.

4.0) I think that the basic process of any person striving to use their own brain to unravel the extremely complex puzzle of how their brain works is, almost by definition and expectation, always going to be extremely difficult. It may actually be that there prevails an automatic, self-protective mechanism deep within our brains designed to attempt to stop this process of understanding from being successful. This thought may seem bizarre to you, but it came to mind as I typed this point, so I included it.

5.0) This thought brought to mind another thought, which I decided not to type, but to leave it to your imagination and comments if ever comes the appropriate moment in our future of us meeting face-to-face! xxxxx xxxx xxx dxxx xxxy.

6.0) I believe that another foundational key to understanding your brain's functionality is to realise that your Master Conductor exists, and without this crucial part of your brain's operation, it would be unable to achieve what it does. Also, without recognising the existence of your M.C., it is impossible to start to make sense and progress through the whole of its integrated and fiercely complex functionality.

All of this complex functionality is compounded by its incredible speed and, in many parts of its operations, the feature of true parallel functionality, where on occasions, if appropriate, many of your brain's different processing activities all take place simultaneously.

In just having re-read this piece as part of another of my many self-reviews whilst coming to the end of completing my book, I had an original, self-enlightening thought. Wouldn't it be wondrous to be able to copy and accurately replicate all of this universally astounding activity and capability that your brain produces/creates in the form of sounds/music?

I can hear the base/foundational multi-faceted sounds of the continuous ebb and flow of the creation of your consciousness running at 250 times every second. Above that, I hear the sounds that connect to the fearsome complexity at equally fearsome processing speeds of the decoding of your Vision Data. On top of and around this, I hear the processing activities of all the other incoming data for each of your remaining senses. Added to and on top of all of these sounds would be the interactivity between most of your departments and your M.C., communicating with phenomenal speed and complexity as it delicately and minimally teases the players as required.

Despite the vast amounts of everything going on, I am sure it would sound in overall harmony and produce many sounds coupled in balance and the same key, replicating the outputs that your brain creates and then delivers. I hope you have enjoyed sharing my imaginational moments of awe with me.

7.0) A significant number of people believe that your brain comprises of a similar structure with comparable details and operates with a similar functionality as that of a computer. I don't believe this at all. The fundamental and detailed differences between your human brain and a computer are profound. Because of these differences, I think that a man-made, robotic, semi-automatic machine or system, be it an autopiloted car or any other machine, will never come near to matching the overall capabilities of an average human being.

NB I use the word *never* quite deliberately, knowing that it means infinitely longer than a very long time.

To understand consciousness fully, there are a number of stages.

a) Firstly, I believe you have to have a feeling and then an understanding of the fundamental purpose of your consciousness.

b) Then, you will be able to progress to have a feeling and then understand of how it is derived.

c) You can eventually then understand the constitution of your mind and its relationship with your consciousness.

d) This will give you the feeling of the existence of something else and an understanding of the presence of your Master Conductor.

e) Then you will learn the makeup and relationship of You, your character and soul to each other and all of the above.

Once you have obtained some hopefully creditable propositions of understanding of the above that form the five key players in how your brain functions, you can begin to delve into more hopefully creditable ideas, proposals and understandings. These will have more and more details and depth of information about the workings of your magnificent, incredible, awe-inspiring brain throughout the whole Universe.

Crucially, during this whole process, constant checks must be made to hopefully conclude that each of the parts of the whole of your brain's proposed, interrelated systems dovetail, connect, support and are compatible with each other. This is essential across all of the different workings of your brain, or parts of the system would grind to a halt, or, worst case, the whole system's functionality would fight itself to some degree or another.

8.0) Additionally, and finally, I believe that it's impossible to define what anything is until you understand how it works. The more detailed you wish your definition to be, the greater the proportionate degree of detail your understanding of its functionality must inevitably be. It is a classic chicken and egg situation, which is fundamentally challenging to say the least.

SUBCHAPTER 6.3: Your sense of self. Why do you have it? What is it? And what creates it?

I believe that your sense of self is derived from your consciousness, which enables you to be fully aware of everything around you and <u>what it all means to you.</u> It is all achieved by you being aware of all details relevant to you as a unique individual in that moment on this earth.

To be aware of your own bodily state and all of the states and conditions in your immediate vicinity and beyond gives you a sense of self from being consciously, fully aware of yourself. You know who and how you are as a person, plus how you relate to other people and the complex world of your surroundings and beyond in each moment of time.

It is also a crucial part of the process that enables you to make decisions and take the related actions required to be made to achieve your optimum intellectual objectives and physical and emotional health and safety.

Your self also derives from your soul, giving you a sense of how you feel about yourself, plus your uniqueness and worth as a human being living in the world you function in and relate to.

SUBCHAPTER 6.4: Do we actually function in a multi-tasking manner?

The term 'multi-tasking' is stated very frequently and most commonly by women, often with the normally implied rider that men can't multi-task, but they can!

Before this question can be answered, I believe we need to define exactly what multi-tasking is.

My definition of true multi-tasking is: **Carrying out more than one task or activity simultaneously for an ongoing period of time.**

This functionality could also be called "parallel operation" conditions.

I think that your brain does truly multi-task in some areas of its functionality but not in others. However, it appears that it does because of the breakneck processing speed that it operates with.

Let's take the entire complex and detailed process of your brain creating/updating your consciousness, making decisions and taking actions in relation to it all. Your brain receives data from your five senses, B.H.S.M.S. and your internally-instigated thoughts.

It processes them all to understand their meaning to you. It selects what data presents a danger to you, decides what does not offer a threat but requires consideration, and deletes the rest. In some parts of this complex process, there are five or seven multi-sub-step processes operating in **true parallel functionality.** In other sections, there is a **step sequence functionality** operating, when all of the data is presented to your M.C. for consideration, one at a time.

Overall, to you, it appears that all of this data enters your brain and is dealt with in the same instant of time, but this is not the case. It is simply due to the ferocious processing speeds plus most considerations taking place way below your conscious awareness that it appears this way.

The embedded and fully-automatic operation of your vital functions within your brain – your heart, body temperature control, etc., all operate continuously, independently and simultaneously, throughout your lifetime. This is without any direct involvement of your M.C., so it is correct to say that your brain is multi-taking in these areas of operation.

But if you consider your brain's actual functionality in responding to ongoing situations, you have to make continual, multiple decisions of objectives and their required resultant actions and implementation. For example, let's consider the range of skills necessary for driving your car along an extremely crowded street.

a)   On an ongoing basis, you are employing many Developed, Semi-Automatic Skills form your many Category 1B departments, including steering your car, changing gear, controlling the speed, deciding when to brake or accelerate, etc.

b) You are employing many consciously-considered and activated decisions to carry out this very complex, multi-faceted process safely and with ease. This includes predicting where the moving people, cars, animals, cyclists, many shoppers etc., will be within your zone of and, therefore, potential danger within the next 2 seconds.

You could argue you are multi-tasking due to your successful control, management and safe passage of your car, through and amongst all of these obstacles and moving articles during your passage of time in this shopping area. You are making decisions and initiating resultant actions in highly complex situations. This is achieved by employing all of your developed, Semi-Automatic skills, each of which is operating continuously.

However, in every miniscule moment, your M.C. is engaging by selecting, one at a time, one of your car-driving activities, fine-tuning where required, to deal with the changing prevailing conditions. It is managing and coordinating all of these skills and activities as required in the process of driving your car safely.

So, whilst you may appear to be carrying out true multi-tasking as you successfully coordinate and employ many developed skills to drive and control your car safely, by literal definition, you are only nominally multi-tasking. However, this does not reduce in any way the incredible capability and power of your brain's performance, due to the number of incredibly accurate, complex processing decisions and resultant activities it is carrying out every second.

A particularly common example is when you are communicating with someone in a conversation, and they continue to read, type, or both. Although they think they are multi-tasking during this conversation, I believe that their brain is actually flitting extremely quickly, to and from reading, listening, typing and speaking. Therefore, they are not entirely focused for long on any of these four activities. Consequently, they will operate in an inefficient and, probably at times, inaccurate manner.

SUBCHAPTER 6.5: Free will. Do you have it?

I have noticed, during recent years, it has become an increasing practice for the media to seek opinions about all sorts of topics without first establishing precisely what something means. So, again, before I can accurately, correctly and properly, in terms of my opinion, answer this question, I must define what I understand Free Will to mean.

Free will is having an *opinion* about <u>anything</u>, whether it be *deciding* on and *implementing* an *action* you wish to take, or having an *belief* about some politically-driven topical rule/ regulation or anything.

The topic could range from fairly minor up to of major importance to you, but the key is that you openly, honestly and genuinely feel that you have arrived at your decisions <u>on your</u>

<u>own.</u> You weren't coerced, directed or pushed to any degree by any person or organisation in any way whatsoever during your deliberations.

As a human being, I believe unquestionably, that <u>theoretically,</u> you do have Free Will, providing you <u>wish to</u> and are <u>allowed</u> to express it. This is compared to a man-made and programmed computer that does only what it has been pre-programmed/told to do, but only concerning questions and situations it has been pre-designed and pre-prepared to recognise and respond to.

However, if you stop and think a little below the surface about the process used to decide what to do or think about at any one time, it depends upon a combination of a multitude of actual and possible influencing factors. These all <u>relate to the situation</u> you have been exposed to, several of which you may have been consciously aware of at the time of your deliberations, and others, perhaps not.

A list of some of these influencing factors are:

1) Your genes.
2) Your character.
3) How you feel emotionally in that moment, in relation to the topic of consideration.
4) Whether you are biased about the topic of consideration.
5) Your vast array of experiences throughout your life to date that relate to the topic of consideration.
6) Whether you have been subjected to related brain-washing of some type: face-to-face, in the media, by advertising tools, whether you have succumbed to it, and whether or

not you have been consciously aware it has taken place at the time.

7) Whether you feel that one or more people you respect have a personal and maybe biased self-interest in the decision you ultimately made, and they may have deliberately tried to influence your judgement.

8) What information you have collected and been presented with about the question you want to deal with, and whether this information is correct, biased or appropriate to use. (This is another minefield – what is correct, what is the truth, and what is a combination of these?)

9) Whether you have previously been faced with making this decision or one very similar and, because of the negative consequences that resulted, you make this current decision accordingly.

10) Whether your current and future ambitions are related to this decision.

11) Whether your age, health, hobbies, the state of your marriage/relationship have some bearing on the decision.

12) Your understanding and interpretation of what you may have heard and seen in relation to the topic of consideration.

So, the fundamentally simple, superficial answer as a human being is yes, **you do have free will**.

But the answer, following some in-depth thought, is not so easy because you could argue that you have been pre-programmed with some, or possibly the majority of your views by other human beings. These could be your parents, family, friends, teachers, work colleagues.

If you look at each item on the list above, **1)**, **2)** and **5)** would almost certainly have influenced your decision. You would probably find that a fair number of the other ones may have, at least to some degree, also affected your decision.

In conclusion, as with so many things in life, if you take a simple, superficial, shallow and narrow view upon each one, you will probably fairly quickly arrive at a response, make decisions and take related actions. However, later you may wonder why these decisions created such consternation and difficulties.

I have come to believe that a significant percentage of decisions made by a considerable portion of people in many walks of life fall short. They have not taken into account the necessary depth and breadth of thoughts and considerations required, nor the multifaceted structures and layers that exist and prevail about the importance of the topic in question.

This invariably results in poor quality decisions, the consequence of which is a long list of avoidable errors and difficulties. There are generally additional financial costs etc., too, resulting in a large expenditure of human hours of effort and money to rectify.

SUBCHAPTER 6.6: Are you the same person today as yesterday?

Does this mean – are you the same person today as you were yesterday, when comparing your emotional and physical characteristics and all of your memories, experiences, knowledge, strengths, skills, weaknesses and fixed views about a large number of topics?

If my interpretation of this topical question is correct, then I would answer no, for the following reasons.

As a fully alive, active and energised human being, you automatically continue to learn, change and develop. The amount of change from day to day as expressed in percentage units over your life span to date will usually be extremely minute. However, sometimes, even one item of transformation may be fundamental to your view of a significant part of your world. Due to continually having new experiences, which may alter previously held views as you learn new facts about a whole range of topics, as a consequence, data in your memories will have modified, removed or added to.

The result of this means that when related to a prevailing situation, say today, at noon, your decision or actions may be different than compared to the following day if presented with exactly an identical situation. You are *not quite* the same person as you were yesterday, regarding all of the data stored within your brain, as a consequence of some or all of the reasons detailed above. You will also be 24-hours older.

SUBCHAPTER 6.7: *All humans have a brain, consciousness, mind, character, soul and intelligence. Do animals, including birds, fish, insects, reptiles and other living entities also all have these characteristics?*

Let's go through each of these points one at a time for ease.

Consciousness: I believe that all living beings and entities mentioned in the title have some form and capability of a consciousness. Therefore, they have a related awareness of their surroundings, bodily state and how their existence within their immediate locality fits into and relates to others.

Living entities are at the lowest level of the capability pyramid, and each having its own form of consciousness is absolutely vital. This is so they can successfully stay safe and obtain food or energy to live and survive, despite the potential dangers that exist for nearly all of them. This is particularly the case for those living lower down the spectrum of size and capability than others who inhabit the same living space or area.

Brain: *Apart from living entities*, I believe that all other living beings mentioned in the title have some basic format and capability of a brain, covering a very wide spectrum. The way that all of these brains function, at their absolute most basic level, is the same or similar to the rudimentary functionality of a human being's brain.

In all cases, the living being's brain's role is to enable them to create and update their consciousness to keep safe. Also, to govern their moment-to-moment and daily ongoing activities to take actions appropriate to their needs. For example, take in food or what keeps them alive, procreate, sleep and rest to recover their physical and mental energies ready for their next wakeful period in their life.

For each different type of animal and bird, etc., the degree, range and depth of capability of their Brain will be related and appropriate to satisfy their ongoing requirements. The fundamental differences are that human beings' brains operate at a far greater range and depth of capability, capacity and understanding than any other living beings' brains are capable of, with human beings at the summit of the pyramid of capability.

Mind: I don't believe that living entities have a mind, but some insects and fish probably have a form of mind. I think all other living beings have a mind, each of which has the necessary degree and range of ability to create and update their consciousness and carry out the decision-making required to survive in their normal habitat successfully.

Character and Soul: I don't believe that living entities or insects have a character and soul, but I think some animals, including birds, fish and reptiles, do have them. I also believe that only those living beings with a greater depth and range of capability have a character and a soul. These living beings show awareness of the emotional state of beings they interact with in their lives. Part of their decision-making contains emotional and soul elements to it at times.

Their degree of character, soul, and the awareness and use of emotional states in comparison to the human degrees of these characteristics depends on how far up the pyramid of capability they are.

Intelligence: I believe that intelligence exists over an extensive range of capabilities in the same or similar cohorts. It is created from the combined benefit of many different factors, skills, capabilities and knowledge. Intelligence can also manifest itself and be utilised in very many different situations in life. I also think it exists in various forms and categories.

An example of **one type** of intelligence's application and benefit is the ability to solve problems or successfully resolve challenging situations that you have not faced or had to deal with before, nor seen the solution by watching others solve them.

I believe that humans generally are obviously blessed with a relatively high starting level of intelligence. I also consider that some forms of animals, including some birds, reptiles and sea animals may have a relatively lower but fair level of intelligence. Some animals, birds and other beings are thought to display intelligence through their activities. However, in some cases, it may be that they have inherited abilities through their genes from skills that their predecessors happened upon. Therefore, it is a combination of luck and circumstances rather than intrinsic intelligence alone, so observing their actions could lead to the wrong conclusions.

SUBCHAPTER 6.8: *When you die, what happens to your consciousness, mind, soul and all of your memories?*

I very firmly believe that, as shown by my definitions and descriptions of each of these vitally important faculties that you have, they each exist, live and function within your brain. While you are alive, with your brain functioning healthily, each of these faculties will be alive, healthy and fully functioning. When you die, a few seconds later, your brain will die, along with all of its vast range of activities. So, inevitably, will your consciousness, mind, soul and all of your memories because they exist and function within departments in your brain.

Some people propose that your soul leaves your body and goes off to heaven upon your death. If my definition of your soul, what it comprises and where it exists are correct, then, if it did leave your body and relocate to heaven, whilst it still existed, it would have to go through a kind of multi-stepped, sequenced process similar to this:

a)   Change its state of detailed existence from being coded within actual/physical neurological sets of your brain cells.

b)   Be copied into another format/state that can retain its new state of existence within its own makeup or structure.

c)   This would need to be capable of coming out of your brain and through your skull.

d)   It would have to travel to heaven, wherever that is located, via some form of transportation energy.

e)   It would be relocated into a suitable medium in heaven.

f) It would be able to function by some form of energy under some form of direction and control.

Additionally, each of the above steps in the process would have to have something or a form of guidance and control. Maybe the Grand Creator has been at work, once again, to provide all of the requirements as above, including utilising some of these astronomical number of celestial bodies that occupy the vastness of this Universe. They must have some purpose.

If not, then when you die, and your brain immediately and rapidly begins to die, your consciousness, mind, soul and all of your memories, probably in that order, will also follow the demise of your brain.

SUBCHAPTER 6.9: Are there other planets with a life-form similar to ours anywhere in the vastness of this Universe?

In this life of ours, I have noted that very occasionally, what seems totally implausible, completely unrealistic and seen to be impossible **actually comes about**, with most people saying – "I just can't believe it!"

But sometimes, what seems absolutely a definite no-brainer, like, for example, at the very least, one other planet similar to ours will exist along with a similar life-form, either more or less advanced than ours, *turns out to be WRONG*.

We have to be wary of the power of wishing for something far too much that, for quite a long list of reasons, we almost crave it, such that we should stop and ponder a little.

It seems to me that most people involved with trying to find data about this big question are almost willing it to be true. Plus, there is the basic percentage aspect to consider. Surely, out of the vast astronomical number of galaxies, stars and planets that we estimate exist, even if a minute percentage of them could maintain a life-form even vaguely similar to ours, this would amount to a substantial number. Therefore, there must, at the very least, be a number of them!

But, my **feeling and instinct** about this big question is that **there are no other planets with a form of life anything like, let alone similar to ours, anywhere in the vastness of this Universe.**

Additionally, this planet of ours is naturally suitable for our human race to inhabit for our basic requirements for comfortable survival. How can we justify spending an astronomical amount of time, money and scientific resources attempting for a minute percentage of our world population to live/survive on these other bodies that are totally unsuitable for us humans to live on? It seems to me that we should spend all of these resources on our own planet and improve and maintain what we have.

As I was carrying out the last read of my book, one more point on this topic came to mind, which was this. Presumably, the Grand Creator, who created the overall process or system from which the observable Universe, which we see and understand today was the result of, surely must have had an objective or a reason and therefore a purpose for creating it. It can't **just be for us to live on our own planet and be alone within the whole of this limitlessly bounded Universe** – can it?

Is it to house other beings, of other forms of life totally and utterly different to ours? Is it where all people from our planet and maybe other planets go to live after dying?

So what is and what can be the purpose or purposes of the whole of the Universe and all it comprises, beyond our planet and our neighbours?

This is a serious question I am posing, and in doing so, it has raised another query in my mind, which is that I don't recall hearing this question raised before. It may have been raised, and I have missed it.

If I haven't missed it, then why has it not been broached before many times in the wonderful T.V. programmes on astronomy, for example? This question has no doubt been raised amongst the philosophers of our world, but surely it needs highlighting more generally. Does the presence of the Universe somehow give the continuing existence of our planet more security? Can the whole of our Universe exist for literally no purpose at all, ever? I find this question creates a strange, uncomfortable and hanging unease!

SUBCHAPTER 6.10: What is reality, and what is the truth? Are they the same?

A former Prime Minister recently stated in a T.V. interview that reality and the truth were exactly the same, and this got me to thinking, was this correct?

SUBCHAPTER 6.10.1: What is reality?

A) OVERVIEW: The simple and perhaps automatic answer to what appears to be an extremely simple question could be, well, that is obvious, isn't it? The reality about anything, or things or any set of conditions that exist at anytime, anywhere in the world is simply that – what is there is what is there – no ifs, no buts. For argument's sake, it is what you see, hear and understand from what is very clearly stated or presented to you, the recipient of all the data or information that your eyes and other senses receive and your brain processes and understands.

But once again, let's give this the appropriate depth and breadth of thought that this question deserves. Consider what we are all presented with approximately fourteen million times every day whilst we are awake, as our consciousness is updated throughout our lives. Bearing this in mind, the answer to this question is far from being as simple as it may first seem.

Example 1 – Different people experiencing ostensibly identical information presented by the same people at exactly the same moments in time.

A large group can be simultaneously presented with information over a period of time, each seeing exactly the same view, hearing identical words, and feeling the same emotional atmosphere at the same time, from ostensibly the same standpoint. For example, there are one hundred guests at a wedding reception, held in a large, open-plan room. Each of the bridal party due to make speeches is sitting on the prime guests' table at the head of the room to be clearly seen and heard by all others. Would each guest report seeing, hearing, experiencing and concluding exactly the same as all of the other 99 guests during the period of these speeches?

Afterwards, if you asked every one of the 100 guests of varied ages and nationalities the same 25 questions about what they had observed and they thought about their experiences, I suggest that you would receive a very wide range of views. This is despite ostensibly having had, received or witnessed an identical set of data, information and experiences.

Question 1 – How could these different people experience different realities from ostensibly the same information?

How everyone's brain responds to and processes the same experiences and information very much depends upon a long list of the combinational effects of the conditions and factors. These are very personal and specific to them and include, for example, their own personal opinions about so many experiences.

So, despite the fact that all of these guests are each exposed to nominally an identical set of experiences, this does not happen at all times, though. Each person, on occasion, will be focusing on different people, other activities and alternative viewing aspects, compared to what other people are focusing on. Therefore, they will be observing different details at certain points than others.

The exact process of how they **relate to and decode** each item of information entering their brain via their five senses, B.H.S.M.S., and internal thoughts, depends upon several things. They experience a combinational interaction to the incoming data based on their personal details of a related and connected selection from the following:

- Their life experiences and memories.
- Their character.
- Their soul.
- Their prejudices.
- Their hidden agendas.
- Their current and future ambitions.
- Their age, health, their hobbies, the state of their marriage and relationships.
- Their relationship to the people presenting the information.
- Whether they wished to be where they were at that particular time.

- Their understanding and interpretation of what they had heard and seen.
- Many more personal conditions and aspects of their life to date

Reality is totally related to what is in the brain of the beholder and is therefore uniquely related to the individual brain of each observer.

Question 2 – Where is reality created?

Reality data is always received, processed and created within and by the brain of each beholder.

The **reality** is that in that moment in time, it is raining, or you are in a situation that presents a danger to you, i.e. reality is something that is real around you, near you, potentially affects you and is available to be processed by your brain. It is only after your brain has processed it that it becomes *your personal reality of that moment.*

Question 3 – Where does reality fit with your consciousness?

I believe that your consciousness could also be referred to as **your reality**. It's exclusively related *to you* with your unique personal perspective, *your unique* view, your unique sense and understanding of the world you are in and surrounded by and how you should best respond to it in each moment of *your* time on this earth.

I think it is essential to know and therefore to be aware that someone standing next to you at any time will ostensibly be experiencing exactly the same views and information coming into their brain from their senses as you. However, despite the aforementioned, they will not have developed *exactly the same consciousness* or describe exactly the same set of reality relating to their senses.

In the same moment, if your consciousnesses could be compared in detail, they would be found to have some significant differences, particularly in some categories of incoming data and also in what incoming data was to be acted upon or ignored.

Two final points:

a)   If someone has directly presented information to you which is actually incorrect, it will still be a reality to you, the direct receiver of the data, even though it is wrong.

b)   I don't believe that people should ask the question – what is the **reality** about something. They should ask – what is the **truth** or the **facts** about something.

SUBCHAPTER 6.10.2: What is the truth?

B) OVERVIEW: The more I thought about "what is the truth" and how you seek to obtain it, the more I realised that it was nominally impossible to get the truth about most if not all things. The more complex/multi-faceted the creation of things, situations, conditions are, the more difficult seeking the truth about them becomes. This is because you are obtaining/receiving/relying upon a wide range of different types/categories of interactive data from other people and facilities. Most, if not all of it, is questionably correct, sufficiently accurate enough for a host of possible reasons.

Then, when you consider/hope that you have obtained all of the required data to decide what the truth actually is, your brain has to process it all and determine whether your conclusions are sufficiently accurate or correct to satisfy your objectives. What is the absolute truth about anything unless it is a very simple, one item, or condition, easy to verify in the moment? For example:

The sun is out, it is raining, or it is windy here, but these examples are more in the category of reality than the truth. These examples could be changed to become less simple by someone asking – How much is it raining? How windy is it? Has the sun been out here all of the time from 2 pm to 5:30 pm? This last example is definitely in the category of the truth.

SUBCHAPTER 6.10.2.1: The categories of the truth

When the truth about anything is being considered, I believe it falls into one of these three following categories.

a) **Category A** – When it occurred in the past and is completed, it is nominally the **Historical Truth**.

b)   **Category B** – When it is in the moment and ongoing, it is the **Current Truth**.

c)   **Category C** – When it is in the future, it is the **Predicted Truth**.

Please note that **Category B** will inherently contain, to some degree, categories **A**, **B** and **C** on an ongoing basis, the degree of which shall be due to the prevailing comments, assessments and considerations being carried out by you or whoever.

SUBCHAPTER 6.10.2.2: Some available tools that can be selected from as appropriate to the requirements for obtaining the truth about a Historical Truth.

1)   Locate, identify, gather and collect relevant available data.

2)   The use of normally dedicated and suitable measurement systems.

3)   Use graphs to display the relevant data.

4)   Utilisation of the knowledgeable and experienced assessment by humans of the relevant collected data.

5)   Establish systems that gather data about the various topics and objectives.

6)   Establish commonly accepted and adopted definitions of conditions etc., that relate to any data required to be logged and utilised. This will make comparisons of the same topics gathered in by different organisations, countries etc., to be sufficiently comparably valid.

7) The utilisation of information from newspapers, films, documentaries and books.

***SUBCHAPTER 6.10.2.3:** Some available tools that can be selected as required and appropriate for obtaining the truth about a Current Truth.*

As above, see 6.10.2.2.

SUBCHAPTER 6.10.2.4: Some available tools that can be selected as required and appropriate for seeking to obtain and support the truth about a Predicted Truth.

As above, see 6.10.2.2 **plus**:

1) Use predictive models with much relevant, realistic and sensible care.
2) The utilisation of graphs depicting the categories, historical, current and future.
3) I believe in the collective power of a relatively small group of:

a) Intelligent, solidly logical with good common sense human beings, not driven by any personal egos or other conflicting forces but by the common objectives of the group.
b) Who are held in high esteem by their peers.

c) They must also have many years of actual experience and knowledge in all of the multifactorial causes of all aspects of the fields in which predictions are required.

d) The power of the experienced human brain in assessing and weighing the combinational factors, concluding with an estimated outcome, is the human brain at its best and most powerful. It produces results that are likely to be the most accurate of any other system or process available to be considered.

NB A crucially important component of this system is having an extremely competent chairperson with good knowledge across all relevant fields of consideration, to control and efficiently manage this group effectively.

SUBCHAPTER 6.10.2.5: Some examples of attempting to establish the truth in everyday life activities.

These are the examples that we are going to explore over the next few pages. As a quick reminder, Category A is Historical Truth, Category B is Current Truth and Category C is Predicted Truth.

Example 1) In an ongoing tennis match, whilst a particular point is being played, was the tennis ball in or out? This is a Category B Truth.

Example 2) In an ongoing football match, was a player on the attacking side in an offside position? This is a Category B Truth.

Example 3) You are asked whether a particular person is honest? This is a Category A and B Truth.

Example 4) The U.K. citizens were asked to vote by the government in a referendum – Should the United Kingdom remain a member of the European Union or leave the European Union? This was basically asking for people to judge whether their future lives would be better remaining within the E.U. or not. This is a Category C Truth.

Example 5) Is the cost of the HS2 project, the high-speed train link, justifiable? This is a Category C Truth.

SUBCHAPTER 6.10.2.6: Examining the examples where the responsible and involved parties make herculean efforts to strive to obtain an acceptable, desired, accurate and truthful judgement.

A GENERAL BUT EXTREMELY IMPORTANT POINT TO CONSIDER FIRST:

A) Every measurement system is never 100% accurate. It always contains an amount of error, albeit occasionally extremely small.

One absolutely fundamental, crucially important fact to be aware of is that any data or information gathered, assessed, measured and then displayed on a meter, screen or whatever, is never precisely 100% accurate or correct, (i.e. in principle, it never has 0% error compared to the truthful, factual, value or actual condition being measured). This is simply because all measurement equipment systems inherently operate over an accuracy range of normally plus and minus a percentage of the **actual value or information or condition** being measured or assessed.

In general terms, a very good to good quality (expensive) equipment accuracy range is nominally between +5% to -5% to around +10% to −10% of the actual value, information or condition being measured or accessed. Less expensive measurement systems operate over +10% to -10% of the actual value or greater/worse. Generally, the smaller i.e. the more precise the accuracy range, the disproportionately more costly the system is to design, manufacture and maintain.

Example 1 – To determine whether the tennis ball landed inside the playing area or not to decide which player won that point.

This is a Category B Truth.

As I understand it, the **Hawk-eye system** used in tennis gathers information automatically from a number of cameras. They are part of a dedicated, custom-designed system to provide visual informational evidence, from which a judgement is made about where the ball landed.

I must make an extremely important point at this stage:

I haven't been able to obtain performance data for the Hawk-eye system. Therefore, I am presenting its principles **as I see them** with my **estimated performance data. I must apologise profusely to Hawk-eye or any other involved party if I am misleading anyone with any of my comments and suggestions**, which is certainly not my intention.

Having enjoyed immensely playing and watching tennis for very many years, I must congratulate the designers and the manufacturers responsible for the benefits that the Hawk-eye system has brought into serious, competitive tennis. It minimised the previous degrees of annoyance, frustration and very heated arguments that prevailed prior to Hawk-eye being utilised.

Here are my estimated thoughts for consideration:

1) Let's say the overall **actual** accuracy range of the Hawk-eye ball detection system is between **plus 3mm** to **minus 3mm** of the tennis ball's actual position when landing on the court.

2) Let's also say that in plan-view, the edge of the tennis ball **was just in/on the line** after a particular rally, i.e. this is the actual/truth condition.

3) However, The **displayed graphic** could have shown/pictured/measured the ball to be in the range of **between 3mm out** all the way to **3mm in.**

As I have already said, I don't have any actual data for the Hawk-eye system, so I am pulling those figures out of the air. This is to demonstrate the principles of how extremely complex and difficult a measurement system such as this actually is to satisfy all main parties who relate to it. Yet, in tennis, I believe they have certainly have handsomely succeeded.

Example 2 – To determine whether or not, in an ongoing football match, the attacking player was onside when the ball was passed forward, initiating an attack that culminated with the ball being projected into the defending side's goal, thus scoring a valid goal, providing no other infringement occurred during this period.

This is a Category B Truth.

Very importantly, please note:

I haven't been able to obtain any performance data and detailed information for the football VAR system, so I must state very clearly that I am presenting the principles and some details of it as I see it. Therefore, I must wholeheartedly apologise to Hawk-eye and any other company involved with the design and manufacture of the system, if I mislead anyone with any of my comments and suggestions. Again, I am trying to give my readers a feel of how horrendously difficult it is for these types of measurement and assessment systems to achieve even slightly better accuracy and benefits for all involved parties than the previous system, let alone a lot better.

Again as I understand it, fundamentally, you have a camera system referred to as the VAR (Video Assistant Referee) providing visual information. It can be used for a number of controversial football incidents, one of which is to review if the offside law is being broken or not.

With the offside situation in football, you have a scenario where one of the judgements required with assistance from the VAR is to answer these questions. Where precisely should the offside line be drawn? Was the attacking player behind this imaginary line when the ball was passed to them, thus allowing them to potentially be able to score a valid goal?

But, additionally, with the football system, you have the crucially added final feature of the measurement system visual display with all of its tools available. It is shown to human beings who study the visual information to decide whether the goal was valid or not, which in itself introduces a potential range of human error.

B) For someone to be able to decide whether these systems in Ex.1 & Ex.2 are acceptably accurate and reliable enough for their purpose, I believe they would, in an ideal world, ask the system designers and providers many questions for each system as appropriate.

In itself, this can create its own potential error and all of which can combine to create a cumulative error. I mention the various points above to show that most measurement systems and particularly those two above have an extremely difficult job to do with others, having an almost impossible one. None of them are easy and straightforward to design and operate with acceptable inaccuracies, such that the recipients of their judgements are sufficiently happy with their results.

I give great complements to the designers and manufacturers of the Hawk-eye tennis System and the VAR Football System for tackling and reducing what had been considerable thorny problems for very many years for spectators, players and their management teams.

C) The principles of the accuracy range applies not only to measuring data with measurement systems comprising of physically existing equipment primarily as in Ex.1 & Ex.2.
It also applies to gathering data about all of the other examples listed in 6.10.2.5 as it involves harvesting existing, actual data from many sources and includes personal opinions relating to some of these other examples.

Each collection part of a system, inherently includes its own degree of inaccuracy. At worst, it can be accumulatively negative or positive, resulting in a relatively very high level of inaccuracy range. Therefore, ideally, to successfully achieve your objective for the other examples listed in 6.10.2.5, you must first decide the approximately acceptable accuracy level you are seeking to achieve.

To form a sufficiently, acceptably accurate, truthful judgement about each everyday life activity that you are assessing, you must seek to obtain information relative to your subject that is:

1) Sufficiently acceptably accurate.

2) (Not easy, but) Presented by people who do not have hidden agendas; otherwise, they will leave important information out, use the expediency of telling lies, or present other unacceptable errors.

3) (Not easy, but) Not presented in a biased way.

4) Presented with all of the information you require to form a sufficiently accurate judgement – this sounds easy, but how do you judge when you have reached this position? You just have to go by your instincts.

5) Not presented to you based upon guesses about future unknowns. It is presented with supportable facts, or the information is at least shared stating it is a judgement without verifiable facts.

Question 1 – How do you establish what the accuracy range is of any data you have collected or been supplied with?

Ask the people who have provided the data and/or who have designed/established the system: What is its accuracy range? How did they or others arrive at these figures, and have they included any educated guesses? You could always ask to see their actual calculations, or estimations, although this could be tricky.

Let's get back to the examples of attempting to establish the truth in every-day life activities.

Example 3 – You are asked whether a particular person is honest.

This is a Category B Truth.

You can't definitively measure honesty. You can speak to the person being judged and ask them many relevant questions, including – would you describe yourself as being honest about everything, some things, etc.? Studying them extremely closely as they answer enables you to be able to commence forming a judgement. You can also speak to several people who have direct, relevant and detailed experiences of how the person has operated in the past and currently and take note of their opinions.

All of the information you eventually collect will be processed within your brain, resulting in an overall judgement. You may think that the person is honest or not, or you may decide you require more information.

Within the process of your investigations, your question may inevitably be broadened or narrowed based on your findings. For example, this particular person is always honest about situations related to themselves but not when it concerns any of their children because they cannot accept anything critical about them. Also, they may be unable to be honest about something that could put their job at risk. This may lead you to realise that their answers and your judgements may require some qualifying attachments.

Example 4 – UK citizens were asked to vote by the government in a referendum: Should the United Kingdom remain a member of the European Union or leave the European Union?

This is nominally a Category C Truth.

This was basically asking for people to judge whether the whole of their future lives would be better remaining within the EU or not.

This requires trying to predict the truth about the future of many different topics, some of which are of extreme complexity and of the utmost importance to the immediate, medium and long-term future of the whole of the UK's population. It is in the Category C truth group, which is the most difficult category of all to consider what the truth might be, compounded by requiring attempted predictions of the truth for many years into the future. Its sum total of difficulty is reflected in the many combined factors detailed in this Subchapter 6.10.2.

It also, requires for example, even minimally reasonably accurate predictions of the highly complex, ever changing, immense number of interactional, multifactorial causes that combine to create the future economic status of the UK's businesses and economies. Plus, to some extent, predictions of other countries' businesses and economies that we may deal with in the future, including probably with all countries currently within the EU.

To equip everyone eligible to vote knowledgeably on such a highly complex all-embracing set of topics that affected all aspects of their lives, their children and many future generations, they should have been provided with more associated information in a fairly easy to understand basic format.

D) A summary of important aspects.

Due to the comments above, the **summary of important points below**, and to receive a sufficient amount of **solid, clear, easy-to-comprehend information, the majority of voters** should have been presented with the following two lists of fundamentally basic information. They should have been given basic facts and basic predictions, such that they were then able to have a reasonably well-informed opinion with which to vote.

E) My suggested notes and information supplied, along with the voting form, are detailed as below:

NB Please read the following before continuing.
- Statements of actual facts are denoted by **Fact**. Statements of **Educated Predictions** are denoted by **Predic.**
- The degree of good and bad shall be indicated with the appropriate word/s Very Good or Bad etc.
- Information denoted by a source and a name or title indicates where the information or opinions came from.

If the UK vote to REMAIN a member of the EU, these are your government-supplied PRINCIPAL consequences, predicted by the sources as detailed:

a) This is the list of all of the **GOOD to VERY GOOD** principle aspects and benefits to the **UK of REMAINING a member of the EU** viewed over a period of the next 25 years.

b) This is the list of all of the **BAD to VERY BAD** principle aspects and downsides to the **UK of REMAINING a member of the EU** viewed over a period of the next 25 years.

If the UK vote to LEAVE the EU, these are your government-supplied PRINCIPAL consequences, predicted by the sources as detailed:

c) This is the list of all of the **GOOD to VERY GOOD** principle aspects and benefits to the **UK of voting to LEAVE the EU** viewed over a period of the next 25 years.

d) This is the list of all of the **BAD to VERY BAD** principle aspects and downsides to the **UK of voting to LEAVE the EU** viewed over a period of the next 25 years.

F) A summary of very important aspects.
This topic of whether to leave the E.U. polarised opinions long before the actual vote and even more so after the vote. The Remainers refused to accept the majority vote to leave, so they argued in public and schemed in the Houses of Parliament in several ways to attempt to achieve their objective. Respectful and useful debates and discussions were almost impossible to have due to the tone, the high levels of emotion in the debates, the

venom displayed and the personal animosity prevailing related to this particular topic.

Also, a significant difficulty that was disturbing to witness was the degree of future consequences predicted, always presented as fact by the Remainers to the Leavers. People, particularly on the remaining side of the argument, made a lot of detailed predictions about many future economic states. They were presented with great gusto and confidence as if they were all indisputable facts and any other predicted opinions were just lies and not worth listening to.

This subject caused serious disagreements between long term friends and within families. The Remainers predicted consequences of leaving the EU were in the order of we would crash out. It would be catastrophic. The economy would immediately fall over a cliff edge on the day we left.

Example 5 – Is the cost of the HS2 project, the high-speed train link, justifiable?

This question is in the Category C Truth.

*OVERVIEW: The major difficulty for the prevailing government regarding correctly answering this question of truth relates to the ongoing challenge UK political parties have faced over many years. Their task is to satisfactorily and successfully ensure that the many **projects of a range of types**, sizes and costs that have arisen, are organised and managed correctly by people put in charge of them. This has failed in the past, presumably because the leaders did not have the required capability and experience.*

To run any project of any type, size or cost successfully, it is vital that a team of suitably experienced and capable people, who have worked in private business, are put in charge of managing and running the whole of the project from start to finish. This team must include a competent chairperson with a relevant, practical background and people who, between them, have experience across all of the aspects of knowledge and professionalism that embraces those which the project comprises.

They need to be able to ensure that the correct processes and standards are achieved and followed during all steps of the project as it develops from conception through to completion. They will finish nominally on time and within/on budget. They will satisfy all of the objectives they were required to set out to achieve as defined in the all-embracing specification of requirements that this team's first job was to develop.

The key and initial part of any project is to establish a fully bespoke specification of requirements, sufficiently detailing what is required. It starts as a blank piece of paper and ends with the: Specified, proposed, costed and quoted, refined, ordered, designed, approved, manufactured, constructed, finished, installed, pre-tested, commissioned and fully working system, over at least, initially, six months of full operation.

If this simplification of the process is followed, everyone who requested and specified it will be satisfied that all requirements, setting standards and objectives in each project area along the way, will have been fully satisfied and therefore be formally accepted by the project team.

One of the key actions early on with any project, but particularly with a project of this immense cost and inevitably quite long timescale, is identifying and separating the different parts or areas of the project. Then, allocate a member of the project team with the appropriate range of expertise and experience to look after each area.

This specification will primarily be sent out as a draft to everyone who requested the HS2 project to ensure all of their basic requirements and objectives have been satisfied within this initial first draft. Part of the process within this first draft of the specification will no doubt have been the HS2 project requesters answering multiple questions that came to the minds of the specification-writers whilst producing their first draft.

When the second draft of the specification has been developed sufficiently, it is prudent to send it to companies capable of satisfying various parts of the project's requirements and schedule many initially probing project meetings with them. From these numerous meetings, a sufficiently accurate total cost and timescale can be developed. A financial benefits justification for the completed project can be drawn up to obtain nominal approval to continue or not with the project.

One of the many repetitive comments made about a project that has not followed the path described above is: "The price and timescale to completion have gone up again." This is generally in the order of at least 30% up to 100% or more each time. The facts are that the price has not gone up. The previous prices stated were **never evaluated correctly in the first place** simply because the project was fundamentally mishandled.

G) The resultant difficulties.

The HS2 project seemingly has not fully followed this process as above, with the prevailing consequences and related difficulties, not the least of which is that the final total costs remain unknown. This is despite work and costs being committed and carried out over quite a long period of time.

In conclusion, this is one example where a facility like the HS2 project, despite being in the future and the enormity of work required to create it over a long period, **the truth of the future costs** of its creation, completion and timescale can be reached **quite accurately.** However, this is only the case **providing it is managed as described above.**

Also, thinking very carefully about **future cost-benefits of the HS2 project,** a truthful estimation of these can be arrived at, but **not as accurately** as the creation of the system project total costs figure. This is due to the multiple actual cost-benefits creation factors being many years in the future when the project is completed and beyond, thus requiring them having to be predicted. Many cost-benefits creation factors are challenging to predict with any reasonable accuracy due their nature of change. For example, the factor of people increasingly working from home as their working base as opposed to daily commuting into their companies' offices has had major consequences in a large reduction in public transport usage. Since the COVID-19 pandemic, this change has become significantly more common.

H) *An overview of any future predictions.*

If you are ever required to predict the future status of any system, topic or condition, I suggest you have an extremely careful ponder about your objectives which are in consideration. Note how far into the future you have been requested to make your assessment, simply because most, if not everything being considered, will be in constant change, as everything it is created from is continually changing.

Try and list out all at least of the different major factors that, individually and in combination, substantially contribute to the creation of the condition or status of what you are predicting. For each factor, decide how stable it is, how many other factors affect its status, the frequency they would normally change, and by approximately what percentage range.

Bear in mind that **it is impossible** to predict the future status of anything in the world at any time or place with **any degree of good accuracy**. At the end of the day, your prediction is always going to be hopefully an educated and experienced one. Occasionally, it may transpire that your prediction turned out to be fairly accurate about something, but that is just some significant degree of luck.

<u>With this in mind, be careful how you present your prediction to others and what you may be held responsible for as a consequence!</u>

Everything, condition or status in this life is never ever only caused by one thing or condition. It is always caused by or is **a result of the interaction of different conditions or factors, which I refer to as multifactorial contributory causes.**

The above applies to extremely simple conditions with a few settings and factors where the resultant outcome creates something of concern, all of the way up to exceptionally highly complex conditions with vast settings, and factors. There is a range of many different causal factors, which are all usually changing, and some can also be interacting with all or most of the other ones. It will normally be the case that there is a relatively small percentage of the most major influential factors, followed by a larger percentage of less influential factors and so on.

I) An overall summary of reality and the truth or facts.
Categories A and B (historical and current) are the two categories of the truth which are about real activities or conditions. They are facts that actually occurred sometime in the very recent or less recent past.

Reality is about real information or conditions that actually exist that are presented, occurred or prevailed in nominally a moment of the present. They are received by people who each process the same information to some very small or, up to a larger degree, differently.

One indisputable certainty about the **Category C** truth (predicted) which is the future about absolutely anything, is that no one knows what it will be, simply because they or it or them hasn't happened yet. They can offer a knowledgeable and experienced opinion or guess, certainly. However, despite this, particularly these days, people appear to believe that their predictions/guesses are actual facts, judging by the total confidence and conviction they deliver their statements with and their complete rejection of any other case presented to them by literally anyone else.

It never ceases to amaze me how often superbly competent, really intelligent, ultra-professional news presenters on the TV say to a wheeled-in expert, "I know it is not easy and is difficult but – what is going to happen about (whatever) in (some future timescale)?"

It is not easy, and it is not difficult – <u>IT IS ALWAYS UTTERLY IMPOSSIBLE</u>.

The opening question was: What is reality, and what is the truth? Are they the same?

From all of the contents in 6.10 above, the truthful reality is that they couldn't be more different!

I rest my case.

SUBCHAPTER 6.11: Is lab-derived data compared to real-life naturally experienced data nominally the same, particularly concerning the behaviour of humans?

*OVERVIEW: I have spent a while pondering this topic and concluded that the objective of trying to establish the details of particularly how your brain and other hidden and extremely complex systems work by simulation in the laboratory etc., will never be 100% identical. Therefore, it will probably not be **sufficiently similar** to the actual system conditions themselves, which are always, by definition, occurring in real-life conditions.*

I believe that the consequences of this are that the detailed conclusions derived will probably be significantly inaccurate. Therefore, when leading *and added* to other similarly derived conclusions due to a compounding effect, they will inevitably take you farther away from the actual truth and facts of the system you are desperately trying to understand the detailed functionality of, plus other aspects.

Some of the differences between the actual occurrence and the sequence of related events in a real-life set of conditions compared to the lab-simulated one possibly include:

a) The real-life one is **totally unexpected** and the lab one is not. You will inevitably be told what will happen regarding some of the elements of the process, probably the overall objective, plus other aspects at some time.

b) The real-life event contains human emotions, particularly adrenalin and probably others. The lab one will likely not have all of the same emotions, nor the same quantity of adrenalin and/or maybe not other replica emotions. In both scenarios, several different emotions will probably be combined, leading to possibly significant variations in the consequential results.

c) The real-life conditions will see the real object contained in a real-world situation, all of which the lab one will probably not contain. Consequently, your response time and other responses will, I believe, not be the same and possibly significantly different.

The resultant, combinational effect of a) b) and c) is very likely to produce conclusions as described at the beginning of this topic.

SUBCHAPTER 6.12: Can your human consciousness be uploaded or copied from your brain into a computer, robot or some other data or information platform and can it operate within this other platform as it does now within your brain?

OVERVIEW: I have noted that this question, which relates to what teams of scientists have set themselves as an extremely serious objective, comes up in various forms of our media.

The initial and primary reaction I have to this view and objective is that, from my understanding of the situation, scientists cannot understand how your consciousness is derived and, therefore, are unable to define what the human consciousness is and its purpose. How can anyone have an opinion and believe that this objective is achievable when they don't understand what they are dealing with?!

I firmly believe that if these people were able to understand and therefore be able to define precisely what **human consciousness** is, how it is derived, what it comprises and exactly why we have it, they would understand the following:

a) Your consciousness exists within your mind in your brain for the purpose of keeping you safe and dealing with each of your unique and ongoing situations throughout the whole of your lifetime.

b)   It is *continually derived/updated* from all of the vast amount of data received from your five senses, your B.H.S.M.S. and your internally instigated thoughts. Your brain formats, processes and understands the meaning and relevance of all this data to you as a unique and particular individual on this earth. It does this by utilising your intelligence, plus your unique, personal, vast amount of knowledge and experiences stored in your multitudes **of** Memory Departments, developed throughout your life *up to that moment.*

c)   This enables you to fully create, update and utilise your consciousness to keep you safe at all times. You also successfully select and deal with each situation and related decision you are faced with and take the resultant actions continuously throughout your lifetime.

So, to get down to the nitty-gritty of answering our question above:

1)   Your consciousness doesn't exist as it is now and continue to exist ever afterwards without change. It is continually changing/being updated when any of the existing data alters or new data is received by your brain via your senses and from within your brain.

2)   I believe that this cycle of updating and taking actions required by your consciousness takes place continually throughout your life at a rate of 250 times per second.

3) People seem to think that you just have to somehow upload a person's consciousness in this moment in time, and then forever afterwards, you have it to use. <u>In my opinion, this is completely wrong</u>.

4) Your consciousness is only of use to the person whose brain is processing it, and only then if it is up-to-date in each moment.

NB In order to update your consciousness, you would have to replicate:

a) All of your brain's many data processing networks and the multitudes of departments in which all of your life's memories, experiences and knowledge are stored. You also need your mind and your M.C. to organise and manage it all to understand the relevance of all the data you are receiving at every moment.

b) Each of your senses' hardware input receivers – your eyes, ears, mouth, nose and touch sensors. You also need all of the nerves and data input converters connecting each sense's data into your brain's data input networks, plus the data formatting networks to configure all the data from your senses.

An absolutely key part of this process is applying your brain's intelligence to understand the meaning and collective relevance to you of all of this data in the context of the moment in time in which it occurred and was received by you.

c)   Your consciousness can only be derived and formulated by having received all of the data derived from your senses, your B.H.S.M.S and any internally generated thoughts. Most of this data is acquired from OUTSIDE your brain, so these facilities have to be uploaded and connected physically and software-wise into your brain as a fully completed and functioning system at all times.

All of this means that you would have to rely upon a man-made replication of the most wondrous and capable processing system and end product functionality, which is the human being, to make the uploaded consciousness be of any worth. You already know my thoughts about the capabilities of bots versus those of an average human being and why I hold these thoughts.

In conclusion, I believe that, for the reasons above, all of these objectives at their fundamental level are simply unrealistic and unachievable and, therefore, they belong in and should remain in science fiction.

SUBCHAPTER 6.13: Will robots ever become equally as capable as or even more capable than humans, thus enabling them to take over the earth and, in the process, spell the end of the human race?

OVERVIEW: The first and extremely important point I must make at this stage is that I am totally supportive of the increasing use of computerised systems, their algorithms and programmed logic in the fields of research, medicine, the day-to-day work of automated manufacturing engineering processes, etc. This work, in most cases, can be carried out much quicker and generally with greater accuracy than by humans.

*What I do object to is that I do not believe that **true intelligence** is being utilised in these systems, yet they are usually presented to and seen by the public as employing genuine intelligence.*

My simple answer to each part of this four-part question is, <u>in principle,</u> no.

I deliberately use the phrase <u>in principle</u> to caveat the risk of what happens if increasingly more people in positions of power over us believe the overall answer to this question is yes. Then, their unquestioned belief puts us all at an increasing risk of this situation, whilst never becoming completely fulfilled, becoming to a troublesome degree, a self-fulfilling prophesy born of unquestioned expectation.

SUBCHAPTER 6.13.1: A <u>simple list</u> of the fundamental reasons why <u>I believe that</u> the answer is *no* to each part of this four-faceted question.

1. Robots are 100% man-designed and 100% man-made with relatively few decades of man-created evolution of all of their software and hardware.

*1-H. **Humans** are 100% designed and made by the Grand Creator, with aeons of years of evolutionary improvements of all of their software and hardware.*

2. Robots do not have a human-like brain. They are dumb machines that operate by following pre-written, pre-programmed instructions that trigger various pre-arranged, pre-required functionalities contained within their pre-programmed instructions. These functionalities are in response to data received by their man-made hardware sensors – cameras, audio devices, position sensors etc., and maybe, over data networks.

*2-H. **Humans** have a brain with genuine intelligence, the **average** power and range of capability of which is possibly the most capable single unit processing system in the whole of the Universe. Humans can operate following instructions where appropriate and necessary, and they can also operate totally and truly in fully autonomous mode where required. Their brain receives all of its incoming data from their five senses, (sight, sound, touch, smell and taste) built within their body, from their B.H.S.M.S. (Body's Health Status Monitoring System) and any internally instigated thoughts when appropriate.*

3. Robots have no intelligence and an extremely limited range of knowledgeable data compared to a human. This immediately precludes them from being having a consciousness which is an immeasurable loss of awareness, capability, understanding of the many details of what is happening around them and how they all inter-relate. They rely simply upon using their pre-programmed instructions to respond to the relatively limited data coming in from various sources and from their sensors. This runs, at times, the very high risk that they may have missed or misinterpreted something that could be vitally important to their prevailing situation and its responsibilities.

3-H. Humans have a consciousness that is automatically and continuously updated from the vast detailed amount of incoming data being received by their brain. They use their consciousness during every moment throughout their life to enable them to keep safe and carry out all of their requirements, considerations and actions at all times. The risk that they have missed some incoming data or misinterpreted some incoming data compared to robots is extremely low.

4. I don't believe that intelligence can be written into the instructions in a **robot's** program. I think that robots have not one iota of even the starting level of capability in the range that human intelligence exists. Therefore, they have to be pre-programmed to be instructed about what to do at all times about their prescribed, expected capabilities and duties.

4.H. Humans, by acceptance, have intelligence. This is their most crucially important capability, particularly when used within the process of creating and updating their consciousness. Even employing the starting level of human intelligence foundationally enables us, humans, to create and update our consciousness. We have the vitally important factor of utilising an extremely high level of understanding of the contextual relevance and meaning of all of the individual and combinational sets of incoming data, some of which we may not have seen before.

Our human intelligence also enables us to create original thoughts when required, to assess and consider the incoming data in the process of updating our consciousness, to be able to take the appropriate actions to keep us safe, etc. This means that we may not have stored memories and knowledge of some of this data or these particular data combinations and their meaning and relevance to refer to for guidance, but, applying our intelligence, we are likely able to make the correct judgements.

*The immense benefit of this capability is that we only require a **relatively** small database of knowledge, which is part of how our consciousness is created and updated. We thus need the relatively small volume of brain we have, as opposed to requiring a brain the size of an elephant's body if we had to store, in memory, the unlimited combinations of all of the data we need to have available with which to manage our life. Employing human intelligence is part of the process which enables the creation and updating of an extremely useful, highly detailed, multi-faceted, in-depth and crucially informed human consciousness.*

Part of this utilisation of our intelligence in this process includes being able to recognise instantly what incoming data is not relevant to our safety or does not need to be dealt with. Therefore, it is not required to be processed and responded to and will be ignored in that moment.

At their best, the power, capability and usefulness of all other living creatures and entities' consciousnesses, are significantly less, compared to that of human beings. Nevertheless, like all other living creatures and entities, humans crucially rely upon the existence, creation and updating of their own consciousness to keep safe and find food and shelter to survive in their day-to-day existence within the world they inhabit.

5. I believe that **robots** are not capable of automatic self-learning. I know that they are attributed with this ability at times, but I believe they are still fundamentally, following a pre-programmed set of instructions at a basic level. This instructs them to look for data, find it and store it for use by some trial and error routine or whatever. It could be seen as a form of self-learning, but it is still essentially following a pre-programmed set of instructions.

Obviously, they can gain some knowledge if they run into a problem or combination of situations that have not been catered for by their pre-programmed instructions, but they will be unable to function. They will have to rely upon their human programmers to note the problematic data and modify their programme etc., to hopefully prevent a future re-occurrence of those difficulties.

*5-H. **Human** brains have the capability to learn from their mistakes and therefore self-improve their capabilities of managing and controlling whatever task they are dealing with.*

6. Robots seek to understand the data they are receiving by reference-comparison to a man-made set of memories or a database of information that has been pre-programmed into their system. Suppose their sensors see or sense an object (moving or stationary), type of person, or anything whatsoever that is a dangerous or troublesome threat to the robot's role due to its position or capability. If this thing cannot be matched with its database, then the robot will take no action, thus possibly leading to a dangerous or troublesome situation.

6-H. Humans *have an extremely large set of memories in their databases within their brain, covering a vast range of categories and topics. It is unlikely that a human being applying their intelligence whilst undertaking a task will be faced with an item, condition or situation that they can't recognise and understand and therefore be unable to deal with successfully.*

The human brain can be presented with a combination of conditions and data from its senses, some of which it has <u>*never experienced before*</u> *and will therefore have no stored memories of it. However, due to the application of its intelligence and maybe intuition, it will generally be able to decode and understand the meaning and relevance of this data. Crucially, in the context of the prevailing situation, it can decide whether you have to take any immediate action regarding danger prevention or other reasons. This objective may require an immediate recourse from an enquiry to Google or another human being if time permits.*

7. Robots have a man-designed and man-made body to suit the particular, specific work or role they are required to fulfil.

7-H. **Humans** *have a body that has been sublimely designed by the Grand Creator, with aeons of years of evolutionary improvements of all of its hardware. It is designed to be able to carry out an almost unlimited, extremely wide range of roles and tasks.*

8. Robots to date, are designed to fulfil a very particular/specific role, i.e. they are only capable of carrying out this role and no other, without major rebuilding, in all aspects of software and hardware.

8-H. **Humans** *are designed to carry out a vast range of different tasks independently and where required, using a vast array of suitable tools, normally without any significant pre-training.*

9. Robots are 100% without any human-like emotional facets, elements or attributes. This is a serious limitation if and when they are required to carry out a role which demands an accurate understanding, consideration and interaction with the humans involved in their situation. Their considerations would need to include aspects of human emotions and their related consequences.

I don't believe that a robot can be programmed to **have** human emotions and a soul. They can be programmed to say the appropriate words and display suitable facial expressions, etc. However, these are simply just artificial and therefore false. The robot will have no inherent, intrinsic, innate, inborn understanding of what the words it may be saying actually mean. Nevertheless, they can obviously be programmed to say what the exact definition of any word they say is. *9-H. **Humans** who are normal and emotionally healthy, by definition, have a set of emotions related to their characteristics and soul. They can carry out roles where having and understanding typical human emotions are crucially important to achieve an acceptable outcome from the situation.*

10. Robots, in proportion to the size and complexity of the programme that decides their functionality, will, upon initial use, probably always have a programme that contains design faults, usually referred to as bugs. This can mean that, dependent upon the role they are carrying out, they are capable of functioning in what could be a dangerous manner to people who are within their operating zone. Some design faults can appear possibly a year or more after commissioning due to a particular sequence of events and/or a combination of fault causal conditions.

*10-H. **Humans** carrying out a role generally don't have to experience any of the above difficulties to any significant degree. They may require a degree of training before undertaking some complicated tasks but they are capable of automatic self-learning due to their intelligence. If there is a particularly difficult and problematic condition within some very complex process they are carrying out, they can automatically provide vitally important data to other professionals involved. Working together, they can solve all of the difficulties relatively easily and quickly and safely.*

Also, whilst humans are being trained, if they are unsure of something they have been asked to do, with their intelligence, they are capable of raising their concerns and assisting in solving the situation.

NB As I see this very commonly raised question, the heading of Subchapter 6.13, as such an important one, please forgive me if I also respond to it with the following information.

SUBCHAPTER 6.13.2: A more detailed list of reasons, presented from a slightly different perspective of why I believe the answer is no to each part of this four-part question above.

A. I believe that two of the awesome capabilities that the <u>average human being</u> is inherently born with and gradually fully develops after birth is their ability to develop a human consciousness. The most important capability is being able to accomplish this with their human intelligence. I believe they are also inherently born with this, and its capability gradually develops as they grow and learn. The third awesome capability we are all also born with is the absolute starting foundational level of developing and utilising our memories and knowledge. We gradually continue expanding these over our lifetimes to cover the immense range and depth of so many topics across the avenues of this world we live in.

B. As each human being's intelligence develops through their experiences, knowledge, and own inherent potential capability, the depth and range of perception and the consequential collective value of their consciousness increase accordingly.

C. What I believe most strongly is that each human being has an ongoing consciousness that, in all of its detail in each moment, is unique to them. It may be very similar, certainly in parts, to other human beings who are nominally experiencing the same experiences as they are, but each one will be unique.

D. I am also of the opinion the human mind primarily functions foundationally upon the existence of the human consciousness. Without this, it wouldn't have all of the data required to respond to in order to keep you safe. It also wouldn't know what situations you are best required to resolve, make decisions about, and take action upon in every moment throughout your life. Your consciousness gives you a highly detailed understanding of everything that is happening around you constantly and forever. From this knowledge, you can make the most appropriate and best decisions for yourself at all times.

E. I don't believe that a pre-programmed list of instructions can ever include the capability of having or creating intelligence. I can't ever envisage any man-made machine itself being able to self-develop to acquire intelligence and a consciousness for all of the reasons and complexities of capability, detailed in this book.

F. It would require making the equivalent of an average human being's software and hardware. Human beings are not man-made; they are **born**. Just because you label a man-made system as intelligent, does not mean it actually is intelligent. All of these man-made systems do exactly what they have been pre-programmed to do – nothing more and nothing less.

G. Although the human mind is always automatically learning, remembering and updating its memories, it will never make decisions and take actions <u>purely</u> from memories of previous situations you have encountered. Even if the circumstances that it experienced before are very similar, some of these details will invariably be different to the prevailing ones, so your M.C. will always make your complex decisions and actions specifically in response to your current situations. It will consistently refer to the actual detailed information your consciousness has presented to you to be acted upon and apply the combinational meanings and relevance in context to the details of your prevailing situation.

It will never make the equivalent of pre-programmed decisions and actions, which is all that a computer programme can only do simply because it does not have any intelligence or a human consciousness. Therefore, how can these man-made machines ever be equal to human beings, let alone become more capable and become their master?

H. The amount of memories and knowledge about a huge range and depths of so many topics the average human brain has is astonishing. Its intelligence and ability to combine items or sets of data items and knowledge across any different issue or knowledge situation to fully and immediately understand the context and relevance to your current situation and its processing speed are stunningly breathtaking.

I. Robotic machine computer systems are only specific to one particular area of activity and requirement. The average human brain can instantly begin to respond and apply itself to an almost unlimited range, type and category of conditions. It may have never experienced some before, but by applying its intelligence, it understands the details and relevance of the situation with all of its interrelated data and commences dealing with it. If a bot was presented with a combination of conditions that were not included in its list of instructions and responses, it would and could do nothing at all.

J. It is true that a computer dedicated to a specific task can carry out this type of investigative role much quicker than a human being. For example, searching through a very large database comprising of a huge amount of medical test samples to identify a set of results that indicate a serious disease present.

This is not what I would call using intelligence; it is simply a computer programme following programmed instructions of comparing each set of actual data with a typical diseased set of data and highlighting each one that is a good match. This kind of comparison exercise can certainly be carried out much quicker by a programmed computer system than by a human being.

The important point is that an averagely capable human can carry out almost an unlimited number of roles, activities and requirements with none or minimum pre-training required.

K. Most of the above has only dealt with the foundational software part of the human being compared with the software parts of a robot. However, let's begin to look at the hardware parts of the human being that detect, receive and deliver your five senses' data, the data from your B.H.S.M.S. and your internal thoughts into your human brain to process and understand it all. When we now compare and look at the hardware currently installed in robots, it begs the following questions:

a) How can the capability, flexibility, manoeuvrability, reliability, clarity of data, precise decoding of all fine details of data from each of your five senses etc., in all horrendous weathers and conditions imaginable from your human body be able to be matched to any comparable degree of accuracy and reliability by a robot with its sets of many different sensors?

b) How can the physical performance of man-made machines ever be remotely equal to the control, balance, incredible manoeuvrability, flexibility, co-ordination and of the awesome range of all of these capabilities of all parts of the human body, limbs, hands, toes, etc.?

I noted that the wonderful, world-renowned, never to be forgotten Professor Stephen Hawking was reported as saying that Robots will take over the earth *if they are allowed to develop themselves and develop intelligence,* which could spell the end of the human race. He was quickly followed by a very prominent observer of the Universe who agreed that many people would bet on Robots becoming intelligent, but he questioned whether that necessarily implied consciousness. He presumably didn't understand how consciousness is created, its role, and the enormous benefits of its value and worth to its human beings. The truth is that without their consciousness, human beings are nothing.

I find it staggering and not a little worrying and disappointing that, as I currently understand this, no one publicly and officially has yet been able to define human consciousness in any detail. This must surely be preceded by understanding what it is, how it is created and its role within the human mind's functionality. Yet, <u>despite this lack of knowledge about human consciousness</u>, which people feel/guess/know is crucial to the functionality of the human mind, people think that:

a) Robotic machines are capable of becoming at least of equal capability if not more *capable* than humans.
b) Robotic machines are capable of **developing human intelligence.**
c) Robotic machines are capable of **developing a consciousness.**
d) Robotic machines are capable of **carrying out original thought.**

e) People believe that all these awesome, human-only capabilities will somehow be acquired/bestowed upon future, initially man-made machines **which will make themselves** at least equal to or more capable than their human creators. This is despite all of these beliefs being from people who do not appear to have any depth of understanding of how difficult original thought is to create and what human consciousness really is, what its relationship to human intelligence is.

How can a machine which does not have human intelligence be able to develop human intelligence? ***Is this the absolute, ultimate no brainer?***

They appear to be obsessively driven by making references to the make-beliefs of science fiction books and films of robots. However, it appears that they don't truly understand how <u>incredibly capable the average human being is</u> and how they <u>actually function.</u>

Example 1 – Describe in great detail the complexities of updating your consciousness, enabling effective decision-making and taking the related actions relevant to driving safely whilst operating your car in extremely challenging conditions.

With human intelligence, I believe that one of the crucially important abilities that it is used for is to significantly contribute to your ongoing, lifelong creation and updating of your human consciousness. During this process, your M.C. engages its **intelligence** by **creating original thoughts** related to incoming data it has received, to consider what appropriate actions are required to process and deal with it.

It does this by always considering the data in the context of the situation it exists. Sometimes, a range of a large number of different types and items of information, which can be complex, interactive and detailed data, is received by your brain. It comes from your senses, B.H.S.M.S. and your internal thoughts about, for example, a highly complex and fast-changing situation as car driving can be, particularly at times.

I will use an example of a situation we have probably all encountered and can therefore relate to – driving a car in extremely busy and fast-changing, interrelated road traffic and pedestrian conditions. This is a description of the procedure whereby your brain develops your consciousness to be able to process and safely deal with all of these conditions.

a)   Faster than you can blink, your brain will have received and processed the data.

b)   It will have understood what each of the incoming data items from sometimes, all of your senses actually is. For example, (this is a lady pushing a pram), (this is a man walking), (this is a vehicle travelling), (this is a vehicle behind me), (this is a lady in front on the pavement) etc. It does this by matching each item it has seen and heard with data stored in its memories.

c) Now comes the crucial involvement of your human intelligence capability, aided, supported and enabled by utilising the incredible processing power and speed of many facilities and capabilities within your brain. There is an enormous quantity of highly detailed data learned and stored in your memory cells from all of your life experiences, all readily available to your mind.

d) Your M.C. also noted in **b)** the following details because they importantly **relate in context** to the fact that your M.C. knows that you are driving your car in highly congested and therefore potentially dangerous conditions. It focuses on providing your mind with information about anything within your driving locality that constitute a potential danger to you, your passengers and other road users and pedestrians. This is so you drive your car with appropriate actions to keep yourself, and all others involved safe, as far as is humanly possible.

To achieve these objectives, the intelligence of your M.C. creates thoughts, asks itself questions, takes note of all the detailed aspects of the types of vehicles, people and all moving and stationary objects in your field of existing and near-future activity. This is to **predict** whether collectively and/or individually they will present a danger **to you** and/or to **themselves**. If the answer is yes, your M.C. considers and creates what options it has, or maybe, in some of these situations, does not have, to prevent these dangers from occurring.

Your M.C. also noted in **b)** above, the following <u>additional finer details</u>, each of which was selected out of an awful lot of other elements that were ignored because they did not constitute or combine with further details to present future danger.

1 – The lady pushing the pram is having extreme difficulty guiding it to keep it safely on the pavement adjacent to your car, and also, her second young child is holding and pulling it onto the roadside kerb of the pram. You hear her shouting with increasing exasperation to tell her son, "Stop pulling us into the busy road!" One of your Category 1B departments has automatically calculated that if you and the pram maintain your speeds and trajectories, the pram will be near the front of your car at a particular point ahead of you. It has warned your M.C. of this danger.

2 – The man walking on the pavement adjacent to your car has a white stick he is using with gusto, indicating that he has much need of it. He is also walking with an intoxicated type of gait, causing him to walk at an angle towards the edge of the roadside kerb. Another of your Category 1B departments has automatically computed and warned you that, again, if you both maintain your current speeds and trajectories, he will be in front of your car at a particular point ahead of you.

3 – There is a moving vehicle, a school bus, on the other side of the road to you. It is travelling over the speed limit and weaving from side to side. It is packed full of small school children, who appear to be screaming with fear on their faces. You notice that three of them are pulling at the bus driver, who is slumped over the steering wheel, as they desperately attempt to obtain some control of the bus. Another of your Category 1B Departments has automatically computed that if your car and this bus maintain your current speeds and trajectories, the two of you will collide unless it alters its path at a particular point ahead of you.

4 – The lady standing on the edge of the pavement is old and frail. She seems desperate to cross the extremely busy road, thirty yards in front of you, to get to the bus stop, to which a bus will soon arrive. Another of your Category 1B Departments has automatically computed that you will be adjacent to her at a particular point ahead of you if both maintain your current average speed and direction.

5 – The car behind you has been tailgating you for the last minute. It is obviously desperate to overtake you as soon as possible, despite the congested and potentially accident ridden conditions, so you keep monitoring its position visually and audibly.

NB The power of your M.C.'s intelligence utilises all of the data detailed above to update your consciousness continually. It presents all immediate/actual **danger and all predicted, possible, future dangers** in your driving locality in the five to twenty metres ahead presented by anything that means danger to you particularly. This distance aspect is variable, dependent upon existing and new, variable changing danger contributing factors and in relation to what they all mean in terms of how you manoeuvre your car in every small moment of time to:

a) Keep you and the occupants of your car safe by avoiding any accidents you might potentially have.

b) Avoid contributing to other road users and pedestrians being involved in accidents from other road users I have not mentioned but are also in the approaching frame of consideration.

c) Keep the lady with the pram and her two children safe by not crashing into them by sounding your horn to warn them they are heading for danger in the road. Also, slow down as much as other traffic considerations allow, plus, consider moving towards the centre of the road if this is an acceptable option.

d) Keep the blind man safe by appropriate use of your horn. Consider stopping adjacent to him if this remains a feasible option by the time you are level with him and he is on the kerb.

e) Keep the school bus in view and hope that it alters its path away from you until it has gone past, but be prepared to take avoidance action if it remains on a collision course.

f) Your primary concern for the lady waiting to cross the road to the bus stop is that she walks into the path of the car behind you if it decides to overtake your vehicle.

Conclusions from the above scenario.

1.0 You will probably never meet all of the extremely challenging sets of conditions described above together, but others with different details and presenting similar challenges could occur. Despite this, the power of your intelligence during everything described above, coupled with the incredible speed of processing powers of your brain, enables your M.C. to do the following. It can oversee the updating of your consciousness, decision-making and resultant actions as the incoming data from your senses changes every moment. These variations are due to the speed and direction of travel of all moving vehicles, people, other vehicles, dogs etc., coming into your area of activity. They all require your M.C. to make many fine-tuning adjustments to many of your car manoeuvring activities, decision-making and actions.

2.0 None of the above actions and decision-making is due to your mind driving in fully-automatic mode and simply repeating precisely and fully automatically what you have learnt by experience and carried out before. It is achieved by your M.C. calling up many of your Developed, Semi-Automatic Skills in your Category 1B Departments to control your car, automatically computing/predicting where in the future it will be relating to the other moving vehicles, people and objects within your area of activity.

All of this time, your M.C. is updating your consciousness from which it will constantly be making decisions and adjustments of actions and objectives, as required by the actual detailed road traffic conditions prevailing at each moment.

The incoming data from your senses will be updated and acted appropriately upon by your M.C 250 times per second.

3.0 The above, detailed example scenario was all about how a human being processes all of the required data in their surroundings, in relation to driving their car safely. The crucial importance of the process and involvement of updating their consciousness and the required power of human intelligence was explained. However, whether it is driving a car or playing any of the sports in the world, or carrying out a thousand and one activities at work, home or play, exactly the same principles and a lot of the details required are the same or similar.

4.0 It was hopefully clearly detailed and noted that the human brain notices each car, person or other moving item as a *basic entity*. But it also, crucially notices and selects all details for each moving vehicle, person, etc. This enables your M.C. to be able to fully understand enough about each person etc., to know the context of how they relate to the traffic conditions. Therefore it can predict whether each particular vehicle, person etc., presents a danger to the car driver, person or maybe all of them.

All other details which have no relevance to danger – the colour of the car, whether it is dirty, what make the pram is, how many spokes the wheels have etc. **are totally ignored by your M.C.** This is because they will waste/cost processing time, causing your M.C. to take longer to make a decision and take actions, therefore possibly leading you and others to be in greater danger as a consequence.

5.0 A robotic, computer-controlled man-made machine, having no human consciousness or intelligence, would see the woman with her pram and toddler exactly as the person who wrote its operating program had pre-ordained them to be seen/registered in their data input region. This would be in conjunction with the cameras and other sensors installed in the robotic man-made machine that detected her.

I imagine it would be that she, with her toddler, may be labelled in its software as a moving person or persons. They would be presented as a particular overall size of object and noted travelling at a certain speed and direction. The software would assess whether they were on a collision course with your car and should be avoided making physical contact with.

It would not understand anything about women, toddlers and prams or notice any of the particular details mentioned above, unless, for some explicit role for a specific robot, it would be programmed with a lot more detail, which would include more than I have mentioned in some areas or categories.

For even a few of the reasons in this section, let alone all of the combined reasons described, can you ever see robots becoming even remotely equal in overall capability of range and depth to one of us humans of <u>average capability</u>?

One very final word on this topic – watch out for this scenario.

Something is, in actual fact, totally wrong, untrue or impossible. However, let's say a sufficient number of people, particularly those who will gain, financially or otherwise, people in the media and our political leaders, frequently keep repeating a statement about something of importance. If they announce that it will happen a sufficient number of times for a long enough period, an increasing percentage of people begin to believe that it will actually happen and meekly accept it as inevitable progress. Please don't believe it!

I rest my case of Humans v Robots.

SUBCHAPTER 6.14: *Man-designed and manufactured auto-piloted self-driving vehicles. In all possible driving and weather conditions, on all conceivable types and qualities of public roads and lanes throughout the UK, can they ever be as safe for passengers to use as travelling with the average, experienced human driver?*

OVERVIEW: Before I commence responding to this question, I would like to make four very important points, leading into and preparing the ground for my detailed answers.

1.0 Firstly, the most important point I would like to make about this whole topic of self-driving vehicles, which is a huge subject with a vast amount of details covering an awful lot of factors. During these many years, the designers of these systems will have made huge improvements, developments and changes, driven by the safety of their vehicles passengers and other road users, systems reliability and, no doubt, many more objectives.

Some of these changes will undoubtedly have had to be kept secret from their competitors and the public, so I would guess that some of my information will be out-of-date, incomplete or slightly wrong. Projects like this are at the very pinnacle of engineering and software design of technical difficulty, requiring at times the development of pioneering areas of functionality and performance. All of this type of work can only be carried out by professionals who are at the very pinnacle of capability in their field. So, I apologise profusely for any information or opinions that I have unintentionally given which are incorrect, in any way, being out-of-date, misunderstood or wrong in some other way.

Bearing in mind my comments above, I may decide to share an opinion about some topic, subtopic or aspect that I stand by. I will always offer an opinion with what I feel are genuine reasons and to be constructively helpful. But a designing and manufacturing company or some other company may hold a different view to mine about some particular topic. This company has every right to hold an alternative opinion to mine, **but** I would ask them to refer to the pointers and notes highlighted in this book. I believe they enable me to call upon my **unique knowledge** of human consciousness, how and why it is created and how and why the human brain operates in relation to it.

This knowledge enables me to make accurate comparisons of the capabilities of an experienced vehicle driver who has a human brain with a vehicle driven by a machine with no human/actual brain.

2.0 Over the last few years, I read about and noted this topic of self-driving vehicles with increasing frequency within the media. More extremely large and experienced companies have been joining forces to develop and produce these systems for the general public and businesses to purchase and travel in. During this period of time it seemed like one company publicised its aspirations, with many billions of pounds planned to be invested when another combining of forces amongst other companies was announced.

I saw them all as charging towards this future expectation of multiples of trillions of pounds of autopiloted annual profits, but also possibly towards a cliff of abject failure. During this time, this all seemed to create an unquestioning expectation amongst the populace at large. Not of if this objective is feasibly, safely and reliably possible, but the anticipation of when will it happen. "I can't wait to go to sleep, read the papers, carry out work on my laptop etc., on the way to wherever, with the utter bliss of no more of that tiresome driving, with zero risks of any nasty accidents or fatalities!!"

3.0 I have the utmost admiration and respect for the power and benefits of employing computers to the increasing limits of their strengths and capabilities, which I spent most of my working life utilising. With the prolific use of computers and the resultant automation and quality of product benefits, companies are able to:

1) Reduce their workforce very significantly.
2) Significantly increase their outputs.
3) Produce higher operational efficiency.
4) Produce better product quality with normally higher profit margins.

As with most things in life, the absolute critical aspect about computers is fully understanding how to obtain the very best that they can offer. Plus, as importantly, to totally comprehend and therefore avoid suffering from their limitations and potential misuses.

4.0 As I get closer to completing my book, and am fine-tuning some parts, as I understand it, some manufacturing companies are announcing they are getting closer to being confident of and allowed to use their self-driving vehicles on public roads. Initially, it seems this will be at level 4 and not level 5, which is the 100% fully-automatic performance selection controlling the vehicle under all conditions at all times.

As I understand it, at least with some companies, with a level 4 selection, the driver will have to sit in the driver's seat and permanently be ready to immediately take 100% control of the car when the self-driving system tells them to take over. I have some grave concerns about the safety, related dangers and implications of this system which are:

a) How long is the list of conditions of which presumably, one or more will cause the self-driving system to tell the human driver to take over?

b) Some of the conditions on this list will be ones that the self-driving system can't resolve. For example, if it detects an imminent accident in a second or two, there is insufficient time for the driver to be able to assess the situation and take over the controls. Others will be that the self-driving system itself has become faulty with hardware and/or software categories of faults.

c) By definition, if the fundamental, prevailing state of the self-driving system is faulty, then it is this defective state that could be absolutely of major consequence all the way through a minor consequence and everything in between. It simply **can't be guaranteed** that it will still be able to instruct the human driver to take over because it is faulty. Also, it may not allow the human driver to operate all of the normal controls of the car to avoid what may be an impending fatal accident simply because one or more of the functions are actually faulty.

d) Assuming that the instruction to the human driver to take over the system works correctly, **how many seconds will elapse** between the Self-Driving System deciding it requires the human driver to take over to when they have assessed the situation, taken over full control of the vehicle and hopefully been able to resolve the situation. The human driver may have been two hours into their journey when the takeover is signalled, and they may have fallen asleep. Fifteen or twenty seconds could easily elapse before the driver is in full control. This could be a lifetime if the car is travelling at seventy miles an hour on a very busy motorway at night with blindingly heavy and blustery rain and is heading into maybe a complex and potentially fatal crash.

The very worst-case scenario is that none of the car's controls will work due to the faulty conditions prevailing, so the human driver is completely unable to take any control of the vehicle.

5.0 I understand that some self-driving vehicle manufacturers have been in deep discussions with insurance companies and legal people about who is held responsible following a severe accident involving a self-driving vehicle and other vehicles, self-driving or not. I can see the benefit to the self-driving vehicle manufacturers that, if at the actual time the accident occurred, the black box recorded data showed the car driver was in full control of the vehicle. The human being would then be deemed responsible for causing the accident and not the company that designed and manufactured the self-driving vehicle system.

However, this responsibility and judgement may very well be unfair because the self-driving system may have created the situation that it passed on to the human driver that became an accident as it was unresolvable at the time it was passed over. Additionally, see the comments in **4.0** above.

NB A very informative entry into the answer posed in the question in heading 6.14 is supplied in my reply to the question posed in heading 6.13:

Will Robots ever become equally as capable or even more capable than humans, thus enabling them to take over the earth, and in the process, spell the end of the human race?

I assume that you have just read my reply to this question above, but if not, **please read that section first** because it not only provides answers posed in 6.13, but most of these answers are also applicable to the question posed in 6.14.

I have included some aspects in my answer to 6.13, which are repeated in my answer to 6.14. However, I have presented them from different perspectives which will hopefully help to achieve a better understanding if required.

I hope this is all clear, and I will continue with what is a short answer to 6.14, with 6.14.1.

SUBCHAPTER 6.14.1: Best practices and basic principles of safety designs when using automatically-controlled computer systems.

OVERVIEW: This section looks at some best practices and best basic principles of safety designs applied in manufacturing and processing industries when using automatically-controlled computer systems. These are required to keep any humans who may be in the vicinity of these automated processes safe at all times, including when any fault conditions occur.

a) Any human beings who worked with the computer-controlled machine system would always **remain outside.** Therefore they were **safely away** from the automatically controlled process areas. These were zones of machines and equipment which were being automatically moved and controlled by the computers, creating potential dangers to humans if they went inside these areas. This meant that not if, but always when, for whatever reason, something went wrong with the automatically controlled machine process, human beings' safety was **never at risk.** They were always being outside the danger zone created by any operational failures or by normal operations and conditions of the process.

Every machine goes wrong at times due to software and/ or hardware problems. However, with autopiloted self-driving vehicles, **WHEN** something goes wrong, human passengers' lives are immediately put at risk because they are inside the process, i.e. inside the vehicle the self-driving system is controlling. When the autopiloted self-driving vehicle is travelling at 70 mph on a multi-lane motorway with all lanes full of traffic, in heavy rain and with a self-driving system software design fault and/or a hardware fault renders the car uncontrollable, what happens to the car and its passengers? **The machine's system has failed, meaning the passengers are immediately potentially going to be injured or worse.**

I would suggest that the total number of potential hardware and/or software faults that could occur with these self-driving systems that immediately render the vehicle unable to be safely controlled would be an extremely worryingly long list, compared with one for a modern, top-spec car made only for human driving.

In fact, human passengers' lives are continually potentially put at risk whenever the car is out on the roads. Additionally, all other road users within the operating zone of each self-driving vehicle are also put at risk when any autopiloted, self-driving vehicle becomes faulty.

As I understand it, it is very questionable that some autopiloted, self-driving vehicle manufacturers have been allowed to test run these cars with the express purpose of finding and exposing any remaining design faults. This has been done on public roads, where, in some cases, unsuspecting car drivers are travelling.

At this time, there are already a number of people who have been killed by these vehicles on test. These are people in the self-driving cars themselves, plus pedestrians and cyclists. I would have thought that one of the primary responsible parties for these deaths, when they were found to be because of a failure within the self-driving system, is the authorities responsible for allowing the use of public roads for this test situation to occur. Also held accountable, I would have thought, would be the chief designers of the teams that have most unfortunately produced these systems that have failed, always with the possibility of people being killed.

b) The automatically-controlled industrial machine processing lines, computer programme control logic, is always presented with input data conditions that it fully recognises, understands, and therefore, responds to correctly and safely.

These input data conditions are from the various sensors on the machine, cameras, limit switches, speed sensors, radar systems, temperature sensors and other types of sensors, etc. These various sets of machine states and conditions are designed by the original equipment designers. Therefore, they are expected and recognised and understood by the computer control programme via its input sensors and circuits at all of the different periods of the machine's process cycles. **The computer is never presented with input data or conditions that it can't recognise.** In other words, it never has to attempt to apply any level of human intelligence or create real human consciousness to try to contextualise the input data to understand what it is and its relevance within the process so that it can take the required, correct and therefore safe operational response actions.

However, with autopiloted self-driving vehicles, their computer programme control logic is presented with continually changing input data. Some of this will not be pre-learnt, pre-prepared and not pre-designed for. Some will not be predictable in its immense and vast array of continually changing sets and different types and categories of input data.

All of this data relates to the highly detailed road environment the autopiloted self-driving vehicle has to be driven in recognition of and in relation to, at all times. Its computer programme control logic receives data from and about very many different sources. It does require full understanding within the context of the prevailing road situation of what it all relates and interrelates to. This is necessary to make the correct decisions of how to control the car safely at all times for its occupant and other people in its locality.

This requires the car control computer system to have:

1) REAL HUMAN INTELLIGENCE.

2) The ability to create REAL HUMAN CONSCIOUSNESS.

3) The ability to apply contextual relationship, awareness and, therefore, related understanding of all conditions, people, vehicles, moving objects etc., all around it, within its zone of potential connection, interference and collision.

Very simply and basically, because these self-driving vehicles are dumb machines, it is impossible for them to have any of these three immensely important and powerful attributes.

c) The automatically-controlled industrial machine processing lines computer must, without exception, always have a **database that contains all of the information, data and knowledge** necessary to operate the machine that it controls in a safe, effective and required manner under all conditions of operation at all times.

Of immense importance, worth and necessity, the average, experienced and developed human vehicle driver has an immense **database of experience, information, knowledge, memories, recognition and understanding** to draw from. It contains all they see, hear and smell whilst they are driving at all times in control of their vehicle. The human vehicle driver is constantly able to draw upon their intelligence to understand the context of what all data entering via their five senses means. Therefore, it recognises what it has to do to control its vehicle to avoid accidents with other vehicles and all other road users, keep its passengers safe and keep all other road users and pedestrians safe from the vehicle it is controlling.

This also requires the self-driving vehicle to have the same **human-type of database with a similar immense number**

of memories. I do not believe this is a realistically achievable objective for an autopiloted self-driving vehicle system simply due to this being a road with no end.

When a fault/accident incident occurs, it could be deemed to be caused by the self-driving system's database being devoid of some particular memory and its related required response. Combine this with lacking the related software required to process this type of knowledge and response to activate the appropriate actions to deal with the situation. Consequently, this road of travel is likely to continue ad-infinitum and probably have a high percentage of resultant accidents to have to deal with and all that entails.

Consider a few of the different moving items, objects, vehicles, etc., that human car drivers will at times, have to take notice of. They have to understand the particular and challenging characteristics they present to make allowances and considerations for and make the appropriate judgements towards, so they can drive their car safely. Here are some examples:

A horse and rider, a rider-less horse, a sheep, cows, tractors, combine harvesters, bicycles, a number of dogs off leads, motorbikes, battery-powered wheelchairs, scooters, pedestrians of all ages, sizes and physical difficulties looking down at their phones etc., blind people and their dogs, gritting lorries, snow ploughs, trams, farmer's vehicles and swinging attachments that take up more than half of the width of the road, etc.

An infrequent situation of a person seen ahead on a motorway bridge about to drop bricks onto vehicles travelling below would, I'm sure, not be understood and therefore be unable to be responded to at all, let alone appropriately and safely by an autopiloted vehicle. You could continue to describe an extensive list of improbable but possible scenarios that add to the dire consequences list of travelling in a vehicle driven by a machine which doesn't understand all of what is ahead, certainly at times. Therefore, it cannot take the required action to keep its passengers safe and possibly alive during these times. The autopiloted self-driving vehicles can't fundamentally achieve these basic objectives as can the human car driver of average ability and experience with a consciousness, intelligence and contextual processing ability and a vast breadth and depth of an appropriate database.

As a consequence, the human driver will understand the individual characteristics for each of these different moving people, animals and obstacles. These must be considered to predict possible dangers and therefore make the appropriate driving considerations and manoeuvres to prevent accidents and keep their passengers and other road-related users safe.

NB Although it is not acceptable to use computers to control processes that contain or encapsulate humans inside or within the process, as described above, there are one or two exceptions where this rule can justifiably be broken. One of these is where a plane is being flown under computer control with at least one pilot on hand. If the computer system becomes faulty, the pilot can hopefully immediately hopefully safe control of the aircraft.

Another situation is to automatically land an aeroplane when the weather conditions are so exceptionally demanding for a human pilot that a computer-controlled automatic landing system can probably do a better and safer job of successfully landing the aircraft. Bear in mind, though, that the pilot is always on hand to take over if necessary, particularly when there has been a loss of critical facilities that may require the application of human intelligence and the related experience and knowledge.

Whilst driving a vehicle, considering numerous moving objects in many different trajectories at various speeds etc., combined with the total number of varying situations and the degree of multiple complexities that sometimes have to be dealt with whilst driving. Hence, this activity is much more challenging compared to piloting an aircraft in most of its conditions.

I know which driver I would place my life and those of my loved ones in the care of every time:

The human being driver with a real human brain, NOT the machine driver with no human/real brain.

I rest my case.

NB If you wish to read the remainder of my case with many more reasons and depths for my beliefs, please read on, but please be aware that the last part may require some extra concentration and fortitude.

SUBCHAPTER 6.14.2: Reasons why autopiloted self-driving cars can't match human driver performance.

This section covers the many specific, particular and sometimes extremely complex combinations of road traffic conditions, all of which are dealt with comfortably by experienced, human drivers. However, they create many additional reasons why autopiloted self-driving vehicles can't match the performance of human drivers.

SUBCHAPTER 6.14.2.1: The more general reasons why autopiloted systems can't match human driver capabilities.

a) Every human car driver has a *human consciousness,* and the key attribute from which it is created is *human intelligence.* They also have an immense range, breadth and depth of knowledge stored in their memories, derived from their car driving experiences and many others.

These combine to give the relevant understanding and meaning of all of the incoming data into their brain, derived within the prevailing car driving situation. Thus continually creating the car driver's consciousness, from which the human car driver makes all of their decisions and actions.

b) A man-designed and made autopiloted system obviously has no human consciousness. It also has no actual intelligence, despite being named as having Artificial Intelligence, which should be called Artificial (non) Intelligence, in my opinion.

Neither does it have the immense wealth of knowledge, understanding and vast range of capabilities that a normal human driver has.

These three crucially important attributes of consciousness, intelligence and a vast range of knowledge and capabilities enable the human car driver to immediately and continually understand all of the safety-relevant details of the continually occurring dynamic situations developing within their immediate driving area. This usually happens within very small fractions of a second of each moment in time, enabling them to accurately predict the **future potential** occurrences of danger within the whole of their driving-related zone.

c) An autopiloted car or vehicle has a total lack of these three absolutely crucially important attributes (above). As a result, it can respond to the same actual situations that a Human Driver has to deal with; however, this response has limits. At best, it is based on the most absolute and minimal basic level of understanding of the input data its sensors present into its computer logic programme, which was pre-written by its computer programmer/s.

If the autopiloted car's logic programme *has not catered for* seeing a situation it is presented with, then the autopilot system will either simply not make any response at all or possibly the wrong response. This will result in whatever the consequences are, which could certainly be life-threatening – not only to the autopiloted car's passengers but potentially also to all other road users in the immediate locality and also possibly beyond.

NB AN EXTREMELY IMPORTANT POINT which attaches to point 1.0 under the Subchapter 6.14 HEADING: Some of the following weaknesses that these autopiloted systems suffer from, as mentioned in the subsequent sections, may no longer be valid. This is due to the improving and additional data made known from the car's status monitoring systems, which would be available to the autopiloted systems. However, I have left them all in because they may still have a degree of weakness/validity that should be catered for within the design of these autopiloted systems where possible.

d) **The human driver** has data from all-round vision via two eyes that can look ahead, around to each side, and look above and behind using three mirrors. They have sound, feeling, smell and taste as incoming data into their brain. Additionally, they each have automatic alarm-type inputs from their brain's immense database of their life's experiences and information to date.

In the car driver's M.C., this alarm-type data automatically informs them if there is a condition that represents actual or potential danger, or concern for the safety of their car, other people or vehicles, etc., in their driving area of immediate relevance.Also, the human driver's vision, via their eyes, will continually be moving under the control of his M.C. in relation to what their consciousness is informing them about. Their eyes will focus on any particular area of detail that is relevant in that moment for the reason of safety etc. The human driver's vision will be available for reading a variety of possible notices, some of which will be temporary and hand produced, but still very relevant to their safe operation and control of the car.

e) **Vision.**

The autopiloted systems will have a number of viewing cameras. In some cases, this possibly limits the view of some areas where, at times, visual data may suddenly yet uncommonly become vital to have but is therefore unable to be part of the cars' driving and position's control logic. Cameras will presumably be mounted outside the car to obtain the best vision data. However, when flying stones and the vagaries of the weather prevail, or they are coated with mud, heavy rain, snow, sleet and condensation, yet 95% of the critical data is your vision, this represents an immediate danger. The vehicle is driving, to some degree, blind from critically required data.

Wipers and heaters can obviously be used, but at times, the quality of the vision would be compromised. Therefore, total and complete safe driving of the car would be compromised.

Each camera-cleaning facility employed represents a safety risk when it fails. There is the potential for a significant loss of vision data and data about other important information required to keep the passengers safe and avoid car positioning errors.

We know the human driver can minimise these weather-related difficulties quite easily with the used of windscreen wipers, heaters, the passengers' help, and the many other ways we all use, including slowing down to suit. It has been found that these autopiloted vehicles' vision facilities have trouble detecting light coloured vehicles against a light coloured background of the sky, etc. This is a situation that a human car driver would not be likely to suffer from to the same extent. If unsure, they would probably take the appropriate safety fallback response upon recognising that something was not quite correct.

f) Sound.

The human driver has sound data to advise and assist him about safety-related issues and related decisions. Here are some examples:

A passenger will shout out – "Watch out (about something)!"**,** causing the driver to take appropriate actions. People outside the car, particularly in slow-moving, congested conditions, may also shout out something related to safety.

The car driver may hear a tyre start to make a bumping sound, indicating a tyre in a potentially dangerous condition to warrant stopping the car and taking some corrective actions.

When worn, some car brakes make a sound to indicate that they should be replaced soon for braking efficiency and safety.

Other sounds may come from the engine or exhaust pipes that should be responded to in some cases very quickly to ensure safety for all.

g) **Smell.**

The human driver has smell data to warn them that brake systems are getting hot and, therefore, they will not brake the car as much as normal. When the emergency stopping requirement could be hazardous, the human driver may decide to get help to get to a garage.

Smells from the engine areas could also indicate that something may need urgent attention, which could be safety-related to the car and passengers.

h) **Touch.**

Feeling vibrations through the steering wheel can relate to safety issues about tyre or wheel conditions or many other possible problems that may require urgent action.

SUBCHAPTER 6.14.2.2: The more specific reasons why autopiloted systems can't match human driver capabilities.

This section covers more specific reasons and situations where I suspect that autopiloted systems can't match the human driver capabilities of responding to the updating of their consciousness 250 times every second to control their car in relation to the following vitally important safety aspects:

a) At all times, in all weathers, keeping safely and sufficiently *accurately* within the marked lane they have decided they require to be in.

b) Keeping a *safe distance* between their car, all other cars and moving items in their locality by relating to their prevailing speed and speed limits. Crucially this is in the context of how busy and what safety situations all other cars etc., and pedestrians are predicted to present, based on their response to their consciousness update.

c) At all costs, avoiding causing an accident or being involved in an accident with any other vehicle, person or any other living creature.

d) Being constantly aware of all the relevant details of everything happening within their immediate area of driving operation, crucially including what their M.C. predicts will occur in the very near future, particularly presenting danger.

All this is achieved by the human driver being able to utilise the combinational results from:

e) Being able to read and understand the meaning and relationship to their situation of the following: all formal, permanent and temporary written road signs; all hand signals made by policemen, roadworkers, and other car drivers on the roadside in accident conditions; all overhead changeable gantry signs; going into and out of garages, and all different and dangerous types of road conditions, for example, black ice, slippery cobblestones, etc.

f) Being able to see the lane markings clearly and at all times has become increasingly more crucial to road safety, and consequently, they are used more often on the roads. This requirement is made extremely difficult but is still vitally important when, as quite often happens, the lane lines are badly worn and very difficult to detect even for a human driver, plus due to weather conditions – snow, mud, poor lighting.

g) Being able to *clearly see* and *accurately judge* to sometimes, because of circumstances, a few inches of clearance between their car and other vehicles and to a few inches up to lane lines when necessary.

h) Being able to have the intelligence to understand why you have to comply with seemingly contradictory instructions with confidence because you fully understand why they prevail and how to follow them. For example, during police-controlled accidents, or where awkward road works dictate that you travel on the wrong side of the road, ignore traffic light signals or the normal rules of the road.

i) Responding and taking actions to resolve the current/prevailing safety related issues, automatically highlighted by their human consciousness 250 times a second when the driving safety-related situations are numerous and are rapidly changing.

j) Having the human intelligence and lightning-fast processing speed of your brain to ultimately decide quickly enough which **one** of a possible number of accident-occurring scenarios you may at times have to opt to enter due to the consequences of that one being the most acceptable.

k) For the human driver and their passengers to be continually safe, the human driver must be able to operate and drive their car under these conditions:

1 – All types of weather, from extremely hot and dry, to freezing, snowy and icy, to exceptionally wet, windy, unusual light conditions, foggy, smoky and dark conditions.

2 – On all types of roads, tracks, motorways, dual carriageways, large motorways and in multi shopping complexes, noting and dealing with extremely deep and dangerous holes in the road, flooded rivers and other high water or hazardous conditions.

3 – Under types of traffic conditions in large cities and towns with serious congestion. Negotiating multiple moving objects of very many different types, horses, horses and carts, farm animals, trams, combine harvesters, motorbikes, bicycles, battery-operated wheelchairs and scooters etc.

4 – With combinations of groups of the above.

l) 100% of every moment in time, having all of the required data relating to every detail of all of the cars, people, other moving items and objects and from some stationary items. All of these things relate to the human driver's driving locality, with the data entering their brain, so that they and all others are kept safe.

In conclusion: All of this crucially required data comes directly into one or more of their five senses, into their brain and their updated consciousness. From this, their M.C. makes each of their driving decisions and related actions to control their body to carry out all required steps to achieve all of their objectives derived from their thoughts and considerations.

This whole *process control* and *operational system* that controls their car at all times is, in principle, beautifully efficient, basic and simple. It is the perfectly proven human driver method of driving any vehicle safely at all times in any places, environments, and in any weathers safely and effortlessly. All of these facilities and capabilities are packaged and contained within the car driver's human body, which encapsulates and connects them all in wondrous harmony and reliability with constant automatic monitoring of healthy/safe operation.

SUBCHAPTER 6.14.3: Comparing the basic chances of hardware and software equipment_failures driven by the HUMAN DRIVER system and the AUTO-PILOTED system. Most of which would probably lead to extremely dangerous situations for the passengers traveling in the vehicle.

NB The failure of any hardware and software **equipment and systems** which are 100% common to a human driver-driven car and commonplace to a nominally equivalent autopiloted car are not being considered within this comparison of failure analysis.

SUBCHAPTER 6.14.3.1: *Considering all the hardware and software equipment potential failures of vision, hearing, smell, touch and brain (software) departments of the human driver system.*

OVERVIEW: The sheer inherent confidence of reliability, accuracy and safety performance of the human driver system is due to the sum total of all of the human driver's supportive aspects mentioned throughout Section 6.14. It is also due to the many years of driving performance displayed by generations of drivers, performing under all driving conditions in all places, nominally everywhere globally. The confidence expressed by these following judgements is based upon 100,000 miles of motoring by a motorist with average good health, ability and experience.

a) The estimated likelihood of the number of times that **any and only one** of the **HUMAN DRIVER'S data gathering senses** (hardware **or** software equipment) would **totally unexpectedly** fail to work correctly whilst driving would probably be **ZERO to ONCE.**

b) The estimated likelihood of the number of times that **all of** the **HUMAN DRIVER'S data gathering senses** (hardware **and** software equipment) would **totally unexpectedly** fail to work correctly whilst driving, would **probably be VIRTUALLY ZERO.**

c) The estimated likelihood of the number of times that the **HUMAN DRIVER** would **totally and unexpectedly** lose some of their capabilities whilst driving, such as only being able **to operate correctly and safely one** of their hardware and/or software equipment abilities required to control their car, would probably be **ZERO to ONCE.**

d)   The estimated likelihood of the number of times that the **HUMAN DRIVER** would **totally and unexpectedly lose all of** their ability whilst driving, to be able **to operate correctly and safely all of** their hardware and software equipment abilities required to control their car would probably be **VIRTUALLY ZERO.**

e)   The estimated likelihood of the number of times that the **HUMAN DRIVER** would carry out totally wrong, unjustifiable, unexplainable or dangerous action would probably be **3 to 4 TIMES.**

NB The judgements above are critically importantly presupposing that the human driver is not driving whilst having become unable to drive correctly and safely for being too tired, ill, intoxicated or on drugs.

SUBCHAPTER 6.14.3.2: Considering the implications of all of the very _basic_ _additional hardware_ and software systems and equipment that must be included in the design and manufacture of an autopiloted vehicle in order to REPLICATE the HUMAN DRIVER's capabilities.

These systems and equipment include:

A) The hardware and software systems and equipment of cameras, sat nav's and radar etc., facilities for steering, braking, speed control and power supplies etc., computer hardware and related software.

B) All of the driving-related **knowledge and processing capabilities of the human driver's brain**, with its immense range of functional skills, experiences and memories, vision, hearing, smell and all of its bodily facilities. These are used to continually assess and decide upon all of the required driving-related conditions to appropriately manoeuvre and safely control their vehicle accordingly.

NB-1 I have mentioned occasionally in Subchapter 6.14 and elsewhere that <u>some principles and details will not all be correct, accurate or up to date</u>. However, they have been mentioned simply to highlight some areas of concern that need to be born in mind when considering the reliability, accuracy and safety performance of autopiloted systems. I fully understand that they are continuing to be tested, developed and improved, all of the time.

NB-2 It is worth noting again, and I strongly believe that to **set an objective brief** for the very best of the best team of hardware and software design engineers, manufacturers and commissioning engineers it would simply be to:

Provide an autopiloted vehicle that:

Can be safely driven 100% of the time, under all of the most difficult to the easiest combinations and types of all moving items and all kinds of traffic with its full range and degrees of conditions. It also needs to manage all possible worst to the best of road surface conditions, plus all potential weather severities and conditions, nominally, anywhere in the world under a fully autonomously-controlled machine system.

This autopiloted vehicle system would also at least have to equal a human driver. If they had committed an unsafe act or if their vehicle had developed a faulty condition, the human driver would instantly recognise the situation and immediately take some mitigating actions to keep all of their passengers safe. This scenario could even include a situation where the most acceptable and safest mitigating action would be to select a crashing of the car the autopiloted system was driving, with hopefully no injuries to anyone, if this option was available.

All of the requirements above shall be fully satisfied whilst sharing the roads with all other vehicles being autopiloted and also with a mixture of human drivers and autopiloted vehicles.

IF THIS OBJECTIVE BRIEF WAS FULLY SATISFIED, THIS ACHIEVEMENT WOULD BE EVEN BETTER THAN MIRACULOUS.

This is not meant to be critical of the capability of the professional world of our engineers, far from it. It is meant to be the recognition of the stupendous competence of the average human being's brain. When allied to the average human being's body, it carries out all of its brains demands, requirements and activities to incredible accuracy and speed of response that is achieved almost every single time, multiples of thousands of times every hour.

NB-3 To set out to achieve all of these basic objectives defined above would entail a gargantuan exercise of:

a) Replicating all of the human car driver's brain's total range and depth of capabilities, knowledge and experiences, for assessing all conditions presented to them and correctly and safely operating and controlling their vehicle under all possible driving condition scenarios.

    I believe that this would certainly take very many hundreds of man-years of the initial software operating control system design and corrective work. Thousands of fault conditions flagged up during millions of autopiloted vehicle miles would need solving. The majority of each fault condition would result in accidents to the autopiloted vehicle, with a significant number of passenger deaths or serious injuries occurring.

    We can all debate numbers here forever, but this scenario is the aspect that concerns me the most in the extreme about the objective of human beings travelling in a vehicle driven by a machine with zero intelligence rather than by a human being who has intelligence. With human intelligence, they will probably inherently have at least a good degree of awareness of all of the different types of roads throughout the world in all kinds of weather, traffic types and conditions.

As the range of capabilities of the autopiloted vehicle system gradually increases, as a consequence of the work described above, the average frequency of faults and related accidents per unit mile of auto travel will slowly reduce. Nevertheless, I would predict that these accidents will be a significantly greater number than with human drivers, when these autopiloted vehicles are increasingly driven more often over the worst weather and traffic conditions. This will particularly expose the many weaknesses of the replacements of the human brain, eyes and ears etc., for what is essentially a dumb machine system.

Also, I believe that the number of accidents will be a lot higher due to the percentage of autopiloted vehicles increasing. Accidents will be caused by the interaction between vehicles driven by dumb machines, without a car driven by a human brain assisting in mitigating a mistake made by an autopiloted vehicle.

b) Another inevitable increasing difficulty will be persuading human beings to take the risk of being passengers in these vehicles whilst they are being tested. This will further increase the difficulties of attempting to establish the actual facts and details leading up to the fault/s occurring. It is essential to be able to review what the sensors of the autopiloted system sensed/saw and then review what the interpretation and functional responses were by the vehicle's control logic to this data.

Comparing all of this data to the actual 100% facts, as seen and interpreted by a human brain, will hopefully establish why faults/accidents occurred, leading to the most efficient and therefore speedy resolution of these issues. If there are no humans still alive after an accident, you will have lost crucially important data from them about which fault causes and potential solutions can be correctly established, leading to safe and correct resolutions being developed and installed.

c) I have been involved with and responsible for monetary costs and pressures bearing down on the engineering teams working to solve extremely tricky fully-automatic machine system faults. Human deaths and serious injuries, with the awful consequences and pressures that follow, plus the threat of a particular vehicle being withdrawn from public use, cumulatively produce the most extreme difficulties. Inevitably, in some cases, I worry that realistically, these problems are unsolvable due to one or a combination of the reasons I have described in my beliefs in these two articles.

Here is another extremely serious aspect of worry and difficulty. For example, there is an accident involving an autopiloted vehicle, a cyclist, a pedestrian and a vehicle driven by a human containing four passengers, two of which are killed. All of the three surviving occupants in the car driven by the human clearly blame the autopiloted vehicle for causing the accident. The autopiloted vehicle is being driven on commissioned testing, with the express objective of trying to flush out any remaining design faults. Who specifically will the relatives of the deceased passengers blame for the deaths of their loved ones?

Also, I see the likely scenario where the ever-growing interconnected web of the software from which the autonomously-piloted vehicle is controlled becomes ever more complex. This inevitably makes detecting the area or areas of the fault affecting control logic increasingly difficult to identify, and until this happens, a successful solution cannot be created.

Additionally, as the interaction and complexity of the controlling software become ever more complex, solving one fault creates an increased risk of creating another different and/or new defect or defects. This is particularly true when the original control logic design was not as solid, stable and 100% without risks of combinational conditions. The worst-case includes a particular sequence of events that combine to cause an operational fault. I have been involved in many of these situations. They are seriously challenging to resolve and require many tools and approaches to be utilised. This includes employing top-notch software design engineers who are 100% honest with themselves and the other members of the design team. Also, extremely importantly, it includes a chairperson who can fully engage all team members with good guidance and understanding, etc. This is highly tricky but immensely rewarding and satisfying when success is achieved.

Question 1 – *One crucially important question is positioning accuracy.*

What is the actual positioning accuracy of the autopiloted vehicle concerning other cars, people, bicycles, lane lines or any other object or thing which it requires to be positioned in relation to?

Refer to Subchapter 6.14.2.2 (where relevant) for more details of required capabilities.

I believe that the autopiloted vehicle's positional control system will decide where it is in each moment on the face of the earth and in relation to other vehicles and lane lines, etc. It will know where it needs to travel along the road to get to wherever its required destination is, whilst always maintaining a safe and acceptable clearance or distance to all other objects. The vehicle is automatically positioned at all times, from the data received from each of its cameras combined with sat nav data, radar data and possibly other forms of data.

As with any detection positioning system of this type, the resultant prevailing accuracy will probably, I believe, be variable due to the accuracy of data received from each of its different and independent systems likely being variable. With a positioning system such as described, the occasional worst-case overall system positioning inaccuracy is when the various systems feeding their data in, are all accumulative, either negative or positive, relating to the actual, true position.

I would suggest that this will lead to having an actual accuracy that could either be dangerously too close to the target or too far away, both of which could, at times, be disastrous for safety of the vehicle and its passengers. For general conditions, I estimate that the human driver system's accuracy range would be in the order of plus 2.5" to minus 2.5" of a target distance. To give an example, if the driver targeted being 8" inside/away from a lane line, his actual car body would be within 8"+2.5" to 8"–2.5". This would result in it being in the range of 10.5" to 5.5" from the lane.

Significantly, the human drivers' positioning system simply comprises <u>one </u>integrated system of their <u>eyes </u>feeding data <u>into one system</u> – their brain's dedicated visionary processing departments. The resultant accuracy and, therefore, the safety of the human driver's positioning would be, as is proven from normal driving standards, excellent and wouldn't create the very dangerous inaccuracy that can result, at best occasionally, from autopiloted vehicles.

Question 2 – A second crucially important question is response time.

What is the response time of the autopiloted vehicles' control system when it has to assess so many things simultaneously?

These factors can include the position of many different moving objects, such as other vehicles, bicycles, pedestrians, dogs off leads, uncontrolled children, etc. Most are travelling at different speeds, directions and changing angles in relation to your driven vehicle. Each has to be assessed individually and collectively by the human driver or the autopiloted vehicle system nominally, in the same instant in time.

This is an extremely difficult exercise to accurately and execute sufficiently quickly enough. However, it is vitally important for the ongoing continual safe and appropriate decision making of how to steer and control your vehicle in relation to all of these other moving objects within your zone of inter-related activities. It is also essential to continually be able to appropriately accurately predict where they will be in the near future, relevant to your vehicle and others.

I believe that this is a crucially important aspect of the **autopiloted vehicles' control system:** to deal with the huge challenge of having a control system's response time that is fast enough to detect, compute/access and respond to any changes in the position of, in some cases, many different prevailing objects safely and effectively.

The human drivers' consciousness update/response time is 250 cycles per second, thus giving a cycle update every 4ms. I believe that this performance would be significantly faster than the autopiloted system's response time. This crucially adds to the human car driver's accuracy and safety of judging and responding to, other vehicles and moving objects whilst controlling his vehicle's position.

I believe that one last crucially important point to make is that the accuracy of vehicle positioning with an autopiloted system when awful weather prevails will inevitably be significantly and dangerously worse than with a human driver. This is for the many reasons given earlier, plus, under the direction of their intelligence, the human driver, recognising the various significant difficulties the bad weather creates, will make adjustments. To still achieve the required accuracy of assessing all visual and audio data to obtain safe driving, they will carry out various actions like slowing down, double-checking some data and maybe slowing down further, etc.

Question 3 – A third crucially important concern is physical manoeuvring.

The human driver's body (under the control of their brain) carries out all of the vehicle's required driving activities of changing speed, steering and braking. With the **autopiloted system**, the vehicle will have to be modified to include three extra electrical/mechanical/hydraulic systems to provide these three car-control facilities. This introduces quite a few additional components, which are potential risks of failure whilst the car is travelling. Any one or more of these facilities, upon failing, could immediately cause the vehicle to go out of safe control, particularly at high speed.

These additional risks could potentially becoming catastrophic for all vehicle passengers and any other vehicles involved with the out-of-control vehicle within a few seconds of failure occurring.

In conclusion, as detailed in Subchapter 6.14.3.2, A) and B), the crucially important aspect is that, in addition to attempting to replicate the brain's capability and knowledge with a huge amount of software design work, the required installation of all of the related hardware necessary to replace the human driver would be immense. Even with the selection of top-quality equipment, it is inevitable that each potential failure within any of this equipment increases the risks of accidents occurring with the autopiloted vehicle's control system.

When I had to make an engineering design judgement about a manufacturing process that inherently contained a degree of risk of system or process condition difficulties which could have led to human deaths, I always asked myself the question – would I be comfortable actually working with this process system design to which my life was potentially at risk from? I always found this rule sharply focused my mind during the solution investigation procedure, eventually enabling me to enjoy a satisfying feeling about the final decision.

I would never put my name to a project like the autopiloted vehicle system because I would feel personally responsible for every death and serious injury incidence greater than that which would have occurred over 100,000 miles of travel with a human car driver. This statement seems rather crude, but hopefully, it clearly conveys the sentiment that I firmly and genuinely feel about this vitally important project to our future world's travellers.

I must apologise to the autopiloted vehicle designers who are reading the views I am expressing. I know that these auto system designers will certainly be of the top, world-level capability. It is just that they have been tasked with what I believe is an impossible set of objectives to fully and satisfactorily achieve. I would guess their targets include an acceptable level of fatal accidents related to an amount of miles travelled with human passengers.

Who is going to be legally held responsible when accidents, including passenger fatalities, occur?

SUBCHAPTER 6.14.3.3: Comparing the autopiloted system to the human driver system probabilities of hardware and or software equipment failure risks, as previously detailed for the human driver.

These risks are discussed in Subchapter 6.14.3.1 a), b), c), d) & e), **and** below.

OVERVIEW: The relative lack of sheer inherent confidence of reliability, accuracy and safety performance of the autopiloted *system is due to the relatively unproven use of these systems and the* **sum total of all of the autopiloted negative aspects mentioned throughout Section 6.14.**

My predicted number of failures is based upon **100,000 miles of motoring by an autopiloted system in all driving conditions and complexities in any location.** The figures would be as follows:

a) The estimated likelihood of the *number of times that **any and only one** of the AUTOPILOTED SYSTEM'S data gathering (hardware and/or software equipment)* would <u>totally unexpectedly</u> fail to work correctly whilst driving would probably be VERY HIGH, **say FIVE to TEN times.**

This compares to the **human driver's** estimated *number of times* of **ZERO to ONCE.**

b) The estimated likelihood of the *number of times that all of the AUTOPILOTED-SYSTEM'S data gathering* (hardware and or software equipment) would totally unexpectedly fail to work correctly whilst driving, would probably be HIGH-ISH, say **ONE to TWO times.**

This compares to the **human driver's** estimated *number of times* to be VIRTUALLY ZERO.

c) The estimated likelihood of the *number of times that the AUTOPILOTED-SYSTEM totally unexpectedly* lost **some of its capabilities** whilst driving, such as only being able to **operate correctly and safely one** of its hardware and/or software equipment abilities required to control its vehicle, would probably be HIGH, say **THREE to FIVE times.**

This compares to the **human driver's** estimated *number of times* which would be **ZERO TO ONCE.**

d) The estimated likelihood of the *number of times the AUTOPILOTED-SYSTEM totally and unexpectedly* would lose **all of its capability** whilst driving **to operate correctly and safely any** of their hardware and software equipment facilities required to control their car would probably be HIGH-ISH say, **ONE to TWO times.**

This compares to the **human driver's** estimated *number of times* to be **VIRTUALLY ZERO.**

e) The estimated likelihood of the *number of times the AUTOPILOTED SYSTEM would carry out a totally wrong, unjustifiable, unexplainable or dangerous action* due to **hardware** and or software **equipment** failures or mal-operation (*not brain processing failures*) would be EXTREMELY HIGH, say **TEN to FIFTEEN times.**

This compares to the **human driver's** estimated *number of times* which would be **3 to 4 times**.

SUBCHAPTER 6.14.4: Summing up with some important principles of the highly complex activity of being in control of driving a car or any vehicle whilst out on the public roads.

OVERVIEW reminder:*Can autopiloted, self-driving vehicles, in all possible driving conditions whilst on the public roads, ever be as safe for their passengers to travel in as with the average, experienced human driver?*

SUBCHAPTER 6.14.4.1: Factors to deal with when driving.

Navigating and driving a car or other vehicle in a safe and proper manner at all times, so all occupants, pedestrians or other road users are not involved in an accident or injured or killed, requires extensive knowledge and skills derived from vast driving-related experiences. It also requires contextual recognition, detailed understanding and dealing correctly with all of the following aspects.

NB The figure in **brackets** is the overall percentage estimation of what degree of capability an autopiloted vehicle has of safely dealing with and satisfying each requirement listed below.

a) All of the different types of roads and road conditions **(70%)**.

b) All different types of weather conditions **(50%)**.

c) All of the vast range of different types of ever-changing traffic conditions **(50%)**.

d) All of the different types of mistakes and misjudgements that pedestrians, children and animals make **(20%)**.

e) All of the interactions of sometimes all of the conditions and details of what is happening around and within the impactive range of your vehicle **(35%)**.

f) All of the vast number of different and unexpected occurrences of a serious situation or condition that requires immediate actions, with some situations also requiring a degree of intelligence **(40%)**.

g) At times, all of the highly complex, interactive decision-making, action-taking and car management manoeuvring, all to be carried out normally within an extremely short period of time **(30%)**.

h) All different types of vehicles, bicycles, transport, animals, people and all other moving items that may appear and affect your responsive actions whilst driving **(35%)**.

i) The car driving system being able to immediately, safely and appropriately deal with a road traffic situation or condition that it had never been programmed to deal with before **(5%)**.

<u>The total/overall capability of the autopiloted, self-driving system for satisfying the list in 6.14.4.1 above is:</u>

= 335% out of 9 x 100% = 900% (the maximum possible)

Therefore the total/overall capability = 37.22%

SUBCHAPTER 6.14.4.2: Reliabilities and capabilities required to drive safely.

For the person or system in control of driving the car or vehicle to carry out the correct and safe responses to deal with all of the conditions on the road as they occur, they must have the following reliabilities and capabilities as listed below.

NB The figures in **brackets** are the overall percentage estimation of how much capability an autopiloted vehicle has of safely dealing with and satisfying each requirement aspect. They are also, where relevant, reliability percentages related to 100,000 miles of travelling.

a)   Be aware of, **sense** and **receive** into their **control system in sufficient detail**, all of the relevant data *representing all conditions and situations occurring*. This will require vision and hearing, and ideally smell and touch sensing capabilities also (**60%**).

b)   Within the **context of the moment** and the prevailing conditions, be able to <u>process, recognise and understand the meaning</u> of all data entering the car-driving control system (**40%**).

c)   Process and be able to <u>understand </u>what the collection of details that each of the aspects covered in a) and b) listed above <u>actually mean</u> in relation to the <u>safe and correct control</u> of driving the car or vehicle (**30%**).

d)   Within the required timescales of each prevailing situation, be able to **decide** and then take the appropriate actions required to deal with <u>all safety </u>and non-safety **aspects**. All other non-safety or non-important car driving situations <u>to be ignored</u> (**30%**).

e)   Effectively and safely respond to nominally all conditions and situations presented to the car-driving system by having <u>genuine</u> <u>intelligence</u> where required, the knowledge and capability equivalent of the capacity, depth and breadth of the **<u>average</u> human brain** (**20%**).

f)   Have an extremely high degree of **reliability** under all weather conditions for all **Data Sensing hardware (60%)**.

g)   Have an extremely high degree of **reliability** of all **hardware for controlling and manoeuvring** the required vehicle control operations for speed, braking, movement, horn, flashing lights, etc. (**70%**).

h)   Have an extremely high degree of **reliability** of being fault-free for all of the **hardware** required for the needs of the **software** circuits for all the necessary operations and activities **(60%)**.

i) Have the ability to create and update **every few milliseconds the equivalent of the human consciousness** from all of the required input data relating to the car driving conditions and situations. This consciousness will allow the necessary decisions and actions to be created to drive the car safely and appropriately at all times **(10%)**.

The estimated total/overall capability & reliability of the autopiloted, self-driving system for satisfying the list in 6.14.4.2 above is:

= **380% out of 9 x 100% = 900% (the maximum possible)**

Therefore the estimated total/overall capability & reliability = 42.22%

The estimated overall capability & reliability of the autopiloted system in relation to the combined requirements in Subchapters 6.14.4.1 and 6.14.4.2 is:

= **(335% + 380%) divided by (900% + 900%) x 100% = 39.72%**

SUBCHAPTER 6.14.4.3: Conclusion of the comparison.

The question raised in Subchapter 6.14.3.1 related to comparing the *autopiloted system* to the *human driver system,* estimation of probabilities of <u>the number of times</u> the hardware and or software failure risks occur over 100,000 miles. As detailed in Subchapter 6.14.3.1 a), b), c), d) & e), the results would be in the order of:

For the autopiloted system:

The number of failure risks totalised over the range of each of the five different types or categories of failure risks = A minimum of **20 TIMES** to a maximum of **34 TIMES**.

For the human driver:

The number of failure risks totalised over the range of each of the five different types or categories of failure risks = A minimum of **3 TIMES** to a maximum of **6 TIMES**.

Comparing these figures:

This shows that the estimated **minimum** number of times a serious failure may occur with the autopiloted system was **6.7** <u>times greater than with the human driver</u>. The **maximum** number of times a serious failure may occur with the autopiloted system was **5.7** <u>times greater than with a human driver.</u>

<u>Crucially importantly to bear in mind is that each failure of both types would likely result in a very serious category of car or vehicle accident.</u>

In sections 6.14.4.1 & 6.14.4.2:

The estimated **overall capability and reliability** for all of the defined aspects and requirements for safely driving a car or vehicle are:

For the <u>autopiloted system</u> = **39.72%** capability.

For the <u>human driver</u> = nominally **95%** capability.

The absolute critical aspect of the autopiloted system's 39.72% capability is that for 60.28% of the driving situations, it has a very significant *lack of total capability* to correctly and therefore safely drive or control the car under the prevailing traffic conditions.

<u>These are likely to be the most complex conditions to deal with and, therefore, are likely to result in the most serious types of accidents.</u>

The overall consequence of the categories of comparisons above are that there will be a vastly greater number of accidents with the autopiloted systems compared with the human driver in charge.

The judgements above are pre-supposing that the human driver is not driving whilst having become unable to drive correctly/safely or whilst being too tired, ill or intoxicated.

These aspects of the human driver have to be controlled by the driver themselves. Fortunately, they can also be managed by the passengers in the car and by other means.

I fully accept that the above estimations of capabilities are just that – estimations. I would stress that I have spent the vast majority of my life driving, and I would like to think that I have a feel for judgements such as these. I have really tried to be reasonable and fair and not be biased against the plans for such vehicles to be used on our roads. I very strongly feel that autopiloted vehicles are not a suitable use for the unquestionable talents of computers.

I would like to say that I approached writing this section by just listing all of the aspects that came to mind. I would finally like to say that these estimated numbers can obviously be debated, but I feel that my developed case against the use of these self-driving systems is sufficiently proven.

For the vast number of reasons presented in the whole of Subchapter 6.14, I know which driver I would place my life and those of my loved ones in the care of:

The human driver with a brain and not the machine driver with no brain.

I rest my case.

SUBCHAPTER 6.15: Your brain looks like a big pudding. How can there be love in there just because of electrical impulses?

OVERVIEW: This is an exact copy of a question recently posed in a short newspaper article recently of part of a very interesting book by Bill Bryson about the wonders of the human body (The Body). I thought it was worth answering, simply because I have also seen and heard this same question asked in some television documentaries and elsewhere.

My answer is:

There is love in there and every other emotion and thought you have ever experienced throughout your whole life. This is simply because these are electrical impulses with a coded, particular and dedicated meaning and purpose. They are not just any odd random electrical impulses.

All parts and subparts of your brain each have a particular purpose and role to play within the whole of your brain's integrated functionality. Every part and subpart of your brain is selectively and appropriately receiving and carrying information, issuing objectives, instructions or information, as required in every moment to satisfy your and its prevailing and ongoing goals.

CHAPTER 7.0 – YOUR MENTAL HEALTH, YOUR BRAIN, YOUR CONSCIOUSNESS, WHAT YOU DO AND WHY.

This section deals with a list of topical questions about different aspects regarding mental ill-health. These are topics and questions that occur in the media that relate to a lot of key points and details that are covered in my book about your brain, your consciousness and about all that you and it does and why.

Before you read on, please refer again to the note in Subchapter 1.1 – **AN EXTREMELY IMPORTANT POINTER** and the paragraph in Chapter 6.0 just after the Overview.

OVERVIEW: Life these days is increasingly challenging for the vast majority of people <u>not</u> suffering from any mental health issues. They are faced with so many new and challenging aspects of their life, each of which has the potential to create separate but additional emotional stress. For those suffering from poor mental health, life is significantly additionally challenging, in proportion to the degree of their stress levels.

There are two all-embracing aspects of consideration that I have noticed, been told about and been requested to include in my book concerning people who are unfortunately suffering mental ill-health and are continuing to live at home.

1) The first aspect concerns those who <u>care for the person</u> who is mentally ill. This is normally their partner, wife, husband, other family or friends and sometimes their children. The longer the person's illness prevails, combined with other fundamental aspects, it creates an <u>ongoing and generally increasing level of emotional stress</u> **for the carers**.

   The carers, who care so much for their loved one, automatically tend to accept their position, so they don't normally speak about and sometimes are not aware of their own difficulties slowly building up. For a number of reasons, this situation has the potential to become extremely injurious to the carer's health.

   Caring for a depressed loved one can be very emotionally draining and stressful. Having an extended, ongoing high level of emotional stress itself can become very damaging to the carer both mentally and physically, particularly if the patient's needs are 24/7. Also, other members of the carer's family can suffer significantly from stress for various possible reasons, including being directly linked to the person being cared for.

   I'm raising this crucial aspect because I feel it is so important to be aware of it in time to manage it and prevent the situation from becoming more difficult for everyone involved, obviously including the patient.

2) **The second aspect** concerns the mentally ill person wishing to talk to another person or other people about their difficulties. Talking therapy is potentially extremely important and beneficial to the patient's future health,

providing the other person or people respond appropriately and helpfully. Even with the best intentions of the person speaking to the ill person, if the wrong things are said and in the wrong way, this can lead to the patient being significantly emotionally stressed and therefore have their prevailing ill health condition degraded.

The reality is that a high proportion of people particularly those who have no personal experience themselves or with family members or friends of having mental health difficulties, do not wish to talk with the ill person. This is primarily because they do not know what to say and are normally extremely uncomfortable about the whole topic. I believe that this is far more so with men than women due to their different emotional characteristics and feelings of embarrassment about not wishing to be seen as weak and incapable.

This is a list of very basic questions that I have noted. I have personally developed some ideas and answers to them based on my understanding of how your consciousness is created, its purpose and how your brain functions.

SUBCHAPTER 7.1 – Why do an increasing number of people, particularly young women, sometimes cut or regularly self-harm in some way?

I firmly believe that the type of person, male or female, who normally carries out this activity, experiences an ongoing, i.e. daily, very unhealthy level of anxiety and emotional stress in their life. No doubt they will have experienced this for a significant period of time before they commence this activity. I call this a situation of having an ongoing unhealthily high Tower of Emotional Stress, comprised of a number of blocks of stress, each of which stack on top of another and is caused by a particular condition or situation in their life to which they react badly.

These frequently occurring blocks of stress normally continue to negatively affect them on a repetitive basis because the person is not dealing with most, if not all of them, in the best possible way and is suffering from depression and maybe other symptoms. I think the usual trigger that causes them to carry out these self-harming types of actions is when their prevailing emotional stress level has become far too high, to the point that they are really struggling to cope with it.

There is a whole process of **thinking** about carrying out this type of action, **planning** and then **carrying out** the actual activity and **experiencing pain** for the period following the self-harm. I believe this focuses their mind such that they are **not thinking the usual swirling set of negative thoughts**, each of which generally creates a block of emotional stress and anxiety.

The net result is that for a number of hours, encompassing all of these separate periods relating to and including their self-harm and including their period of actual pain, their stress level, which had been running unhealthily high, is significantly reduced. Their life becomes calmer, relatively peaceful, less stressed and simpler, thus giving them **significant peace and respite from their normal merry-go-round of emotional turmoil within their mind.**

One aspect worth mentioning is that, because of the person's character and the blissful escape from their usual emotional stress they experience when self-harming, this could lead them to self-harm more frequently, simply and additionally because it has become an addiction. An additional possible reason, at times, for any person self-harming is for it to be a call for help that say, 'I am in serious emotional difficulty. I must talk to you about it all.'

One final aspect to mention is that, in some cases, the person involved may have extremely low self-esteem. This could trigger their inner demon to turn against them, causing them to self-harm and maybe worse.

I believe that the increasing percentage of recorded, self-harming people who are **female** is due to several combinational factors. The following elements cause them to become anxious and stressed, leading them to **self-harm** and appear in escalating figures.

1)   Women are normally a lot more concerned than men about their looks, body and facial aspects and how many friends they have. They are more likely to be involved with social

media voting pressures etc., amongst their peers, causing them to suffer an increasing number of blocks of significant anxiety from these activities. Though I have noticed that a growing number of males presented in the media are, to a degree, self-worshipping their bodies and facial looks, so this factor is spreading its coverage.

2) The characters of women compared to men are more emotionally sensitive and therefore more reactive to situations in life. This leads them to become more easily anxious and emotionally more stressed than men.

One final and most crucially important point I must make is that anyone who is suffering from the conditions above or any other mental illness conditions that are not clearing up must seek help from their GP without delay.

SUBCHAPTER 7.2 – Why do people suffer from disorders such as Asperger's syndrome, which is a form of autism, and A.D.H.D., and what can be done to help them?

OVERVIEW: My firmly held belief is that the fundamental cause of autism in someone is that one of the most crucial parts of their brain's processing system for **establishing and updating their consciousness and taking actions from is**:

a) *In the extreme/worst cases of autism,* **not working at all.**

b) *For those with a lesser degree of autism difficulties, it is only* ***partially working correctly in proportion to their degree of difficulty.***

Refer to Subchapter 2.3 – <u>B i) and ii) with particular reference to B ii)</u>.

NB There are other chapters describing the cycle of the creation of your consciousness with additional details, but Subchapter 2.3 is the most basic and best one to read first regarding autism. The others are Subchapters 3.1.1, 4.1 and Question 3 in Subchapter 6.1.1.

In autistic people this faulty part of the process of **creating their consciousness** occurs when they **should be deciding**, in the context of that moment, which **incoming data** mainly from their senses (but also from their internal thoughts) poses **no threat to their safety**. At this point, they **should also decide** what incoming data does **not require any other/non-safety action from them** at that time.

When your consciousness creation/updating process is working faultlessly, your M.C. immediately identifies each item of incoming data that has no safety implications or other relevance to you. **Your M.C. deletes all of these from your consciousness updating** process and only deals with the remainder of data. This could be 20% of all of the incoming data in that moment, dependent upon the busyness of your setting.

The most serious, monumental consequence of this faulty part of people's multi-part consciousness creation process is that their brain is not ignoring data. It is not filtering out **any incoming data at all** or, in some lesser cases, is not filtering out a significant percentage of incoming Data that it should be filtering.

1.0 Other important factors in relation to people who have autism are:

a)   I believe that, one crucially important causal factor that will significantly add to their difficulties is the state of the patient's <u>prevailing, ongoing Tower of Emotional anxiety and stress.</u> On days when this Tower of Stress is extremely high, the person suffering from this disorder will suffer proportionately worse than normal/usual. The significant worst-case consequences of the person suffering from Asperger's is that they are already suffering from a very high Tower of Stress. They are attempting to process *100% of the incoming data 100% of the time.* In busy environments, with an awful lot of data coming into their brain from their senses and internal thoughts, they will have to deal with serious data overload. This is swamping their brain as the information floods into it. Their **brain desperately attempts to process it all and will probably end up not processing much, if any of it!**

    At times, this will create sheer total confusion and panic for some patients, creating the consequences of your brain being unable to deal efficiently, effectively and correctly with much if any of the incoming data that is flooding into it. This will lead to the person suffering from functional difficulties, feeling highly anxious, emotionally stressed. They are desperately attempting to consider and deal with all of this incoming information they feel requires attending to, but extremely frustrated, embarrassed and anxious with their inability to do so.

b) These are worst-case scenarios but potentially a possibility.

In extremely busy incoming data settings, some sufferers may at times be seen charging about from one area or situation to another. They seem out of control and to be achieving nothing of any worth as they attempt to process all of their incoming data. They will no doubt have frustrated teachers, parents and others, adding to their already highly anxious and stressed states by sometimes, through sheer frustration, receiving criticism for their bad behaviour and all sorts of other criticisms. They will suffer from maybe self-destructive feelings of inadequacy, embarrassment, anger, lack of self-confidence and utter bewilderment. This leads to even higher levels of anxiety, depression and even worse behaviour and performance of their incoming data processing.

c) Again, these are worst-case scenarios but potentially a possibility.

All of these challenges will be in addition to their difficulties in processing their consciousness, leaving them facing an ever increasingly bleak future, undoubtedly a frightening proposition for anyone. These sufferers will require an enormous amount of careful support, understanding and constructive, helpful actions to give them belief and hope for a better future. I believe they can have this, particularly with the help tailored to and most appropriate for each individual's particular difficulties.

Every person is unique when considering all aspects that combine to create who they are and what they do. I believe that each person needs to be carefully studied by assessing their particular autistic difficulties to create a plan based upon the best way to help them improve the processing of their consciousness.

d) I think that some people who have this type of disorder and are attempting to minimise their difficulties are likely to try and significantly reduce the amount of data coming into their brain. This is particularly related to their sight because this is normally by far the most amount, followed by their sound. I can imagine they will adopt various strategies to attempt to lessen the degree of difficulty and frustration they experience in their moment-to-moment, daily life.

They will probably try and minimise their amount of close interaction with other people because, the brain is extremely busy working on many different aspects and topics whilst directly connecting with others. Because of this, even if they attempt to carry out these activities, which will be bound to be making them anxious already, they will be unable to or wish to deal with this process effectively. Unless, perhaps, it was with one person they knew really well, liked, trusted and therefore felt relatively comfortable in the presence of.

e) I would guess that, where they have the opportunity, they will try and spend a lot of time on their own or with a few other people they are close to. They probably read and write a lot as both of these activities allow them to control the rate at which the data is coming into their Brain for creating their Consciousness and thus will be very therapeutic for them.

My book's basic and very simple objective is to inform and help people wherever they have very significant difficulties in their lives.

I believe that the younger anyone who has this disorder begins to get help to minimise their difficulties, the easier it will be for their brain to hopefully modify and improve its functionality.

*Helping people with autism by working with them appropriately to help them minimise their difficulties, if done correctly, should produce significant benefits **with absolutely no risks at all**.*

SUBCHAPTER 7.3 – Are the desperate, mentally ill people who commit suicide simply making a cry for help?

OVERVIEW: *You very often hear these comments made about a desperately mentally ill person following their successful suicide and all too often, particularly in relation to a railway line suicide: "What a thoughtless action to take when the consequences for others are they are late for work," they pronounce. "Why don't they think of the* *trouble their actions will cause countless others?" say the railway passengers affected.*

There are always exceptions to every situation, but I don't believe that generally, this is the case. I think that they feel they have reached a pit of their deepest despair. They see no way out of a life of constant and deep difficulties. They feel tired and worn out with their ongoing battles. They may have decided they have no value to anyone. They won't be missed and don't see any light at the end of their tunnel of darkness. They just wish it all to stop, and so they commit suicide.

However, I see other aspects to bear in mind, which are:

a) When anyone is in such mental turmoil as described, they will be completely unable to make the best and most logical decisions for themselves about anything. The last thing they will be able to consider is the disruption to other people.

b) If they intended to make a cry for help, it would always be too late after a successful suicide.

c) If the situation is one where the person has not made a determined effective effort to end their life. Instead, they carried it out unsuccessfully and in seemingly half-hearted manner, then this may very well be a case where it actually was a cry for help.

d) In a significant number of cases, the person involved may have extremely low self-esteem which could trigger their inner demons to turn against themselves, causing them to commit suicide.

e) A significant percentage of males are too embarrassed to admit suffering from mental illness. They soldier on, keeping their difficulties to themselves, even from their wives and partners, and they sometimes self-harm for the reasons above. Some finally resort to committing suicide, thus making the ultimate escape from their troubles.

One final and most crucially important point I must make is that anyone suffering from the conditions above or from any other conditions of mental illness which are not clearing up is that they must seek help from their GP without delay.

SUBCHAPTER 7.4 – Is the placebo effect real? If so, how is it created, and how does it work?

OVERVIEW: *I believe that the placebo effect is real and it does work. However, this is providing the patient or the recipient of its benefit totally and wholeheartedly believes in the process they are embarking on to achieve something <u>significant to them</u>. When this is the case, they are open and receptive to its creation. Therefore, they will benefit from the* **additional help** *the placebo effect provides towards them achieving the successful outcome they wish for.*

I believe that your brain's sixth fundamentally important role is the utilisation of the incredibly powerful, effective, indicative and corrective tools it has available, which are:

Pain, discomfort and/or functional disabilities and additionally, prompting and guiding you to self-help and inherently engaging your placebo effect.

Your brain employs *each of* these tools individually and collectively, as appropriate, to every set of your circumstances to assist you in recovering from physical ailments and poor mental health.

For example, to encourage you to resolve your poor mental health, your brain itself will deliberately create symptoms of: **Headaches** of many types and/or **dysfunctionalities** of many kinds – you can't talk, see or think clearly, etc. This is not because you actually have an individual physical and/or chemical cause, related to these symptoms. Instead, it gives you these symptoms to deliberately force you to slow the pace of your life down. It wants you to stop you daily/regularly carrying out some activities and engaging in stress-creating attitudes because it knows they are each contributing to your ongoing poor state of mental health.

Your brain will know that your M.C., from its past experiences, will recognise that the functional cause of these symptoms is far too high an ongoing Tower of Anxiety and Emotional stress. This is caused by several separate, underlying causes of anxiety in your life, most of which you have not been effectively trying to resolve.

A) The sequence of the process above could flow like this:

1) Your **brain** is very worried that you have a damaging, very high ongoing Tower of Anxiety and Emotional Stress that has existed for far too long. This is causing you to increasingly suffer from a prevailing consciousness dominated by suffocating anxiety, emotional stress and the all-too-frequent resultant negativity.

2) Your **brain** knows the <u>functional causes</u> of this worrying condition are:

a) That you have far too many unresolved situations in your life, each of which is creating a block of Emotional Stress within your total Tower of Emotional Stress.

b) You are far too busy in your work and your home life, causing you to suffer from a high number of individual stress blocks that appear as part of your Tower of Stress.

3) Your **brain** deliberately gives you symptoms of a bad headache and some dysfunctionalities. This is to make you <u>less able to continue carrying out the activities in your daily life that contribute to your very high level of stress.</u>

4) Your **M.C.** recalls from its memories <u>what created these symptoms</u> in **3)** before, and therefore knows what actions require taking to resolve the whole situation.

5) Your **M.C.'s** <u>strong belief</u> in knowing what the causes of your ill health are, <u>combined with knowing</u> what actions need to be taken to cure your ill health, creates a very strong <u>PLACEBO EFFECT</u> within your **M.C.'s** mind. It is now confident that your ill health will be resolved.

501

6) This <u>PLACEBO EFFECT</u> immediately <u>reduces your overall stress level in your Tower of Stress.</u>

7) Your **brain** notices this, and because it is pleased that your stress level is dropping, it reduces the **degree of your headache and dysfunctionalities.** This immediately creates a further <u>reduction in your overall stress level in your Tower of Stress.</u>

8) Your **M.C.** commences its campaign of tackling your condition and its causes as detailed in 1), 2) a) and b) above.

9) Your Brain is very pleased to see these activities taking place and responds again by diminishing the **degree of your headache and dysfunctionalities,** which immediately creates a further <u>reduction in your overall stress level in your Tower of Stress.</u>

As the causes of your mental ill-health are reduced, in terms of their damaging effect, and some of them eliminated, your Tower of Ongoing Stress will reduce. In turn, the degree of your headache and dysfunctionalities will lower, culminating eventually in your mental health being fully restored to tip-top status!

Make sure that you keep it this way – permanently!

IN FINAL CONCLUSION:
Your placebo effect is potentially involved in literally everything you do in the whole of your life at all times in all places, at work, outside work – ALL PLACES! This may seem strange,

but it is true. Many people think it is only involved with you having physical health operations etc., which it certainly is, but that is only one area or situation of your life. What is of prime importance is that you create your placebo effect with every objective, every job or project you have, whatever the aim happens to be.

If you do not create your placebo effect fully, you will probably not have the best of outcomes. If you create it fully, you will have the best possible outcome that you are capable of.

I believe that the placebo effect is very complex, multi-faceted, interactive, extremely powerful and beneficial when fully engaged and utilised by you. The creation and utilisation of the placebo effect in the example above will occur due to your M.C.'s previous experiences and utter belief in the benefits of all of its actions as detailed.

To read **many more details than above** about the placebo effect, please refer to Subchapter 2.5.2, sections ROLE F-9 and F-12.

SUBCHAPTER 7.5 – For people suffering from chronic deep depression and other severe mental conditions, why does passing controlled electrical currents through their brains sometimes achieves startlingly beneficial results when all other treatments have completely

failed? Are there any possible downsides to this treatment?

OVERVIEW: This treatment regime for people with extreme mental health problems is called ECT or Electro Convulsive Therapy and has been applied to patients since the 1970s.

I believe that the primary foundational reason for what I would describe as this quite extreme treatment being successful in some cases, is due to the ongoing very deep depression, caused by the extremely unwell state of mind that the unfortunate patient has experienced for an extended period. During their wakefulness, their mind will have been full to saturation at times with a swirling, continually cycling set of emotionally draining negative and psychotic thoughts. Most, if not all of these, they will have been unable to quell or control to any degree during a long period of time.

In this quite extremely unwell state of mind, no other form of help has been able to even begin to penetrate through this impenetrable fog of draining negativity. The resultant oppressive despair they feel has worsened due to no treatments they have received having given any relief or hope for a better future.

During sleep, their brain will have been desperately attempting to resolve their considerable difficulties by considering their issues. This has probably frequently led to poor quality and insufficient sleep, thus exacerbating their mental health difficulties.

They are presented with this electric shock treatment as the solution to their predicament. If they believe that this treatment will help them, the placebo effect of this thought will be added to the actual effect of the treatment itself, thus benefitting the patient two-fold.

I believe that the effect of this treatment of sending electrical currents through several broadly-selected departments of their brain stirs up the **prevailing state, contents** and, therefore, thoughts in their mind within those departments. This creates epileptic-type fits with the consequence of hopefully eradicating most if not all of these continual negative thoughts.

a) The **best possible results** of this type of treatment are:
- The patient awakes and thinks – 'I can't believe this.'
- Their mind has not been this calm and free of all of these extremely disturbing thoughts for a very long time.
- Their mind is consequently, with major significance, now open to various forms of help that their mental health professionals are offering them.
- The patient feels as if they have been re-born, and they now have a relatively blank slate to work with.

b) The likely results of this type of treatment are:
- The patient awakes and experiences a reasonable degree of the range and depth of the results as **a)** above. However, after a number of weeks, which may have included other forms of treatment, the effects of the ECT have worn off, and their extreme emotional state returns as before.
- The patient receives further ongoing ECT sessions. Each time, due to the reasons given in **d)** below, there is always

a risk that they will suffer some of the serious symptoms described.

c) The **disappointing results** of this type of treatment are:
   • The patient awakes and feels pretty much the same symptoms as before, goes home, and after a few days, still feels exactly the same symptoms as before.

d) I believe that the **worst results, which are unfortunately quite possible,** are due to the basic nature of the crudity of the treatment method. There is a lack of detailed knowledge – a lack of depth of understanding of the complex functionality of our brains and the detailed uniqueness of each person's brain. These outcomes can include:
   • The patient awakes and finds they have exactly the same symptoms as before but also suffers **new** possible symptoms of:
     ◻ Memory loss
     ◻ Difficulties of speaking, reading, walking,
     ◻ Feeling suicidal
     ◻ Brain damage

Some, if not all, of these new difficulties, are consequences of the aspects stated in **d)** above.

Based on this information, I believe that there is a very loud question prevailing. Should this type of treatment continue?

SUBCHAPTER 7.6 – Is there a primary, underlying cause for the increasing, high percentage of the population

who suffer from significant, ongoing poor quality and quantity of sleep?

OVERVIEW: You have no doubt seen highlighted in the media over many years the headline – at last, the recipe of what you must do to achieve a good quality night's sleep. The list containing these silver bullets type solutions is extremely long.

I firmly believe that for the **vast majority** of very poor sleepers, their **one primary underlying functional cause** is suffering from far too high an ongoing level of **anxiety,** resulting in **an elevated Tower of ongoing Emotional Stress.** By ongoing, I mean the height of their Tower of Emotional Stress is unhealthily high most days, over a long period of time. It comprises many blocks of stress, each created by anxiety about some particular situation in their life.

Unless this underlying cause of far too much anxiety and stress is seriously identified, tackled and gradually reduced to a low and emotionally healthy level, their sleeping difficulties will continue. Tinkering about with a few of these, what I call non-primary causes, may help have some better quality sleep for a short period, mainly due to the placebo effect. However, for the vast majority of people, their extremely poor-quality sleep will re-appear and continue.

In addition to considering and dealing with the factors above, for the younger generation particularly, there are two other potentially additional causal factors to check out. If they are applicable, they must also be addressed.

a) Whether they are getting sufficient regular physical exercise every week, especially if they used to get a lot. Regular exercise is highly beneficial to very good mental health.

b) The other question is, are they emotionally addicted to playing games on their computer, including gambling? This comprises two intertwined, very serious addictions and normally entails playing against people around the world until the early hours of the following day. If they are gaming, they will certainly have awful sleep quality.

Whilst attempting to sleep, their mind will be full of thinking about a long list of repetitive, unresolved anxieties, plus what I call repetitive negative thoughts will be swirling around. This doesn't allow their mind to settle to a calm, peaceful and reflective state, thus preventing them from getting to sleep easily and fairly quickly.

Then, after eventually getting to sleep, their brain will be desperately attempting to find solutions to the long list of the different unresolved situations in their life, each causing them significant anxiety and emotional stress. Some of these concerns will be re-created during their sleeping processes during dreams and thought processes.

Also, some of the other tidying up activities their brain needs to carry out during sleep, re-processing their memories, etc., may not be completed. This will result in them suffering additionally from not feeling refreshed when they awake in the morning, due to their brain not having put its own 'daily processing activities house' in good order. Consequently, its processing operational efficiency will be very poor, causing them to feel mentally jaded and sluggish right at the commencement of each day. In itself, this is just the worst feeling to have, especially if you have to get to work and face some particularly challenging issues.

Based on the **underlying functional cause** of their sleep problems being **far too high an ongoing level of anxiety, resulting in an elevated ongoing Tower of Emotional Stress,** to tackle and finally solve their sleep problems, they need to carry out the following fundamental actions.

a) Firstly establish a list of all of the <u>**underlying causes**</u> of all of the different issues and situations that are **each** creating anxiety and emotional stress within any areas of the whole of their life.

b) Establish an understanding of why they are reacting so anxiously to each of these <u>**underlying causes,**</u> which involves searching for the <u>**underlying root causes**</u> that create these anxious reactions.

c) Armed with this knowledge and understanding, acquired by hard work, decide how to **deal with and eradicate where possible, or at least minimise,** each of their Emotional Stress Creators on the list.

A list of some of each person's possible <u>**underlying root causes**</u> will likely be from a combination of some of the following:

a) Personality.

b) Lifestyle at work and at home.

c) Habits, with all of their attendant details.

d) Relationships with each of the key people in their life.

e) Prevailing and future life objectives.

f) Views about themselves and generally, other significant people in their life.

g) State of their all-round health mentally and physically.

h) Difficulties from having their sleep problems.

i) Biased attitudes to a number of life's aspects.

The above process and its aspects sound simple. However, it requires an awful lot of discussion, honesty, sometimes brutally honest, constructively critical, time and hard work, particularly by the patient, ably guided and supported by their counsellor.

I believe that the process above and continued below, **must be managed and led** by a professional mental health counsellor experienced in the use of Cognitive Behavioural Therapy, normally arranged by a GP.

If the patient is not guided by their counsellor in the best, most appropriate and empathetic way for them and their needs throughout this, particularly at times, delicate process, the consequences could be alarming for the patient's mental health.

These ideas I've mentioned could be part of the patient's counsellor's regime. They would apply actions and plans in an order and way that would be appropriate to their view of the patient's situation and their own individual preferences. It is so important that the patient and their counsellor work very closely together to develop a mutually trusting and respectful relationship. This will support the patient to achieve the best possible outcome for improving both their quality and quantity of sleep and their related emotional health.

One very important point to be aware of is that not everyone who is too stressed is aware that this is the case. They have been in this state for such a length of time it has become normal and accepted by them.

Another vitally important point is to check that the patient is not making too many changes, alterations and deletions that are all being processed at nominally the same time. For a number of different reasons, this would probably cause a significant degree of de-stabilising in their life, causing a significant degree of additional emotional stress.

It is essential they work with their counsellor to review the list of all contributing issues, conditions, situations and other causal factors relating to their stress. Then, in order of priority, note the major contributors, but also include some easier and quicker ones to solve. Agree on an initial shortlist and upon actions to eliminate or reduce, as realistic, each item by an achievable completion date.

Regularly review your progress and current objectives with your counsellor. During this exercise, presumably, most people will be carrying on with their busy working life or whatever. Therefore, it is vital that the sets of aspects they set themselves to work on are comfortably achievable.

You and your counsellor establish, work through, modify and solve each of the issues and causal factors adversely affecting your life. This crucially important exercise of assessment, actions and changes will gradually and effectively be the potential key to slowly and controllably opening the door to the quality of sleep you desperately need and so wish to enjoy.

Adding to the list above, you will probably be including quite a number of changes for example, to your lifestyle, at work and home. You will be modifying your attitudes, objectives and ways of approaching them, plus dealing with people and many different things and situations in your life. You will have to make the required changes in the appropriate areas of your life to be able to achieve your basic objective of reducing your ongoing anxiety and emotional stress levels.

Generally, the longer your sleep difficulties have prevailed, nominally the longer it will take to solve them completely, but as you gradually lower your anxiety, your sleep difficulties will reduce.

There is no quick, simple solution to your problem. You have to come to realise that only you can <u>gradually improve your emotional situation and related sleep problem</u>. It is so, so important that you believe in your counsellor's ability, keenness to help you, and the process they have outlined, which you are following together. The completed application, combination and belief in the benefit of all of these elements will fully engage your placebo effect. Consequently, you will gain a very significant additional benefit along your road to eventually achieving excellent quality sleep every night.

The above gives one simple framework of a system to pursue.

SUBCHAPTER 7.7 – Panic attacks – What causes them? Can we do anything to prevent them? Can a person recover a life that is becoming increasingly suffocated by them?

OVERVIEW: *More people are suffering from panic attacks as our world becomes increasingly infiltrated by activities, situations, practices and electronic facilities. Each of these has the potential, particularly with some individuals, to trigger individual anxiety and emotional stress, leading to an increase in the ongoing Tower of Emotional Stress they are already carrying.*

We all carry, to some degree, an ongoing Tower of Emotional Stress which may be a low/safe/healthy level most of the time or not, as the case may be, for each individual. More people than you would probably guess regularly suffer and, in some cases, daily from panic attacks. In extreme cases, this is to the extent that they feel they have to manage and arrange their activities, including work, around what situations would trigger a panic attack to avoid being exposed to them. Even some people who have very high profile jobs feel they have to operate in this manner.

The basic cause of a panic attack is when someone is about to, or has just commenced doing something which makes them extremely anxious. They become highly emotionally stressed, adding to the stress level they were already carrying.

Here are several examples of a few basic activities and/or situations that may induce panic attacks in some people:

a)   Going on to a stage to perform some form of activity.

b)   Taking extremely important exams.

c)   Being exposed to heights in many and various types of situations.

d)   Being exposed to confined and cramped claustrophobic conditions in many situations.

e)   Being in large, maybe busy and maybe noisy crowds of people or exposed to not so big groups of people.

f)   Being the sole focus of people's attention; not necessarily a lot of people and not necessarily on a stage.

g)   Being assessed in a job interview, within your working environment or many other environments.

Depending upon the prevailing circumstances, the brain of the person suffering a panic attack can become so concerned about the degree of stress their person is expressing. It fears for the consequences of their decision-making and resultant actions due to being driven by their increasing level of sheer emotion and panic. Because of this, it may make their panic attack even worse, so they, the person themselves, or someone else who is there, removes them out of the situation they are reacting to. This enables them to start to recover their emotional unbalanced and, in some cases, potentially dangerous state of mind.

As a reaction to a commonly practised activity, some panic attacks can become a standard/habitual reaction due to habit and the person expecting one to occur. Let me give an example of how the principles of a previously, commonly practiced activity with no history of triggering panic attacks can develop into a panic attack creator.

A person's normal route to work involved driving their car along an extremely busy section of the motorway. One day, whilst on this hectic motorway section, he experienced a relatively low level of panic attack. He was able to continue driving to work on the motorway, arriving there successfully, albeit a little stressed from his unnerving experience. He thought no more about this occurrence and life went on.

A few weeks later, the same situation occurred. However, this time, the panic attack was so severe that he had to leave the motorway, which he, fortunately, could do almost immediately. He became extremely concerned about this situation and set about attempting to solve the cause of his difficulties. His focus of attention was on the motorway-driving activity. He theorised about why driving on the motorway could be so emotionally stressful to suddenly create severe panic attacks after many years of no problems whilst regularly driving on motorways. Unfortunately, his musings did not throw up any conclusions.

For a few months, general driving on motorways continued without any problems. But then, again, whilst driving to work it re-occurred and also whilst not driving to work. He could give no logical reason/s why he would be particularly stressed whilst motorway driving.

Again he questioned himself about, whether historically he had experienced some significantly unnerving motorway situation that may have created a deep-seated emotionally bad P.T.S.D experience cause. No. Neither he nor his father could remember such an experience, including him being on the motorway as a passenger in his father's car.

Eventually, after much thought and discussion with friends, he developed a theory of why he was very occasionally experiencing his difficulties. It revolved around his ongoing Tower of Emotional Stress. He would get up in the morning, along with his wife and his young children. Whilst watching the clock, he would carry out a long list of activities: waking his children, organising showers, getting breakfasts, school stuff and his work stuff ready, helping with general tidying up, dealing with very occasional children tantrums and a very occasional slight tiff with his wife.

Each of these many activities would create their own relatively small block of stress, adding to his fairly comfortable Ongoing Tower of Stress building up before he left home.

On most mornings, he would get up comfortably early and carry out all of these activities efficiently and without any particular stressful incidents. Therefore, he arrived at the motorway with a relatively low ongoing Tower of Emotional Stress and would not experience any panic attack issues at all.

However, on the mornings where he had maybe got up a little later and experienced stress from some tantrums etc., by the time he left home, he would already be carrying a higher than normal Tower of Emotional Stress. On top would be dumped a pre-exposed, but initially not too high a block of stress, due to him having developed a degree of expectancy of suffering a panic attack on the motorway. As he got closer to the motorway, if he could see and hear a higher than normal density of traffic, this would trigger the existing motorway-caused block of stress to grow significantly. Unfortunately, the traffic conditions and the increased risk of being late from work were a big stress creator for him. Therefore, it was not surprising that, due to the aforementioned combination of conditions, he would occasionally suffer a panic attack.

He theorised that the motorway-driving activity itself was not the root cause, but the 'final straw that broke the camel's back' type cause. The risk with such situations developing as described is that the final straw activity is **not seen as the cause.** So, from then, any time motorway driving is necessary, even beginning with a very low Tower of Emotional Stress, the anxiety-combination of the pre-exposed expectancy and substantial belief that a panic attack will occur, actually combine to creates one. This is an example of the extreme power of your mind but operating in a negative way.

What is so important with such experiences is that the underlying cause is identified as soon as possible. This way, the appropriate corrective approach is applied, thus enabling the difficulty to be carefully and confidently removed. Additionally, it is essential that efforts to significantly reduce the person's unhealthily high ongoing Tower of Stress are made, with all of the many resultant benefits being obtained.

It is imperative to be aware that a person may increasingly and eventually become so emotionally reactive to a particular activity or situation that, as this activity approaches, the block of anxiety and emotional stress created within their mind grows quickly and spontaneously. Even if their ongoing Tower of Stress was relatively low, they would still experience such a significant increase to their immediate Tower of Stress that they would suffer a panic attack of some degree of emotional disturbance.

One last example of an extremely worrying chain of events that occurred in recent times is a lady who reported her difficulties live on the radio. She described herself as having worked as a psychologist. She also described herself as having had treatment for stress and depression and, as a consequence, was currently out of work.

This lady increasingly came to dislike being in crowded conditions. One day, she went to the checkout in a large superstore to pay for her goods and suffered such a serious panic attack, she ran out of the shop leaving her shopping behind.

She saw the shopping/crowd scene as the root cause of her panic attack and changed her shopping habits to only shop in relatively small shops. Eventually, this changed as she also became uncomfortable in these situations, and she changed to only shop online with home delivery.

She became increasingly uncomfortable whilst visiting friends in their houses. She didn't suffer actual panic attacks, but suffered what I would surmise as very low level, potential beginnings of panic attacks. She stopped going to her friends' houses and invited them to her house. However, they became uncomfortable visiting her due to the conversation predominantly being centred upon her panic attack difficulties and her worsening state of mind about it all.

The ramifications of this sequence of events and her decisions to remove any activity in her life that would cause or risk causing a panic attack was that she found herself increasingly isolated from people and the real world day-to-day activities. She also felt increasingly anxious and emotionally stressed that her life was in turmoil, which it most unfortunately was. As she had not been able to reduce her ongoing emotional stress, and it had been increasing, she had not been able to begin facing up to and individually tackling the activities that gave her panic attacks. The compression of her basic day-to-day life was gradually emotionally suffocating her.

As noted from this poor lady's circumstances:

It is crucially important for anyone who begins to experience a panic attack brought on by something, and they cannot deal with it successfully themselves or with the help of their partner, to enlist the appropriate professional help as soon as possible. I would strongly advise them to seek help from their GP. I firmly believe that, in most cases, once a panic attack (P.A.) occurs as a reaction to the **same triggering activity or situation** and is repeated, the more times this happens, the elimination of it becomes proportionately more difficult.

NB It is vitally important to correctly identify what type of P.A. trigger activity and/or situation the cause is. If you look at the list of different P.A. triggers **a)** to **g)** above, for the majority, they can relate to and be created by a lot of different actual activities and/or situations.

It is like many things in this life of ours. Most are not as simple as they appear from a superficial view of only the tip of the situation's iceberg.

Lastly, it requires a great degree of courage to deal with the causes of your panic attacks, particularly some of them. It is vitally important that you are aware of this and gird up your loins to face up to them, look them in the eye and face them down. After this first biggest hurdle is overcome, it becomes increasingly easier. You can enjoy the satisfaction of gradually grinding your monster into the dust of the past and open yourself up to your new life.

One final and most crucially important point I must make is that anyone suffering from the conditions above or from any other conditions of mental illness which are not clearing up must seek help from their GP without delay.

SUBCHAPTER 7.8 – Jet Lag – Why is it so disruptive to your state of mind, and what causes it?

I believe that jet lag is far more disruptive to most people's physical states and their functional and emotional health than they are aware of due to the combinational effect of each of the following factors. The cumulative amount of disruptive jet lag experienced depends upon: your flying times, length of flights, when you eat and when you return home, the quality of your seating arrangements, your body's position whilst you are sleeping, each person's prevailing emotional and physical states during your entire flight and their unique characteristics.

Add to these things the following factors:

Factor **a)** When you experience jet lag disruption on your outward journey because your normal time to go to bed is altered, so you are fighting against your body clock's regular sleeping regime.

Factor **b)** When your usual eating and possibly consuming alcohol times and quantities are probably significantly altered.

Factor **c)** When the total time of relative, good quality sleep is significantly less than normal. It will also probably comprise of short periods broken by toilet disturbances, exercise to prevent D.V.T., not sleeping flat or in your normal most comfortable positions and being in close proximity to many other strangers.

Factor **d)** Before you have probably fully recovered from the negative effects of far less quality and quantity of sleep you require every night, you return home.

Factor **e)** Your natural/automatic body clock may be altered to some degree, so getting back to your normal sleeping pattern will take some time to achieve.

Factor **f)** You experience jet lag disruption on your homeward journey, with the basic repeat of the factors above. Additionally, if you are returning home from a lovely holiday, you will be less emotionally buoyed up than when you travelled out because it has ended. In contrast, on the way there, you had all of the great expectations you subsequently enjoyed.

The cumulative negative effect of all of the above, I would propose, is far greater than most people are aware of. It will probably require a few weeks to fully recover from, dependent upon a number of jet lag related factors unique for each individual. I firmly believe that for most people, the most significant and disturbing single negative factor above is the degree of the disruptive effect of extremely poor quality and quantity of sleep they have suffered. Having a very good night's sleep comprising of the number of good-quality sleep hours you ideally require is the primary foundation of living an emotionally, physically and healthy, happy life.

SUBCHAPTER 7.9 – Fibromyalgia – Is there an underlying cause, and if so, what is it and how best to treat it?

OVERVIEW: *I believe that **in some cases, for this horrible condition**, which may have attached to it the phrase – is the cause in the patient's mind or body, with all of its many related extremely unpleasant and disruptive symptoms, there is a **<u>functional cause.</u>***

*For too long a period of time and for a significant percentage of the time nominally each and every day, the person is suffering from **far too high a level of anxiety,** resulting in **<u>an elevated level of their Ongoing Tower of Emotional Stress.</u>***

NB Due to each of the many symptoms, a few of which can be experienced by patients with this condition, they will therefore suffer a very high level of emotional stress. This **includes** the stress caused by each of the anxiety creating factors, conditions or difficulties referred to below.

The **underlying causes** for their ongoing **high level of Ongoing Tower of Emotional Stress** will no doubt be a consequence of quite a long list of *unresolved* factors, conditions or difficulties in their present and possibly earlier life. These factors or situations create their own block of emotional stress, all of which combine to create the unhealthily **High Tower of Emotional Stress** within the mind of the person suffering the consequences of each of these unresolved, worrying and problem-causing disruptive conditions in their life.

The consequences of the combination of the above are that the poor suffering person experiences the following:

a) They feel over-stressed most of the time.

b) They will experience various degrees of depression.

c) c) Their mind regularly feels foggy, cloudy and unclear.

d) d) They struggle to make sensible, good quality decisions and actions due to their very high emotionally stressed state of mind, which spirals around the elements of their current, primary difficulties.

e) e) They make decisions and take actions based upon emotion and very little cold logic.

The consequences of this are that the poor person suffers from:

1) Extremely poor quality and quantity of sleep which very significantly adds to their difficulties above.

2) Each of the many typical symptoms related to this crippling condition. Their **brain is desperately trying to help them by giving them pain and many other dysfunctional conditions to attempt to slow the person down and stop doing what they are currently doing.** Each of their activities, and in some cases, lack of activity, is creating anxiety and stress, which adds to and maintains their **ongoing, unhealthily High Tower of Emotional Stress.**

It is one big circulating sequence of events with its problem causes, the consequences of these and their brain's reaction to their cumulative effect is its attempt to reduce the person's prevailing emotionally stressed state.

What can be done to address the patient's difficulties?

The patient needs to seek Cognitive Behaviour Therapy from a counsellor who practices this type of help, arranged via their GP.

The following is a basic simple process along which the counsellor may begin to gradually help the person get better. What I think is absolutely imperative is, whilst proceeding along this path, they must do frequent reviews with their patient. They need to discuss how they are progressing and decide what to do next, which depends on how the patient has reacted to date, is reacting currently and making changes to their original basic plan accordingly.

It is so important that the counsellor's patient feels very much involved and participates in this journey. Consequently, they understand the logic of their counsellor who should listen to what questions and ideas their patient may have. All of the time, the patient should support and feel confident about what you are doing as a team.

To begin the process to help the patient out of their quagmire of emotional and functional difficulties of the whole collective, interactive and interrelated state of all of these conditions requires the very simple, very thoughtful, cool and calm approach.

Sit down with the person and have a quiet talk about their difficulties. How long have they existed? Are they gradually getting better, or are they getting progressively worse? How do they feel about their life?

Very carefully, explain what you think the **functional root** cause of all of their difficulties and symptoms is (as above), and see how they respond to all of this. Do they think that your theory of what is causing their symptoms is correct? See if you can help them to buy into this plan of assistance. Lay out how you would proceed to identify what situations in their current life are creating undue anxiety and explore if some of their anxieties are caused by past experiences.

For best success, one crucially important factor for the patient to begin to minimise and eventually solve all of their difficulties is that they actually have faith and believe in the benefits of your proposed system. Once you can get them to acquire a genuine belief in all of these elements of your process, they will engage the extremely beneficial power of their placebo effect. The power and contribution this will add to all of the work you and they put into improving their mental health and will aid it enormously.

It is also very important that they have confidence in the person helping them through the process of treatment. They need to be totally committed to engaging with it all and making their absolute best efforts to see it through. Hopefully, as they gradually identify what situations they are anxious about, decide how best to deal with each one and begin to take the appropriate actions, their level of anxiety will gradually reduce. It will continue to do so as they continue what is effectively a healing process for them.

Also, the degree of their symptoms of dysfunctionality will reduce as they gradually take more control of their life. As their brain sees them dealing effectively with their situation, it will proportionately further reduce each dysfunctionality. They may have been taking drugs to assist in dealing with their difficulties. In this case, I strongly suggest that, as their condition improves and their confidence in this corrective process increases, the counsellor discusses the treatment plan with their patient and their doctor. The aim would be to very gradually reduce the dosage of medication until hopefully it is completely removed, with their emotional health remaining stable and in good order.

Part of this process should include the patient learning how to spot any signs that they are beginning to become anxious and stressed again. They should learn how to deal with this situation and gradually re-establish good emotional health and control of their lives once again.

SUBCHAPTER 7.10 – Epileptic Fits – Is there an underlying cause? If so, what is it, and how is best to treat it?

As I understand it, one of the prevailing theories is that the patient suffers from epileptic seizures simply because <u>parts of their brain have become faulty.</u> When the treatment of drugs fails, the foreseen cure is to establish the location of these faulty brain parts and surgically remove them with as minimal damage as is possible to other parts of their brain that do not require removal.

I pose the questions of:

Are the underlying functional causes that the person is suffering from as follows?

a) A far <u>too high</u>, ongoing level of anxiety and emotional stress, thus:

b) Causing them to suffer from a prevailing consciousness that is dominated by **suffocating anxiety, emotional stress and the resultant negativity**.

c) A very high <u>rate of increase</u> of anxiety and emotional stress due to a very stressful incident suddenly being experienced by the person.

I propose that: Because their brain is so concerned about these conditions above, it provokes an epileptic fit to shut their disturbed functionality down totally. With directed floods of electrical energy, their brain washes their prevailing repetitive negative and worrying thoughts out of their consciousness, thus giving them a relatively higher degree of emotional peace than they were used to when they recover from their fits.

Their brain is then hoping that their consciousness will recover, reaching a much healthier emotional state than before their fit and will continue in this state.

If my beliefs are correct, I propose that the fundamentally best treatment and nominal cure is for the patient to have Cognitive Behavioural Therapy to:

a) Establish the <u>underlying causes</u> they are being stressed by.

b) Establish the <u>underlying root causes</u> of why they are reacting so anxiously to each of the <u>underlying causes.</u>

c) Resolve each of these <u>underlying causes</u> of their <u>elevated</u> ongoing level of anxiety and emotional stress. Consequently, they will acquire a normal and far healthier state of mental health, plus, in doing so, banish these horrible epileptic fits from their life.

As always, the principles of the solution required to manage their difficulties are simple and straightforward. However, carrying out the whole protracted process requires a lot of effort, fortitude, courage, work and stickability from the patient and their mental health therapist.

Ultimately, by the initial end of the process, the patient will have gone through a lot of hard work with their therapist. They will have acquired knowledge and understanding of why they had been so stressed, including establishing the **underlying causes** and **underlying root causes** of **all of their stresses.**

Most importantly and additionally, much discussion will have taken place to decide what alterations to their ways of life they should make, to contribute to a much less stressed life and a much more enjoyable one.

Everyone's life should be lived with a good percentage of **enjoyment** and **satisfaction**. It should not be a continual daily battle for survival. If this is your basic situation, step back, review it all and carefully make changes before it is too late. Life is to be enjoyed. If it was 100 % perfect every day, you would not be able to appreciate it, and I also think it would be totally boring!

Please don't waste it.

The patient will have been given tools to recognise if they begin to travel down the road of becoming too stressed again and address their situation themselves. At times, they may require a little aid from their therapist to recover their situation.

SUBCHAPTER 7.11 – Are crosswords, sudoku and many other brain games good for keeping your brain healthy, warding off dementia and other diseases of your brain?

OVERVIEW: I think that this question is far too limited and narrow. It is posed towards utilising a small percentage of the total vast number of your brain's Category 1A and 1B departments. It is carried out without any physical exercise and normally in isolation from any other human being, for numerous hours per week in many cases. It is also carried out in achieving an extremely self-

related benefit when you have correctly solved the challenge of each particular exercise.

The achievements are normally of no use to other human beings unless you compare notes with a friend, and generally, other humans don't benefit from your achievements. This pastime requires a relatively low amount of Brain processing detail per cycle of updating your consciousness.

These comments aren't meant to dismiss this pastime, but to highlight other aspects that relate to this hobby. I know many people partake in it with great gusto and enjoyment, with normally the prime reason being to keep their brain healthier than otherwise, particularly after retiring. This hobby tends to create an inward focus into oneself, which can be unhealthy if carried out over too high a percentage of every week.

Let us expand the question.

How can you keep the whole of your brain healthy, keeping it in excellent working order and, consequently, best ward off dementia and all of the other brain diseases?

I believe that the key focus of importance within the question is the part – *the whole of your brain*. I would further expand that to include the whole of your brain and body.

I consider the functionality of your brain and body to be inherently intertwined. They each depend upon and need the other simply to satisfy each of their/your ongoing needs throughout every second of your life. Your body, with all of its integrated parts, is kept alive, healthy and fully functioning 100% of the time by your brain via all of its process control output signals, commands and requests from all of its departments that are dedicated to such roles.

Your brain could not be fully healthy, at optimum temperature, fully alive and fully functioning without its required blood flow, sugar/energy and oxygen supply, all of which come from your heart under complete control of your brain.

Your brain could not achieve all of its objectives unless your body was in excellent order and fully able to respond immediately to carry out every command as directed from the prevailing requirements of your consciousness and all of your Category 1 department's activities.

The human brain has such an immense degree of capabilities. For example, its awesome range and depth of skills and expertise, plus the extreme speed that it processes data from the vast number of it different, specialised and dedicated departments as it utilises those needed to deal with all of your second-by-second, ongoing necessities as you navigate your local world within your requirements of the larger world we all inherit.

Your body, with all of its moving parts, sinews, bones and muscles, is permanently responding to the commands and directions of your brain. It adopts an astronomical range of controlled movements with the requisite precision, power and sensitivity to satisfy the detailed requirements placed upon it.

So, to fully answer the question above, to keep the whole of your brain fully healthy, you must also keep the whole of your body fully healthy. Do this by keeping both usefully busy, carrying out the following regular ongoing activities, thus keeping your brain's cellular state healthy and all of its departments functionally healthy.

1.0 Ideally, utilise the whole of your brain's enormous range of skills as often as possible and to the limit of each ability. It takes a long time to develop each of your Developed, Semi-Automatic skills gradually. If you use them less often and to a lower level of skill, each of these will slowly lose their ability to perform, commencing at their previous highest level and reducing downwards in capability.

2.0 Keep your brain and body working hard doing useful tasks at work inherently and at home, for yourself and others. The satisfaction of a job well done and giving to others for no financial reward are uplifting and engender a healthy mind and, therefore, good mental health.

3.0 Make daily contact with friends and other people, not just within your family. The brain is extremely busy when socially interacting with other people, so this activity, for many different reasons, helps to keep your emotional health in good order.

4.0 Ensure that you maintain your sense of humour. If you have lost it, you are probably far too stressed. You must sort this out and regain your sense of humour. If you realise you have never had a sense of humour, work at establishing one. It is one of the most powerful tools to stop becoming too anxious about things and taking things too seriously. It allows you to see things at their inherent level of importance to you. It automatically keeps things in an emotionally, practical and realistically healthy perspective.

5.0 Learn new skills and pastimes, hobbies and sports. It will help to keep your brain and body healthy and your zest for life active and well.

6.0 Sensibly practice monitoring and being aware of your ongoing level of anxiety. If you realise that you are too anxious and stressed too often and therefore experiencing poor emotional health and sleep, take steps to identify and deal with the causes of each of the situations that are creating your anxieties. If you are still struggling, seek the help of your GP.

7.0 Get a sufficient amount of exercise at a brisk physical level, ideally in the fresh air every day.

8.0 Regularly review your life and goals within it, set realistic but challenging targets, and work to achieve them. *Once you feel too old to dream, you will wake up in heaven too soon afterwards!*

9.0 Getting a sufficient amount of good quality sleep every night is indicated by waking up, feeling refreshed and ready to embrace the day with vigour. If you do not feel like this other than the infrequent occasion, sit down and make a list of all of the different things in your life that make you feel anxious, which are ongoing and not being addressed.

Work out a plan to tackle each one and eliminate as many as possible. Work at dealing with the rest to regain and maintain control of your life such that you don't end up with the same situation being a frequently recurring one in your life.

10.0 Ensure that you ideally have an hour or so most days where you enjoy a quiet, emotionally chilling out period on your own or with your spouse/partner, ideally near the end of the evening.

Review certain aspects of your life, appropriate to your situations. This practice keeps your life focused on the objectives you should consider and prepares your mind for healthy sleep.

Ensure that you can sit and have peaceful control of your thoughts, look at your outstretched hand on the end of your arm and see that your fingers are not shaking at all. If they are shaking, you need to work at calming the anxieties in your mind.

11.0 It is important to include coffee breaks and lunch breaks at home and work, giving your brain a chance to chill out a little, particularly if you have been working it hard. This regime will allow any emotionally stressed parts of your mind to be de-stressed, ready to get back to work, in an emotionally healthy and refreshed state, after your break.

12.0 Whilst awake, it is very important that your brain does not functionally and emotionally **switch off** too much. If your brain is not sufficiently and usefully busy enough for continuously long periods, I believe it will become sluggish and functionally inefficient, with you feeling emotionally mildly depressed and zombie-like.

Being awake and looking at your TV, for example, where you are **just viewing and observing in a switched-off emotional state, without carrying out much self-determining and calculating activities** for too long, creates the existence of these states. If this state becomes the norm for too many hours per day and days per week, your brain is at risk of becoming increasingly less functionally capable in some of its departments of functionality.

If this state continues over a very long period, your brain will become degraded, resulting in you suffering emotional, functional and physical health difficulties. The degree will be dependent upon the emotional health of yourself, your daily circumstances and the degree and frequency of your periods of unhealthy states.

13.0 Whilst you are of working age and have to work to earn money, I feel that it is extremely important that you have a job that you really enjoy most of the time. You feel satisfaction from your work and feel appreciated by your boss and that your job is worthwhile. Be realistic that nothing in life is perfect all of the time. You spend a significant time of your life at work, and it's so important for your self-esteem, satisfaction and mental health that you enjoy it. If you are in a job where you don't have any or very much of these returns, carefully and seriously consider changing.

14.0 Try and lead a life of decency towards others, say thanks when appropriate and where you have opportunity, always try and help others. These values create a solid emotional foundation of a very healthy state of mind.

15.0 It is also extremely beneficial for your brain's health to learn new skills, probably the best of which is dancing, including learning new dance styles and steps. This inherently involves social contact with other people and relating to wonderful music, which keeps your whole machine, i.e. your brain, its coordination of your entire body and your overall physical, emotional fitness and health in the best of order.

16.0 Always maintain the ability and willingness to laugh at yourself within situations and be able to see the humour even within dark and difficult times. It de-stresses the mind and soul, keeps the mind clear and balanced and enables the path of the best solution for you to be seen and clear to travel along.

17.0 When anyone retires, and for various reasons, for men particularly, it becomes more difficult to adopt all of the healthy activities listed above. The most difficult objective to satisfy is keeping your brain working hard enough and challenged sufficiently with a wide range of useful activities. Therefore, this will cause a decline in brain processing performance and a loss of emotional satisfaction from a job well done.

Going to live in a retirement home presents greater risks of not keeping sufficiently mentally and physically active. This leads to their brain and body losing their fitness and vitality; thus, their whole machine begins to age quite quickly, with their medical health and enjoyment suffering accordingly.

18.0 If it's one of your hobbies, by all means, enjoy sudoku and crosswords, etc. But please also consider other activities.

There you have it. Without spending much money at all, if you regularly practice the above, most of the time, you will stand the best chance to keep your entire machine fit, strong, and in good working order whilst enjoying a full, happy, long and satisfying life to near the end.

SUBCHAPTER 7.12 – What is creating the process where taking painkilling medication usually necessitates having to take ever-increasing strengths of painkilling medication?

OVERVIEW: Let's say you have cracked or significantly injured your ribs. Your brain gives you pain in the injured area to help prevent you from doing anything physical that will further physically stress and risk additional damage to your injured area. It also does this to assist in promoting healing in the quickest possible time. I believe that your brain also gives you pain before you commence to exert your injured area. For example, when it notices that you are about to physically stress your injured area say when preparing to get out of bed in the early days after your injury. It does this to remind you to get out of bed with appropriate care not to overexert the injured area. If you then proceed to overstrain the injury, it will give you a higher level of pain to get you to reduce the degree of strain you are subjecting your injury to.

If you take painkilling tablets, as advised by your doctor, as these reduce the previous level of pain your brain created, you automatically begin carrying out greater degrees of exertion of movements that you wouldn't have done before the medication. This physically aggravates your injury, thus increasing the recovery time. Your brain is aware of this situation and increases the level of pain above the capability of your painkilling tablets to re-establish its ability to give you pain when required, to prevent you from aggravating your injuries. This situation normally causes you to request stronger painkilling tablets, resulting in the above process repeating with you taking increasingly stronger painkilling tablets. The consequences of this are your healing time will be extended, and you may suffer side effects from the increasingly more potent drugs.

SUBCHAPTER 7.13 – How to help/treat unfortunate patients who suffer severe pain levels, even after the amputation of the painful limb.

OVERVIEW: *I saw a short documentary on TV that left me feeling extreme anguish for the poor people suffering from the not uncommon situation in the title.*

The situation was about a woman who had a slight walking disability. However, the overriding condition she suffered from was experiencing extreme pain levels from one of her legs below the knee. She had followed a path of taking increasing strength painkiller medication without success, so had finally resorted to requesting the amputation of her painful lower leg.

She had a consultation with a doctor who had a lot of experience of her type of condition, but she did not recommend amputation. This was because there are a lot of similar cases where after amputation, the pain continued either above the point of amputation in the same leg or sometimes it appeared in the other leg. Despite this advice, the poor lady went ahead with the amputation because she was desperate to try anything to rid herself of the pain.

We were not shown the post-operative results in the documentary, which unfortunately suggests they were not good.

As a consequence of the above story, I sat down and pondered what process could maybe help these poor unfortunate people extract themselves from the desperate predicament they find themselves trapped in. Is there a way to avoid resorting to amputation of a limb that is nominally in good order and then having to deal with a situation that is significantly worse than before their fruitless amputation?

I considered my beliefs of why we experience pain, the extreme and confusing and maybe conflicting symptoms the patient is suffering from, plus the prevailing risks. I believe it would be prudent to evaluate and clarify the medical conditions the patient is currently suffering from and review all of their prescribed medications.

For a number of reasons, I think it would be very beneficial that the patient's doctor carries out the following process with the patient being fully informed and involved. Any unanswered questions must not be ignored but noted and have a second opinion sought from another doctor if felt appropriate.

My first step would be to:

a) Set out to step back and review the whole of the patient's current health from scratch. It is important not to automatically continue to retain any previous assumptions or keep any previous diagnoses and medicines.

b) b) Carry out a complete review of all of the patient's symptoms and conditions. It would be prudent for this review to cover their mental and physical health plus that of their brain's physiological health.

c) Compare all the patient's original to their current, prescribed medicines and their symptoms and conditions that prevailed before and after this review.

d) Due to the patients suffering extreme long-term pain and other difficulties in their life, e.g. poor sleep and many other worries, they will inevitably have been suffering extremely high levels of ongoing anxiety and emotional stress. These are no doubt being treated with very strong pain killers and anti-depression medications. As part of the fundamental objective of trying to help the patient obtain a significantly better quality of life than currently, I believe that the above process should include Cognitive Behavioural Therapy. This would focus on **identifying the aspects of their life that create anxiety and tackling them as detailed elsewhere in this book.**

Once this all-pervading factor can begin to be tackled, it will greatly assist in gradually lowering the level of pain and anxiety being suffered, allowing the quantity and strength of painkilling and anti-depressant medication to be reduced proportionately. This will lessen or maybe eliminate any bad side effects from medications, which will reduce levels of pain and anxiety. Consequently, this is beneficial in the inter-related wheel of causes and effects, thus allowing further medication reductions.

The eventual target of attack within the above process is to reduce or, if possible, eliminate as many different medications historically being taken, creating an overall far less complex inter-related set of symptoms and medication side effects. The additional and major benefit of these prevailing conditions is that it makes successful diagnosis and outcomes far more likely.

Other benefits are a much-reduced complexity of worries and confusion and increased patient confidence in their treatment regime and for their future physical and mental health. One very important aspect to remember is that the more different and, particularly strong, medicines a patient is taking, the proportionately greater the risk of the patient suffering disabling side effects from the complex interaction between them all.

With the above process of involving the patient, which achieves their understanding, support and belief into the processes, activities and objectives, one major, additional benefit they are helped with is the placebo effect. For more details, refer to **Question 7.4**, earlier in this chapter.

I believe that if any doctor is treating any patient for an illness and their assessment and treatment process does not include the doctor's full understanding of the placebo effect and the patient's belief in this process, the success of the treatment will be significantly reduced.

Hopefully, the instigation and continuance of the above process will greatly benefit the patient. The process is relatively long and slightly complex, but this is born out of necessity from attempting to deal with a very challenging situation that prevailed originally. Hopefully, as the patient is taken through this process and is kept fully informed and involved, their medication will gradually be rationalised. Their anxiety will lower and their emotional stress levels will reduce. They will enjoy improving health, which will, in turn, help them to increasingly engage the benefit of their placebo effect, which in itself significantly aids their improving mental health.

SUBCHAPTER 7.14 – Post Traumatic Stress Disorder – P.T.S.D. What is it? What can cause it? Who can suffer from it? How best to deal with it?

OVERVIEW: *What is it? The condition called Post Traumatic Stress Disorder is where someone has been directly involved in or witnessed a situation that has caused them to have suffered a significant level of emotional psychological trauma, up to what could be described as an absolutely extreme degree of psychological trauma. The functional, visual, audible and other details of the situation will be stored within the person's memory department. Crucially, what will also be stored will be the memories of each of the different emotional* *feelings experienced, including the degree of emotional stress felt for each emotion.*

Perhaps the person recalls the event which occurred, for no particularly emotionally beneficial purpose, other than to inform someone about what happened. Even so, these very significant emotionally stressful memories will be relived and re-experienced to the same intense feelings as when the event first occurred, causing them great discomfort again. Some of these emotional memories can be, for example, of fear, anger, anxiety, hopelessness or confusion, experienced singly or collectively.

I believe that the length of time these emotional memories remain with their original level of intensity of emotion depends on several factors. These include the strength of their original memory installation when they were memorised, the total number of times and the frequency they were recalled afterwards, why these recalls were being made and how the patient emotionally reacted to them.

The patient will probably experience recalls whilst asleep. Their brain is reviewing aspects of what experiences and issues they are being stressed and anxious about, searching for resolutions, and maybe working to reduce their emotional strength.

What can cause it?

People often associate P.T.S.D. with soldiers fighting on the front line, who, most days, are exposed to the risks of being killed by a bullet, an explosion, or being captured and tortured.

Being in these conditions for long periods of time and frequently being subjected to these conditions will expose the soldiers to very high levels of ongoing anxiety and stress. This, in itself, is bad for their overall mental health and, ultimately, physical health.

This unhealthy exposure will continue for the long length of each duty period. During that time, they are likely to experience occasions where they see death and horrific injuries to their friends and, to some degree, themselves.

This first exposure of P.T.S.D. being caused is pretty certainly going to create the most extreme degree and quantity of emotional and psychological trauma. However, I believe that many other experiences in life can create a sufficient degree of trauma to cause the experiencing person mental health problems unless they deal with and process these experiences correctly afterwards. This is dependent upon the nature of the person and the state of their prevailing and ongoing anxiety level and mental health.

A few other causes of P.T.S.D. are:

a) Suffering the sudden death of a loved one without any pre-warning symptoms at all.

b) Being raped.

c) Being involved in a very serious car accident in which there were fatalities.

d) Seeing your loved one being killed in an accident.

e) e) Being involved in an accident yourself that left you with permanent, disabling injuries.

f) Experiencing a very serious and prolonged physical assault in which your life felt threatened.

g) Living in your family home where, for years, there is/was regularly bad arguments, violence, serious drunkenness, maybe drug-taking and ongoing emotional stress. This is particularly relevant for young children who are old enough to understand the significance of what they are being exposed to.

h) Having a serious and genuine learning disability where your low-grade work is regularly held up in front of you and your class by your teacher, who proceeds to ridicule your work. The consequences of these experiences are that your self-esteem and self-confidence are reduced to zero. They remain very low and your academic achievements are proportionally reduced. This quite extremely emotionally disturbing experience has the propensity to be remembered in later life when related difficulties cause you to recall the academic damage you suffered. Each time you recall these ridiculing memories, you feel and re-experience the awful emotional traumas attached. In such a case, the person is likely to bear serious anger and resentment towards the teacher, even many years later.

i) i) A child can grow up feeling that their parents didn't love them because the parents spent most of their time dealing with their elder sibling. This may simply be due to their sibling always being in trouble and consequently requiring their parents to provide an awful lot of help and attention. This feeling of being unloved can be so strong that it can linger within the child well into adulthood and beyond with their related experiences and emotional feelings being regularly recalled. The disturbed adult can exhibit negative attitudes towards one or both parents to punish them for the trauma they are seen to be responsible for by their son or daughter.

j) Being treated extremely unfairly and unjustifiably by being dismissed without the opportunity to defend yourself. For example, from a job that you cared about very much, had put your heart and soul into for many years, with an unblemished record and service. The justification was based upon extreme lies you were unable to be allowed to expose effectively. Most unfortunately, this type of situation contains extreme degrees of utter unfairness and frustration, which can eat away at the state of your mind, creating damaging emotional conditions and their related P.T.S.Ds.

Who can suffer from it?

Anyone old enough to have sufficiently understood and therefore be affected by what has occurred, who has experienced, been involved in or witnessed a situation that has caused them to suffer from a *significant to an absolutely extreme degree of emotional, psychological trauma* can suffer from P.T.S.D.

How best to deal with P.T.S.D.?

Some initial, preparatory basic points to bear in mind are:

1) The causes and the degree of emotional hurt and stress of P.T.S.D. will differ for each patient. This is due to the actual details of each experience being different, plus the

character and prevailing emotional health of each patient is diverse. Therefore, each person must be carefully assessed and treated appropriately to their unique circumstances.

2) The first objective is to establish whether P.T.S.D. is **part of the causes** of why any person is suffering from mental ill-health problems. I propose that a lot of patients will not be aware that they are actually suffering from P.T.S.D. because many people think that only frontline soldiers suffer from it. They will remember the incident or incidents that caused them great stress if you asked them, but they may not be aware that they are suffering P.T.S.D. as a consequence. This can only be established by the person being carefully assessed with Cognitive Behavioural Therapy as the first action of help.

3) When a patient says they have experienced a highly significant emotional trauma in their life, I firmly believe that it is not good enough to advise them to move on, leave it behind them, cut it off, let it drift away and look to the future. Certainly, look to and create a better tomorrow, but the patient must go through a process to emotionally clean up and remove their damaging memories to have a far healthier future.

4) During this type of help, the patient will hopefully be assisted with creating a list of things in their life that cause them significant anxiety and stress. It is during here that their therapist should be asking the question, "Does any particular period in their life of exposure to stressful

conditions still give you significant anxiety and emotional stress when you recall these memories?"

If the answer is yes, whatever the causes or length of time the patient has suffered the degree of emotional stresses they have locked up in their memories, I believe the fundamental objective is to gradually reduce the emotional degree of intensity of feelings they have locked away. Hopefully, this will be to the point where they have been banished from their memories forever, just leaving the functional memories without the emotional, hurtful ones.

The process of assisting the patient to recover from the emotionally damaging consequences of P.T.S.D.

OVERVIEW: There are a number of strategies that can be helpful to engage when dealing with P.T.S.D. Each strategy selected, depends upon the details of the patient's characteristics, their prevailing mental health, the case details and the stage of recovery they have reached.

What is critically important when engaging with your P.T.S.D. patient is to remember what they are suffering from. Tread extremely carefully, particularly in the early stages of getting them to recall these horrifically disturbing memories, so they don't become too traumatised again.

a) Ask the patient what they know about **P.T.S.D.** Ensure that, at the end of your discussion, they fully understand how important it is that you work with them to gradually remove all of its damaging elements.

b) Establish whether they experienced only one episode of their P.T.S.D. experience or whether they experienced more.

c) Carefully explain the whole process you will engage in eradicating the effects of their P.T.S.D. At times, repeat this information to your patient so they are always aware of why you are doing what you are, ensuring they remain comfortable with and beneficially focused on the process which you are employing.

d) Establish whether the patient experiences dreams about their P.T.S.D. If so, how often and what are the details in the dreams? This information may be very useful in helping the patient's recovery.

e) Get the patient to describe the whole of their P.T.S.D. experience carefully, including the build-up to it, plus all of the details and circumstances it comprised of. Ensure that you keep a careful eye on their emotional state and call a halt to the proceedings if they are emotionally struggling too much.

f) One question to ask the patient is, "Do you feel that you have any degree of responsibility for having created or caused your horrific experience?"

g) At the end of each session, ask the patient to describe how they felt when re-living their P.T.S.D. experience. Make a note of what they said in order to assess what progress is being made.

h) At the end of each session, ask the patient how they feel the process is going and again note the answer.

i) Sometimes, if it is a viable and available option, and if the patient is comfortable with it, you could suggest that the patient meets the person who may be the primary or only person responsible for their P.T.S.D. experience. This could be risky and needs careful judgement, but it could be very beneficial to the patient's recovery.

j) Asking the patient to describe in writing, all of the details of their P.T.S.D. experience could be very helpful to their healing. They may produce more detail than with a verbal recall, which will promote a better release of their damaging emotional memories.

k) Speaking to someone about your P.T.S.D. who didn't actually carry out actions against you but may, by their inactions or other actions, have contributed to your P.T.S.D., will greatly benefit you recovering from it by hopefully removing the degree of blame that you attributed to them.

l) P.T.S.D. can be created by the sudden and unexpected death of a loved one. However, the emotional stress and anxiety are totally different to that created by the bereavement which occurs, and they must be treated differently.

m) Speaking to, say, the family of someone killed in a road accident caused by yourself would be tough, but would hopefully assist in your healing process if dealt with correctly and appropriately.

n) By speaking to a person and trying to understand why someone didn't treat you well, thus creating your P.T.S.D. has the potential to assist in it being significantly reduced.

Therefore, it is always worth considering this action if it is appropriate, safe and practical in your circumstances.

o) Suffering from P.T.S.D., particularly repeated episodes of it, fundamentally the same experiences as front line soldiers have, but not sufficiently facing, considering and coming to terms with them as they occur, can cause big mental health problems later on. Especially so if they tend to go back to their base and with their comrades and have a good few drinks to help anaesthetise their experiences of the day whilst keeping their experiences locked away in their memories.

This large quantity of horrific and similar P.T.S.D. experiences mount up without being dealt with, reviewed, considered and discussed sufficiently to reduce the degrees of stress they collectively create. Each separate P.T.S.D. experience will be very similar to many others, so they tend to combine to create a very significant emotional stress level.

When a soldier leaves the services to return home, they leave behind the comradeship of their service comrades in arms, their collective umbrella of emotional support, understanding and the ability to ignore the difficulties of their experiences. Sometime later, their mental health difficulties begin to surface. The combination of these stresses will create an awfully large degree of P.T.S.D. which will have to be finally dealt with to be able to begin to recover their individual mental health.

p) Another additional aid to recovery can be speaking to other people with similar P.T.S.D. experiences to yours.

This should significantly help your recovery process because you are speaking about and thus bringing out in the open and facing up to memories of your horrific experiences. Additionally, because you are helping each other deal with their P.T.S.D., it gives you lots of personal satisfaction and, therefore, additional help in actually making some use of these horrific events you have experienced.

q) The patient must ensure that whenever they recall their P.T.S.D. experiences on their own, they do this to continue coming to terms with them and gradually reduce the emotional hurt they are experiencing from them. It is so important that they are not reliving these experiences, for example, perhaps before they started treatment when they were reacting with anger, etc. They must strive towards reducing the level of emotional hurt from them. Maybe they complete this process with a view that they have been hurt too many times since the initial experiences and have come to the idea that life is too short for this to continue indefinitely. "In the near future, when the time feels right, I will move on from this experience and banish its memories forever."

r) It is very important for someone to desist in reviewing their difficulties on their own if this practice is proving troublesome for them.

s) If you are engaging in the process of taking someone to court that was responsible for your P.T.S.D., as a consequence, you will regularly be thinking about and speaking about your difficulties. As this process has a focused beneficial

objective for you, you will emotionally benefit twofold
from:

1) The gradual release and running down of your locked up
emotional memories.

2) Punishing in some appropriate way and maybe eliciting a
formal apology from the person who has been the cause of
your troubles.

t) It is vitally important that whoever the patient is talking
to about their P.T.S.D. experiences shows the appropriate
understanding, care and concern about the patient's
situation so that the patient gathers maximum benefit from
each of these experiences.

u) I believe that it is crucial that the patient gradually runs
down the degree of emotional hurt and emotional stress
they are suffering, from their P.T.S.D. memories. They
do this by consciously facing up to them in a courageous,
correct, effective and safe manner and not having them
processed by some form of hypnosis, taking drugs or the
use of alcohol.

SUBCHAPTER 7.15:The internet – the Good, the Bad and the Ugly – which is it?

OVERVIEW: *The simple answer to this question is that, unfortunately, each of these descriptions applies. Not including the COVID-19 pandemic, the internet, I would propose, is the single functional facility, system or tool that has affected the whole of our* *world more than any other in the history of mankind to date and is likely to be so in the future. It has not only affected one facet of our lives; it has affected, to some degree, every facet of the lives of all humans of all creeds, ages and sexes living on this planet of ours. It has fundamentally allowed people to connect or communicate with such efficiency and detail to vast numbers of others of their choice and sometimes not of their choice. Like every system, tool or facility, it has the ability and potential to be used for good and bad. As usual, the type of use applied comes from within the mind of the user.*

SUBCHAPTER 7.15.1: The Good internet

This is a list of examples of the principles of the Good:

1) It has utterly transformed everyone's ability to be able to communicate with everyone else. People can connect and communicate with ostensibly anyone else in the world, providing they are connected to the internet, at any time and increasingly in virtually any place, with minimal costs, almost immediately.

2) It enables vast amounts of detailed data to be sent to other people almost immediately within their social and work-related activities.

The resultant benefits of the Good:

a) The internet has enabled all previously existing businesses to operate in a significantly more efficient and therefore profitable manner, providing for their customers' needs dramatically quicker than ever before.

b) It's possible to send and receive even extremely large amounts of data in a very short time as opposed to in the past when days or a lot longer would be required.

c) It enables people to obtain information, help and assistance within the medical field, their working field, at home, etc., and into virtually any other area of requirement, far quicker than ever before, with a vast array of potential benefits resulting.

d) It has allowed a large number of people with no particular work experience or qualifications to set up their own business fairly quickly from their bedroom or home. In some cases, these are unique and make profits of vast amounts of money with relative ease, relatively no costs and relatively no financial risks.

e) It has facilitated people who are unable to meet face-to-face for a variety of possible reasons to at least be able to connect visually with their friends and family over the internet via Skype and Zoom, etc.

f) During the height of the COVID-19 pandemic lockdown of the UK and other countries, when people instructed to stay at home and minimise contact with most others. The immensely increased use of the visual and audible connectivity of the internet was extremely beneficial. It kept a lot of people occupied in carrying out a whole range of new and additional activities than before the pandemic. It was instrumental in keeping anxiety, emotional stress levels, related mental health and, in some cases, physical health in a much healthier state than it would have been without these original and new internet-based activities.

g) Within the benefits listed above could also be listed details of a multitude of additional advantages derived.

SUBCHAPTER 7.15.2: The Bad internet

As with most things in this life, **big** benefits normally come with big costs or losses to some. **Here are just a <u>very few</u> examples of the Bad:**

1) During the height of the COVID-19 pandemic lockdown in the UK, and I guess in other countries, many people took up the habit of becoming gamers as part of occupying their time being stuck at home. The downside for most of these new gamers is that they have become emotionally addicted to playing these games. They were specifically designed to make the gamers become addicted once they started playing them, with the added addiction of gambling included in some of them. Once they start the habit, most of them can't stop, with the usual consequence that it ruins their quality and quantity of good sleep, thus causing significant mental health problems.

2) Also, during the COVID-19 Pandemic, the new and increasingly used Zoom facility, and others, enable virtual

business meetings, medical consultations with doctors and physiotherapists, choirs, orchestras, concerts and other virtual gatherings. These gave a lot of people great pleasure, mental health benefits and zero risks associated with visiting surgeries and clinics and of contracting the COVID-19 virus. The adverse consequence of starting to and continuing to use these facilities is that the media sites that provide them have a frightening amount of very personal details of new categories of data about all of these people, which they can sell or otherwise use for financial benefits.

3) It has become increasingly common for people at work to receive emails from people within their own work's location – not just for receipt of a lot of information, but in place of face-to-face discussions. Some bosses and others send someone whose office is next to theirs an email rather than pop next door for a conversation.

4) Increasingly, emails have become the method of having conversations and communicating work requirements to other people. Sometimes, they are used as the work initiating activity, thus possibly bypassing a crucial pre-stage of, for example, obtaining someone else's approval prior to carrying out some activity.

5) People go on holiday and return to hundreds or more emails, representing a mountain of work. Each work item carries an expectancy of a relatively quick response and following actions. Increasingly so, people are receiving emails whilst on holiday via their mobile phones.

6) Prior to the coming of the internet, if someone who had no public, national or media platform wished to complain about anything or set out to accomplish an objective seriously and effectively, they had to stand on a soapbox in some public place such as Hyde Park Corner, and shout with a microphone to anyone who may care to listen. The results were predictably sparse to zero.

But the internet has the potential which enables everyone to pass on their views about anything to an ever-increasing number of almost unlimited other people within an extremely short period of time. If this communication includes the backing of a nationally or internationally recognised celebrity, sportsperson or actor enjoying great following amongst the general population normally, the weight and noise of support can very quickly grow to almost stellar levels.

If the bandwagon appears at the top of the 10.00 pm national news that evening and the bandwagon applies pressure on to, say, the P.M., its objective has the possibility to be achieved extremely quickly.

<u>The resultant consequences of the Bad</u>:

a) People are having increasingly less physical, direct face-to-face communication with others. They are not gaining the benefits of the quickest and best quality way to agree on a meeting date or any other required decisions affecting a large number of other people, which is to meet as a group. Everyone in attendance can hear the views of all others at the same time, giving them each an opportunity to share their views as appropriate.

b) What is also lost is the opportunity of solving particularly tricky situations. These are most effectively, calmly and efficiently resolved with face-to-face contact, when each party can monitor and decode what the other parties are feeling. It creates the additional potential for establishing healthy, inter-beneficial relationships.

c) When people meet, informally or formally, face-to-face with a group of other people, the brain of each person participating in the meeting is working extremely hard. This process is also much more restrictive when communicating via the internet:

1) Interpreting what each person is saying.
2) Thinking about why they are saying this.
3) Analysing if they have a hidden agenda.
4) Thinking about how to respond to what is being said.
5) Studying the other person's body language and facial expressions to assist in understanding the objectives above.

d) Young people particularly are increasingly only making contact over their smartphone or over the internet. The consequence of this is that their brains are not developing the range of social skills or the confidence required to be able to function effectively as described above. They are also losing the pure joy and satisfaction derived from face-to-face interactions, not just within a work environment but purely whilst socialising. Human beings are inherently born to enjoy direct interaction with other human beings.

e) Emails were not designed for conversations but for passing data and information.

f) The practices above have resulted in many people checking new emails on their laptops and/or smartphones after work, at home and whilst on holiday. These practices have inherently increased the ongoing workload and hours spent on work matters of employees. Consequently, having less restful time away from work has significantly added to their emotional anxiety and stress, thus creating mental health issues for them.

g) The highly significant, potential downsides of the extremely effective and efficient creation of internet-processed bandwagons come when the bandwagon is, unfortunately, created by someone who is driven by personal, emotionally-twisted zeal. It gathers a lot of support but has consequential ramifications that cause significant difficulties for very many people.

If the bandwagon has been developed and grown into a state in which it has gathered its own momentum, it becomes almost impossible to contain. It can sometimes inflict an awful lot of damage to a considerable amount of people and their country.

h) The ever-increasing percentage of communication between human beings is being carried out over the internet and mobile phones and not by direct, physical contact as it used to be. Because of the immense power of people's statements on social media and their effects, with minimal accountability for their views and pronouncements, I believe people have become increasingly more arrogant, aggressive, ruder and far less tolerant of someone else's view being different to theirs. Before the popular use of the internet, some people would struggle to get other people to listen to their beliefs. However, with the connective efficiency of the internet, these individuals suddenly found they could reach a relatively large number of people who not only listened and took notice of their opinions but actually agreed with them. I believe that this changed these people into becoming narcissistic, resulting in them being even more ingrained into this attitude and behaviour.

These combined factors have made it virtually impossible for reasonable, constructive and respectful debates to prevail. Short, argumentative communications have become the norm, where people shout opinions at one another rather than present their views and carry out a respectful debate of different thoughts.

I think this aspect of our lives is of the highest order of concern. I have seen it become normal for extreme and unacceptable behaviour and attitudes between human beings in more and more situations in our lives today.

Another very powerful factor underlying those I have already mentioned is the increasingly high levels of ongoing anxiety and the resultant ongoing emotional stress that more people are suffering in these modern and difficult times. This very high level of emotional stress causes the suffering person to react to the prevailing situation, with, on or approaching, 100% of raw emotion and not with any or at least sufficient, mitigating, basic common sense and knowledge learned by them.

i) Extensive, extremely efficient communication and pre-planning is carried out, normally by highly intelligent, very capable human beings over the internet and supported with smartphones to selected recipients regarding planned public demonstrations. This makes it extremely difficult for the Policing personnel to keep control of these public protests. The consequences of these elements are that the Police struggle to prevent them from getting out of control and turning violent from both parties as they react to the protesters' actions, so physicality ramps up.

As the frequency of demonstrations and the levels of violence increase over time, there prevails an expectancy of increasing violence each time, which adds to the likelihood of it happening. These protesters also make their points with increasing aggression, threats and disruption to other innocent people by preventing them from going about their daily routines of travelling to work, etc. They also make increasingly dangerous and worrying threats, for example, of flying drones into passenger-carrying aircraft, which risks downing aircraft and killing hundreds of innocent passengers with each incident. I think it's a great shame that the protesters don't use their intelligence and other skills to try and obtain their goals with non-aggressive, low-key debates and tactics.

j) The downside of the situation where many people became gamers during the COVID-19 pandemic will, I guess, be that they fell under the addictive spell of these games and continued to play afterwards. Therefore, they will be suffering the very serious adverse sleep and mental health consequences of these seriously addictive activities.

SUBCHAPTER 7.15.3:The Ugly internet

As with most things in this life, large benefits normally come with large costs to some. **Here are a few examples of the Ugly:**

1) Historically, outside work, people used their phone when they wished to speak to someone for whatever reason and normally, the time on the phone was relatively short. When at home, they usually only used their house phone a few times per day, unless some particular situation required some extended usage and, on some days, there was no phone usage at all.

2) Since the advent of the mobile phone, followed by the smartphone with internet access, more and more people of all ages are connecting to other people on their smartphones virtually the whole of their waking hours. They are speaking and/or text messaging about all kinds of topics and details, reporting about what they are doing, what they have done,

voting on who currently is the prettiest in their group of friends etc. etc. etc.

3) The ages of people employing excessive use of these devices is going down and also up. They are on their smartphones at bus stops, on buses, walking on pavements, crossing very busy roads, on their bicycles, driving cars, in restaurants etc., on social media sites, on apps, whilst at work in large shops, etc. These activities are carried out by an explosion of an increasing percentage of the world's population who are literally living their lives on the other side of a screen.

They are having less and less face-to-face contact with other human beings. This is simply because all of these new communication facilities, by their use and ***detailed, designed emotional addiction***, have effectively encouraged non-face-to-face communication to take place.

4) They are on their phones in the evening, responding to people phoning or texting them up to and whilst in bed. They meet up with friends in a café, for example, and don't always directly communicate with each other. They are corresponding with other people over their phones and sometimes with the person next to them.

5) They are on their smartphone Googling an item of information they require, and in some schools, this activity is encouraged.

6) They boast about how many friends they have, as judged by the list of people they have regular contact with on the various social media sites.

7) Under the instructions of the owners of these social media sites, these smartphone facilities were designed by the software design engineers to be seriously emotionally addictive to the user. Once they start using them they cannot stop, **due to the seriously high addictive level that users are trapped by**.

8) Historically, people used to play card games or board games with other people at home in the evening for an hour or two and then go to bed and sleep. They played these games once a week or less and usually as a family unit.

9) Particularly **at present,** younger people are playing so-called **games, or e-sports** at home, in their bedrooms on their laptops at every opportunity whilst not at school, every day. They continue into the evenings, late at night and into the next day, playing against other gamers in other countries in different time zones, commonly to game completion at 5 am. They play in teams at times and boast about how good this is for practising and developing team tactics and unity, etc. They are attempting to justify to themselves and other doubting people, how beneficial playing these games is to their development. The very last person to be able to see and accept that they are addicted to something is the addict themselves.

10) A recent, additional element contained within these games is the activity of gambling for money. An extremely addictive pastime in its own right, it has been added to the already extremely high addictive level of which gaming is in that category.

11) Point **7)** above very significantly prevails with these games.

12) Gamers who are still at school spend most of their out-of-school time in their bedroom playing on their games and not outside in the real world.

13) Recently, gaming tournaments have been established, attracting gamers from around the world to take part. Prizes are won for around 1 million euros and sometimes very much more. This further significantly adding to the summative level of addiction and the degree of self-justification to the gamers themselves. Unfortunately, this increases the concern for their ever-worried parents, who see their extremely capable child throwing their potentially high-achieving life away.

The resultant consequences of the Ugly:

a) The **serious mental health consequences** of the examples of activities listed above are that these gamers, gamblers, social media site users and smartphone users can't stop their highly excessive and frequent, daily practice of all of these activities. This is simply due to them each being **extremely, seriously emotionally addictive**.

They are trapped by their addiction, as all other addicts are trapped by their alcohol and gambling etc., which is exactly what the designers of each of these systems were told by their company to set out to achieve.

b) Good quality and sufficient quantity of sleep is the foundation upon which excellent emotional health and excellent physical health stems from. But unfortunately, the other extremely serious **consequence** of these addictive activities is that those who do them do not have sufficient good quality and quantity of sleep. This results in their **mental health** being negatively affected, which makes their sleep quality and irregular sleep patterns even worse, which then makes their mental health even worse. This lifestyle package creates a lot of additional anxiety and resultant emotional stress, making the difficulties of getting to sleep and even then getting sufficient good quality sleep increasingly difficult.

All of this creates a monumentally damaging downward spiral of worsening mental health. It bottoms out at a level, dependent upon the characters of each individual, their overall personal life details, any ongoing help they may receive for their difficulties and how effective this is.

These people will probably receive medication as part of their ongoing help to reduce their anxiety. The degree of assistance this obtains makes their overall state of mental health tolerable. Despite the medication tackling their symptoms and not the underlying causes of their symptoms, they accept this state of affairs.

It can be though, that with some people, they just find an acceptable life balance, and they bumble along with good or bad days. Their life continues based on emotionally unhealthily bad habits which persist out of sheer habit and their life's own inherent momentum. Meanwhile, the people who care about them continue to worry, get angry or give up, praying that one day they will see the light and be able to change to realise their potential. Unfortunately, this lifestyle can result in the person self-harming, having a mental breakdown, or committing suicide.

The consequences of combining of these factors will normally result in the person's **mental health becoming seriously damaged**. Eventually, their physical health also seriously suffers.

c) The other **serious consequences** of their difficulties are that if they are still at school, their schoolwork suffers badly. They get into trouble at school with bad behaviour, poor attendance, and threats to be excluded from school. They have bad relations with their parents, other people and themselves. Their mental health continues to worsen.

d) Other consequences are that their brain doesn't develop in a healthy way with respect to learning and developing the many skills they still require. This includes developing the extremely complex social skills required to interact with other people whilst engaging in face-to-face contact. They don't have many close, good, real friends. They don't feel comfortable dealing face-to-face with people they have some relationship difficulties with, so they attempt to resolve their issues by text messaging only. They don't develop a sufficient and normal range of knowledge within their own brain due to "Googling information" as an easy option. They don't develop the vitally important ability to be able to totally focus on something for extended periods when this very necessary skill is required.

e) Women, in particular, suffer from **serious mental health** issues of low self-esteem, feelings of inadequacy, and high levels of emotional stress and anxiety. This can be due to receiving negative votes from their peers regarding their look, figure, lack of popularity with their peers etc.

Children from eleven years old down to four years old are suffering serious mental health problems of self -harm, erratic and bad behaviour with an increase of 50% with these difficulties over the last three years.

f) I believe that the increasing rise of the percentage of the population suffering from serious mental ill-health is vastly outstripping the number who are trained, experienced, capable and available to help these patients. It is important to be aware that the number of patient hours required to successfully treat mentally ill people is vastly greater than that required to treat to completion physically ill or injured patients.

g) These e-sport tournaments draw many more gamers into this addiction with the promise of making it their work/ money earning method. This develops in their minds the supportable justification that this is to be their future way of life.

The inclusion of effectively gambling for money within the format of games has significantly increased the accumulated addictive element contained within playing. Therefore, it ties the gamer ever more into being unable to stop practising this frightening major part of each day of their lives.

h) The general lifestyle of these excessive smartphone users and gamers is one of very low physical activity and poor physical health. They become incapable of going anywhere without speaking into, texting or looking up something on their smartphones. The gamers can't be without participating in their gaming activity for very long. I believe that these physically and emotionally unhealthy lifestyles are breeding a generation of zombie-like people, living or existing inside so little of what this wonderfully exciting, exhilarating, fascinatingly complex and varied life has to offer on their planet.

i) These high use practitioners of the phones etc. spend a very high percentage of their time inside their bedrooms. They are usually lying down on their backs, creating a lazy-type attitude and a sense of entitlement that others should give them what they want. This habit of lying on their backs on their bed and keeping mentally active whilst awake is very unnatural and counterintuitive. I believe it creates a <u>contrary reaction</u> from their brain, which wants to go to sleep in this position and functional situation. These unhealthy habits don't apply 100% to all of our current generation of youngsters, but I suggest they apply to a rapidly increasing majority.

j) Some parents of these addicted phone users and game players can be very aware and highly concerned of the serious downsides of their children's behaviour. However, as their children become older, they find they just can't put any degree of healthy control into their activities. Having attempted to modify their children's usage and suffering more frequent family arguments as a consequence, they reluctantly back off and worry silently with much increasing concern.

k) Some parents have been brainwashed etc., into believing that this is the new enlightened world of today, tomorrow and the future. They wholeheartedly support their children's activities and engage with them at every opportunity. These parents can also be seen speaking into their phones, walking down a busy street etc., just as excessively as their children.

l) If you are a parent worried about one of your children's excessive use of a smartphone and/or of playing games, test their level of addiction by threatening to remove their phone etc., for one month. Step back and witness their immediate and probably emotionally raw explosive reaction. If your concern has any degree of merit, you will be left with no doubt about the truth.

m) The level of addiction that some gamers have acquired has become so severe that to cure them, they have to be sent to a specialist clinic to treat this particular addiction.

IN CONCLUSION TO SECTIONS 7.15.2 & 7.15.3:

The **sum total of the Emotional Stress and Anxiety created** and the consequential **damage to the emotional health of the seriously-addicted users of smartphones, games and social media sites is immense.** I believe this has contributed an astronomical amount to the explosion of the percentage of the world's population currently suffering from severe mental health illnesses. Unfortunately, due to the difficulties and pressures of the COVID-19 pandemic, the frequency and hours of use of these activities has increased very significantly since the pandemic exploded onto our world stage, thus creating even more current and future mental health illness.

I would postulate that if the internet and all of these facilities had never existed, this frightening growth in serious mental health problems, experienced particularly over the last fifteen years, would not have occurred.

SUBCHAPTER 7.15.4: Other negative/Ugly uses of the internet.

OVERVIEW: This is a very brief description of other types of negative and Ugly consequences of how the internet allows each of these activities to be carried out in some cases, multitudes of times every day around our wonderful world.

1) A criminal can steal money from your account anywhere in the world without even getting out of bed. Before the internet, they would have to get out of bed and break into a bank, etc.

2) The ever-worsening aspect of cyber-crime is that it continues to become more aggressive. The percentage of large and small companies exposed to cyber-attacks continue to rise.

3) UK firms are very concerned about serious cyber-attacks originating in other countries seeking to steal trade secrets from them.

4) In early 2021, a former Cyber Chief, who pre-qualified that he was not a digital pacifist, stated very emphatically: "We weaponise and militarise the internet at our peril." His remarks follow reports of the use of offensive cyber techniques by nations, including the UK.

5) The retired elderly with big pots of retirement money are being particularly targeted by online criminals. They are scamming them out of their money, mainly by using fake accounts that the sites they appear on are struggling to detect and therefore deal with. The scale of online financial fraud is continually increasing at an alarming rate.

6) The many uses of the internet allow companies to gather data from and about their users. These companies make vast amounts of money from selling it, using and misusing it. This data is being gathered in from an increasing number of ways and means, mostly without the data-related people knowing about it, let alone giving their permission for it to be collected.

7) This personal data about people can be harvested in an increasing number of ways, from smartphones, watches, televisions, fitness trackers, speakers installed inside people's houses, sex toys with cameras and WIFI connections, etc.

8) A TV manufacturer has told all homeowners who have their TV to carry out certain checks on them every few weeks to prevent malicious software attacks.

9) Criminals hack into other people's databases to steal data about them and sometimes about thousands of other people that they sell on or misuse for financial benefits.

10) Recently, Bulgaria, with a population of 7million adults, had their tax data stolen in a cyber-attack on the country's tax agency.

11) Governments from countries around the world are able to influence other countries' elections for Presidents, P.M.'s, etc. This de-stabilising practised ability has the potential to de-stabilise democracy and possibly be a party to cause another World War.

12) The increasing existence of lies/fake news has the potential to create difficulties of the most worryingly dangerous kind.

13) Internet sites provide platforms to the worst types of individuals of our human race to communicate to whomever they wish, with ease, efficiency and effectiveness, their views about anyone else, about any topic whatsoever at any time. They carry out these horrific, hateful and maybe lying criticisms towards anyone they choose, with impunity and absolute zero accountability. Again, before the internet, these people would have to get out of bed to go somewhere, speak in public, write down and publish etc., but they would only connect to a limited few others by these previous means.

14) The use of re-tweet and share buttons has allowed the frighteningly efficient and high-speed spread of bullying, hate speech and fake news.

15) One government requires all of its internet users in its country to install a certificate that will allow the government to read anything they type or post – talk about Big Brother personified.

16) National electricity supplies and power station electrical-generated supplies are all at risk of being shut down by attacks over the Internet. If successful, these activities can cause the most serious disruption to a whole country's operational infrastructure, which relies heavily upon electricity to operate and basically function at all. I have thought for many years that these systems and services should never be designed to operate, be controlled and even monitored over the internet in the first place because of the ramifications of being hacked.

17) One of the big social media sites recently admitted that they can't keep up with and stop/prevent criminals from setting up fake accounts. These extremely clever criminals keep one step ahead of them. The site was forced to retrain its A.I. bots so they would hopefully autonomously be able to detect these unacceptable accounts.

18) Wider use of technology over the internet by criminal gangs is posing increasing challenges to Police forces. Europol is currently tracking 5,000 separate international organised crime groups.

19) The spread of child sexual abuse over the internet continues, with the making and sharing of sexual images and videos involving children. Also, live streaming of sexual assaults occurs. The spread of porn over the internet is creating

seriously unhealthy levels of addictions never before experienced, particularly with children. It is one of the main factors that is creating a rise in sexual misconduct towards girls at school.

20) A porn-troll-lawyer has been jailed for 14 years because he shared pornography films with people online and then sued them for copyright infringement.

21) Computer systems used in public services for a host of uses have been attacked by criminals with what are called **ransomware attacks**. The criminals demand very large sums of money to clear the hacking problems they created. These attacks have already virtually stopped all English NHS hospitals from fully operating. Doctors had to resort to paper files and walking to other departments to express verbal information due to these attacks.

<u>Update on the ransomware attacks, which are growing in total disruption and concern with no apparent ability to stop them!!</u>

A ransomware cyberattack targeted a very large software company that serviced one million separate firms (yet to be confirmed), thus enabling the attack to be on a huge scale of total disruption. The gang demanded $70 million to release the locked files. It is confirmed that 800 Swedish Co-op supermarkets and eleven schools in New Zealand have been affected.

22) Patients are automatically supplied with crucial medication by machines operated by computers on hospital computer networks. These machines are vulnerable to hackers who

could make changes to doses that could kill patients. They could also disable alarms on patient treatment machines, putting patients' lives in danger.

23) Recently, UK finance firms' cyber incidents and consumer bank accounts' incidents both increased by over 1000% in the last year.

SUBCHAPTER 7.15.5: A very brief list of the consequences of the list in Subchapter 7.15.4.

1) So much of the list in 7.15.4 is globalisation/connectivity where connectivity (the mantra of social media sites) prevails with zero accountability: dangerous bedfellows to the population at large.

2) I found a behind the scenes view of one of the huge social media companies was truly fascinating. However, I was left with an overall view that the people who worked there were obviously all highly intelligent and capable. At the same time, they appeared like zombies, brainwashed by their employer's mantras and desperately trying to justify their company's activities towards their defined objectives as beneficial to mankind.

3) There are constant criticisms in the media and from unfortunate individuals who have fallen foul of the negative uses of the internet about many harmful activities, most of which are on my lists above. The oft-repeated response is that legislation must be brought in to make the offending

media giants, sites or organisations accountable for the unacceptable misuse of their facilities. Why don't they engage their often-triumphed A.I. bots to immediately and automatically delete the offending activities and posts, thus solving the problems in that instant of unacceptable actions?

I just don't think legislation will ever be effective for a number of reasons. As far as A.I. bots are concerned, I firmly believe, as I have often stated in my book, they have no actual/real intelligence. You can't include real intelligence into written instructions for a dumb machine. You would need an army of human beings, each of which requires an average level of real intelligence and general knowledge to recognise and immediately delete offending material and activities with ease.

They would require the simple directives of not allowing material such as hate-promoting encouragements and material encouraging self-harming or suicidal action glorification, etc.

These media giants seem to hide behind these A.I. bots when these bots have not taken down some information or statement which has appeared on their site. The active software functionality of these A.I. Bots will have been written by the software engineers. They have been instructed and guided by an employee, both of whom work for the media giant itself, so they are clinically responsible for failing to take down this offending material. It is not acceptable to blame anyone else but themselves.

4) With all of the accumulation of activities detailed, these Tech Media Giants continue to grow in wealth, communicative power and resolution of how our world should function. Countries are trying to hold them to account with insufficient taxes paid and other activities that are questionably acceptable. It seems, though, that their immense wealth and power make them impenetrable.

5) 5) It is interesting and worthwhile noting that prior to the advent of the internet, it took many years to create a new company that offered real and measurable added value to the world. One had to gather and develop a team of suitably capable people to build, create, design and manufacture products that the real world wished to buy and use. It took a lot of ability and major financial risks to do all of these things and to ultimately make a profit of possibly, at best, 10% to 15% net.

But, with the arrival of the companies that feed off the internet's interconnectivity, they are able to very quickly grow their business into a vast empire. The owners of the empire make enormous profits of billions of pounds, basically by harvesting detailed data about a vast multitude of people and making money, simply from selling and/or using or misusing this knowledge.

Also, since the internet, individuals can, from within their own home, build up an increasing following of people and gradually turn this into a very lucrative and successful business. It could be anything from simple communications to satisfying the sexual needs of their followers and a multitude of many other activities.

Recently a **seven-year-old** YouTube star who has 21 million subscribers to his Toys Review channel was recently named YouTube's highest earner. What on earth is this world of ours coming to? Where is the measurable and real added-value to the world from these types of businesses, other than to the people who own them from which they make a considerable amount of money?

6) I have noticed that, with the ever-increasing use of communication over the internet, particularly in the last ten years or so, there has been a serious degradation of basic manners, attitudes and behaviour displayed generally between human beings. I believe this is due to more and more people communicating via the internet, a vast amount more than in the history of the human race. I think the consequences of this are:

a) People express their personal views about whoever or whatever, in an extremely determined and vigorous manner.

b) They used to normally prefix a statement of – In my opinion, I believe that so and so and then state their view, but not now.

c) Now, people state their views with no prefix – 'in my opinion.'

d) If the other person or people dare to have a different point of view to theirs, they can't accept this at all. They just don't accept that **everyone has the right to have their**

own opinion about everything, all of the time. So, it becomes an argument rather than as before a pleasant and constructive discussion.

e) If the discussion is about things that would take place or appear in the future, they present these future aspects and occurrences to be in a matter-of-fact mode rather than theirs or others' educated guesses. They just don't appear to understand the unarguable fact about any topic you care to consider is that no one knows – actually knows, what it will be like in the future. Certainly, they can have a guess, maybe an educated one, but it always has been and will remain just that – a guess.

f) There has come to pass what I consider a frightening ploy of getting people to believe some important aspect of life by brainwashing them with constant high levels of repetition of a particular view or opinion or change wished to be brought about. This is done to the extent that people eventually, just believe it without question and then constantly repeat the brainwashing statements themselves to others. This ploy no doubt has been used by leaders of the world since the beginning of time, but in recent times I feel it has become quite prevalent and extreme, particularly about very important matters.

g) There has grown an increasing lack of respect shown towards other people, which is demonstrated by the lack of use of their Christian name and just using their surname.

h) There is an ever-increasing chase towards measuring people's worth in terms of the money they earn/have and how many friends and followers they have on social media sites.

i) Peoples' increasing frequency of communication with an increasingly wider range of other people over the internet-enabled media has resulted in them communicating less and less via direct, face-to-face communication. Whilst communicating, their standard of behaviour and attitudes towards others has become increasingly less acceptable. They are also not developing good face-to-face interpersonal skills whilst growing up, or they are losing them even if they already had them.

I think a significant factor in causing these phenomena is the same as what causes some car drivers' awfully aggressive behaviour on motorways but not on ordinary roads. This, I believe is because, on the motorway, the aggressors won't soon have a potential close encounter or a face-to-face meeting with the other party to have to deal with, after their aggression. However, they run a high risk of having this on ordinary roads. The communications over the internet are disconnected and remote and don't run the risk of the aggressor having to deal face-to-face with the person they targeted.

7) People responsible for the creation of the internet and parts of its functionality and those who own these media giants harvest increasingly vast sums of money off the Internet's existence and usage. However, in recent times, they have noticeably made public criticism and voiced public concerns tinged with embarrassment of the damage done by the internet uses and missuses. The cat is out of the bag, and what's to be done?

8) You hear the constant comments made by people who offer their professional services about tackling and preventing the hacking of people's financial accounts to steal money, personal data and carry out ransomware activities, etc. The fact is that the internet is an open system, and as such, it is nominally open to anyone who wishes to use it. You can make hacking your systems more difficult to achieve, but if the criminals have the technical knowledge and determination, which most certainly have, they will still carry out these criminal activities without the smallest morsel of concern.

9) A final concern is using the internet for military purposes. This type of scenario is depicted many times in the James Bond films, which I feel almost legitimises it and justifies it as an inevitability. This use/misuse of the internet is the most likely activity that will directly lead to the Third World War. Is there anything more frightening and concerning than this?

I worked in engineering the whole of my life across a wide range of many different types of systems employing fully automatic systems, with the best of technique, technology, installation quality etc. Even when employed by the most competent, experienced professionals, it is realistically impossible to avoid, even at best, the extremely rare fault from occurring in such systems as above. So, a country automatically (and even following some manual or other validation checks) under perceived attack sets out to blow up these oncoming perceived nuclear missiles. It also sends an armada of nuclear missiles to counterattack the perceived aggressing country. This scenario just fills me with absolute utter extreme unadulterated dread!

MY OVERALL CONCLUSION ABOUT THE USES OF THE INTERNET ARE:

I believe that when it comes to the sum-total consequences of the uses of the internet, **unfortunately, the benefits are utterly overwhelmingly outweighed by the negative uses and their negative consequences**.

I find it very seriously disturbing that most negative activities **only exist simply due to the existence of the internet,** followed by the type of people who use it in this manner. If the internet had not been invented, our world would have virtually none of these damaging activities with their seriously damaging consequences. Far too high a percentage of the human race has succumbed emotionally and addictively to using and practising these internet-related habits and facilities.

These people **are living life inside their smartphones and games**. They are very infrequently directly connecting with other human beings and **not physically and emotionally connecting with enough of the activities that this wonderful world with its immense diversity has to offer.**

Natural life on this planet of ours is centred on human beings, their work, pastimes, their **direct and real interaction** with **other human beings**, and **all living creatures**. It is naturally centred and created to comprise of living an **authentic life** with all of its facets – meeting **genuine people** outside in the **real world**, visiting all of the real, **physically existing countries**, their fascinating histories, buildings and different nationalities. Yet all you hear, see and are exposed to is VIRTUAL THIS, VIRTUAL THAT wrapped inside Artificial Intelligence.

The human race should aspire to go back to **ACTUAL REALITY**. Have we all forgotten that we all live on a **REAL PLANET** habited by **REAL PEOPLE** and populated by existing **REAL, FASCINATING THINGS TO VISIT and participate in?**

Life is also centred upon humans being challenged to accomplish difficult tasks and the satisfaction of enjoying a good job at work well done, all with the achievement of a hard-earned income and spending it as they wish.

Even when these internet world users are outside their bedroom and house, and nominally in the real world, walking along the pavement, they are still emotionally and functionally inside their universe of smartphones and all of their addictions. They cross-support each other functionally and effectively in their addictive usages and almost glorify them as they continue to live in our world, but remotely within their own false unreal and unhealthy one.

If the internet's existence and usage continue as detailed above, which I judge will be what happens, this world that I see and describe will increasingly be the newer/more modern world that eventually all of us humans will inherit/move further into. In my opinion, change is good, providing it is beneficial and better for the vast majority!!

In my opinion, the internet-related damages to the majority of its users' mental health are of the highest level of seriousness. They significantly contribute to the increasing percentage of the world's population's worsening mental illness level, coupled with the combined and connected worsening sleep problems. The rising mental illness rate is further exacerbated by the emotional stress and anxiety caused by the sum total of most of the misuses listed above.

I believe that the present number of people in the UK who have significant mental illness is many times greater than the number of people within the UK's Health System who can treat them effectively.

If the current numbers of people with significant mental illness continue to rise due to the described internet usage, I consider the long-term future and continuing existence of an emotionally healthy human race to be in unquestionable jeopardy.

How will the world manage to be in a sufficiently stable, healthy and therefore sustainable state to survive if the vast majority of the population has become significantly mentally ill? This includes a number of world leaders and other significant and primary decision-makers and shakers throughout the controlling structures of our world.

I believe that the <u>future health of our planet itself</u> is of equal importance to the <u>mental health of its occupants.</u> **Both aspects must be addressed simultaneously.**

These comments are made with the utmost gravity and serious concern, following a great deal of consideration.

In addition to my comments above, in my overall conclusion about the uses of the internet and dealing with the crucially important topic of people's worsening poor mental health, I present the following Subchapter for the utmost vitally important and extremely serious considerations.

SUBCHAPTER 7.15.6: The inherent consequences of the negative uses and the negative creations of the internet.

I very strongly believe that the basic changes in this chapter must be proposed, accepted and maintained by the collection of <u>all world leaders</u> of <u>all of the countries of the world</u> from the <u>very big to the very small</u> in order for:

a)   Our planet and the continuance of our human race to each enjoy a **permanent, developing, repairing and healthy future.**

b)   The **complete cessation** of all of the extremely worrying, damaging, disruptive and law-breaking practices happening far more frequently around the whole world and within individual countries.

c) The **complete cessation** of practices that are attacking the very foundations of what used to be a far more stable, balanced, law-abiding, fairly well-ordered and decent world.

d) All of the required changes that must be made to recover and to protect our planet's future climate, nominally enabling it to survive healthily forever.

The most important, significant and serious question ever considered by and for the continuance of our humanity and the planet that we all live on is:

Is there any other way? I don't believe so.

OVERVIEW: The overwhelming and driving principle of each of these rules is the total and utter acceptance that all countries live on and share this wonderful planet of ours.

Therefore, it is essential that all of these countries collectively recognise that it is in all of their interests that our **planet's resources** and **climate are maintained and recovered** where necessary.

NB In terms of climate change, which unquestionably requires addressing urgently, I have one note of caution that has been bugging me for some time. As I have previously described in my book, with some degree of detail, every single condition or thing that exists in this changing world of ours is never caused or created by only one thing or condition. It is always caused by the combinational effect of many different things/factors that combine to create the prevailing condition.

With sufficient or perhaps absolute confidence, can any individual or a small group of people:

a) *List out at least each of the separate primary factors that combine to create our planet's climate?*

b) *Can they describe how each factor interacts with the other factors and what these resultant consequences are?*

c) *Can anyone say what the consequence **is** of the combinational effect of all of the aforementioned consequences?*

I also worry that if you don't know **all of the conditions making the patient sick,** you may alter things or give them treatment that makes them <u>worse</u>!

Let's return to the following basic changes that must be proposed, accepted and maintained by the collection of <u>all world leaders</u> of <u>all of the countries of the world</u> from the <u>very big to the very small</u>.

It is important that our planet's resources are shared as equally and as fairly as possible relating to each country's size and needs and that there are never in future any wars <u>at all</u>, let alone another major world war.

This collective and fundamentally new way of life for all countries living on our common planet will not allow any country to continue its historical waring with any other country, state or creed from now on. There will be absolutely no exceptions to this rule from all of the other countries of the world.

Why do countries ever have to make war against any other when they can live alongside each other in peace and harmony if they really wish to? Abolish these aeons' old rituals of fighting and controlling other countries. It is essential that all country leaders regularly meet face-to-face to form human friendships, understanding and real, strong and trusting interrelationships.

All of this, no doubt, will seem ridiculously unrealistic and will never happen.

Hold on.

It *must* happen.

It just has to happen to fully achieve all of the primary objectives. It is not acceptable to achieve 50% or even 70% of the objectives. 100% of the objectives must be achieved so that our common home will enjoy a permanent and healthy future. It is utter madness to continue these centuries-old customs and practices just because they have always existed!

These changes will require the ability to and the acceptance of compromise. Leaders will have to see the other countries' views and objectives and merge them all to end up with fundamental changes accepted by all for the good of all for the rest of time.

It will be totally unacceptable for the rest of the countries living on our planet if only one or even more than one country ops out of these new rules. Every country must accept and completely buy into the new regimes of life in order that the maximum benefits are realised and enjoyed by all.

1.0 All countries must accept and respect that each other country has the right to follow their particular country's different religious beliefs, including their God. Therefore, there is never any threat from a country attempting to impose their religious beliefs or their God on any other country or people in any way possible. Also, there is never any attempt to make fun of or project any other insults towards any other different faiths at any time or place ever. Live and let live. Give respect to all others and receive respect from all others.

2.0 Each different country's cultures, customs and practices must genuinely be respected and accepted by all other countries. There must be a common attitude and belief that it is in everyone's interest to get on with everyone else and achieve this. For example, forget the history of what some other country did to your country or try to forget what another clan or religious following did to yours 500 years ago.

Continuing to promote and foster this extreme relationship and striving to attack the other party at every opportunity, means this relationship will go on forever/ad infinitum. The hatred is passed on from father to son to the extreme degree of being quite prepared to take the lives of the other side when every opportunity arises.

3.0 The attitude required by leaders representing each cult, party or country is to constantly remind people of the new objectives they will live under. Emphasise all of the different attitudes, objectives and ways of life required to genuinely forgive the other country, cult or party. Promote being able to forgive and forget and therefore change for the better the day-to-day lives of all people living on this common planet of ours.

4.0 In addition to all of the above, I believe that one vitally important remaining objective is to focus on improving and developing the existing human quality, capability and resourcefulness of the human beings currently living on our planet. This is so they live their lives in a more meaningful and worthwhile fashion and, wherever possible, help other human beings they meet in whatever way is appropriate to the needs of others.

5.0 To help achieve all of the above, I believe that the focus should be totally concentrated on improving the immediate and long term health and development of the planet we all can and do live on. Additionally, I think we should seek to improve the human status and the skills and capabilities of all of the humans that currently live on this planet that we are blessed with. Stop focusing on other planets, the universe at large and other possible civilisations, spending vast sums of money and an inordinate amount of time and expertise on the immensity of this research.

I propose we spend all of this time, money and expertise on improving our own planet. It desperately requires the appropriate changes and expenditures, the sum total of which will hopefully achieve all of the required objectives.

IN FINAL REVIEW AND CONCLUSION:

The vision of how I think the world's countries should very fundamentally change and work extremely closely together with all other countries will no doubt be seen by the vast majority of people as theoretical perfection, pie in the sky, sheer fantasy.

It will never be implemented anything like fully, and also, no doubt the majority of the world leaders would like to continue as they always have done as is the want of most human beings.

I have reviewed the frighteningly rapid rate of decline of increasingly more and more countries and states. I have seen what I believe is the particular worrying trend, promoted and being copied in principle by others, of the storming of the US Capitol Building in Washington in 2021, by an anarchic, murderous, well pre-organised and ongoing marshalled army of thugs. They attacked the temple of American authority while the whole of America and the world looked on with total disbelief.

There has also been a very large horde of armed, well-marshalled and extremely aggressive, dangerous and incensed protesters in the streets, demanding reverse changes to the recent fuel price rise. There have been street protests demanding the removal of politicians they blame for this, that and the other. These lawless mobs dislike something with the utmost intensity and attack with serious intent any police who attempt to restore law and order, resulting in deaths and many injures.

This trend demonstrates a total lack of respect for the law of the land, the police and their inherent authority. Respect for the laws and rules that govern all life and behaviour in the country you live in maintains fundamental safety and stability in everyone's daily lives, providing a country that is nominally safe to live in. When these laws and the required actions, for example, to combat, contain and ultimately get on top of the COVID-19 pandemic are ignored, anarchy and serious trouble prevail.

The whole world is progressively becoming more and more unstable. Increasingly more countries and people within countries towards each other, automatically, more regularly and viciously, take to the streets with extreme anger, trying to force their wishes upon their elected leaders, about more and more aspects of everyday life. There is an inherent momentum of worsening change that is frightening to behold!! The sooner we take the impetus out of these changes, the sooner we can begin to reverse these trends.

I am sure the immense collective power of all the world's leaders, plus many committed and supremely competent additional new movers and shakers, all working in unison, following the simple rules and objectives detailed above will win the day.

All for one and one for all!!

SUBCHAPTER 7.16: Example of the absolute power of the mind, being aware of and managing it.

This section covers a very noticeable, world-aware example of the absolute and utter immense power of the mind. We will look at the vital importance of being aware of it, managing it knowledgeably and engaging its placebo effect, to utilise it fully to achieve important goals and to promote mental or physical healing requirements you may have.

OVERVIEW: *In the 2019 Rugby Union World Cup Final in November, England were very comprehensively beaten by South Africa in terms of the scoreline, having far less game control and fewer opportunities to score points throughout most of the game. All of the predictions were that England would beat South Africa.*

Immediately after the game, England's coach Eddie Jones was asked what had gone wrong – why had England lost so comprehensively? He simply said he didn't know. A while later, he added that sometimes you lose a game, have an exhaustive de-brief, and still don't know what was wrong. It just happens sometimes. It wasn't because of lack of effort made, which the players confirmed, saying that they couldn't have trained any harder or prepared any more. Eddie also said that throughout the whole week, everyone was pumped up, and he felt the players were in the right place. "We just didn't do it tonight. The players will hold the hurt from their defeat for years to come. We're going to be kicking stones for four years."

Interestingly, Eddie, made one singular point that I feel was within touching distance of the underlying cause of their failure, which had maybe come from out of **the depth of his subconscious**. "In rugby, in any sport, there is never an entitlement. Just because of what we did last week (thrashing New Zealand), we were never entitled to come here and do the same. We've done everything to try and win this. There is never an entitlement. Tonight we just didn't get it."

After the match, knowledgeable spectators pointed out areas of the game in which England were relatively poor but did not point to any underlying cause/s of these poor performance factors.

Soon after the game had finished, I was as shocked and disappointed as anyone who had witnessed the demolition of this particular England Rugby Union team. I sat down and stepped back from the immediate game. I went through the following processes, the objective of which, hopefully, was to identify the underlying reason or reasons for why it went so horribly wrong for England.

Here are my thoughts for your consideration.

SUBCHAPTER 7.16.1: The process of the build-up for the South African team as they approached the World Cup final.

At its core was their captain Siya Kolisi. He was South Africa's first black rugby captain, the kid from the township who only thought about how he would get his next meal. He was acutely aware of how he was looked upon as an example to so many South African youngsters of what to aspire to achieve in their life. Kolisi admitted before this particular final that the captaincy had weighed heavily upon him. He was acutely aware that he was not just a rugby skipper for the South African team, but a symbol: a beacon of hope for so many throughout the whole of South Africa.

The team were particularly inspired by references from South African rugby stars from the past, including Bryan Habana, and when Francois Peinaar collected the Rugby World Cup from

Nelson Mandela. South Africa's current president publicly greeted Kolisi saying, "You carry the pride of our nation."

Back home, the entire South African nation was going barmy with support for their team. The team coach said to the team that they were not playing for themselves anymore. They were playing for all of the people back home; to give them pride in themselves, in their country within the world and to look forward to a better future.

The South African rugby team were fired up by the cumulative effect of each of the different elements described above. Additionally, they were playing at the pinnacle of importance and of achievement – in the World Cup final. They were also impassioned because they were playing a team that had demolished the New Zealand team in the semi-final. This New Zealand team was hailed by some as not just the best rugby team but the best team of any other sport. So, they knew that they had to be at their absolute best to stand even a small chance of winning.

If you just take a little time to read again from the start of this section, try and emotionally absorb each of the separate, individual motivators that prevailed. Gradually, automatically and inevitably, they fed into each of the South African rugby team's player's minds as they approached this World Cup final.

As a cumulative consequence of all of the above, I believe the South African rugby team performed at a level significantly higher than the collective sum of all of their players' capability, and then even more, such was the empowerment prevailing. In this type of situation, with such an extremely emotionally charged environment, there is always the risk that the players/ team can be overwhelmed and struggle to cope. This is where the team coach/manager and the captain play a key role in being aware of this risk and ensuring that this negative response doesn't prevail.

This South African team were a very strong team in terms of their number of world-class players, their physical strengths, their combative style of play, and they were in the final on merit. However, there are additional benefits when the human mind is switched on and fired up to a super-controlled, efficient, super-focused and determined manner. The physical power and control over the body lead to the mind/body connection and co-ordination being razor-sharp, super-fast, super-efficient, super-strong and determined.

When you add the players' own placebo effect factor to all of the elements detailed above, the accumulated emotional effect in their team as they went out on to the pitch to do battle in the final would have been off the scale if it could have been measured by a suitable meter.

This was the opposition England faced when they walked out on the pitch – some adversary!

SUBCHAPTER 7.16.2: The journey of the England team from when Eddie Jones took over, their approach to the

World Cup tournament, their progress during it, all the way to the World Cup final.

In the four years after taking over as England's coach, Eddie Jones had lifted the team from the depths of despair. They had gone from failing to emerge from the pool stage of the 2015 World Cup and from a world ranking of N.8 to No.1.

To date, Eddie Jones has developed a squad and a team that has become very confident. The players are extremely keen and proud to become part of the team, and the nation is very proud of it. The team play an exciting, pacey style of rugby and the manner in which they play puts bums-on-seats at England rugby matches. The prime mover for this immense progress was, I think, Eddie Jones, and I admired him immensely for gradually building up and creating this squad of players.

As the England team developed, they had a world-record equalling winning run followed by a dip in form. Eddie Jones' position was under fire but the team's performance recovered and, leading into the World Cup Tournament, England were expected to do very well. They made their way through the rounds with competent performances, the minimum of drama and expectations of the ultimate success quietly grew.

England then played New Zealand in the semi-final of the world cup. This New Zealand team was hailed by some as not just the best rugby team in the world but the best team of any other sport. Despite the quality and record of success of this New Zealand team and the resultant aura and confidence that they exuded, England not only beat New Zealand, but they also demolished them, apart from the scoreline. They were prepared brilliantly by Eddie and by the team actually believing they were very capable of beating New Zealand. Their super standard of play and their super determined will to win obtained a very well-deserved win.

Eddie brilliantly worked the psychology on the opposition in the build-up to the match and effectively put an emotional mirror up to their Haka just before the start. England exploded out of the blocks with a two-minute try and never really let New Zealand off the hook for the rest of the match.

The team who had spent ten years at the top of the world rankings were, at times, reduced to running around in circles like headless chickens. They just weren't used to being treated like this. They emotionally succumbed, with England keeping up their relentless pressure of tight, fully-focused, effective, determined, super-quality rugby for the whole match.

After this superlative performance, the media was awash with immense and worthy praise. Even the colossus and the most admired but not easy to please, World Cup-winning captain Martin Johnson, was raving about all aspects of the England team's performance. Due to this prevailing situation, the classic risks are there that can so easily arise, thus jeopardising England's chances of winning the world cup.

During the week between the semi-final and the final, **was when for the first time, the final came truly into focus.** The

England team had to prepare themselves for the ultimate prize of winning the Rugby Union World Cup final.

I say this simply because, **before they had actually beaten New Zealand**, they couldn't really focus/think about the final. New Zealand were seen by all rugby players and followers as by far the best team in the whole tournament and, therefore, the biggest hurdle to overcome to actually win the World Cup.

So, here were this England team, which many were saying, compared to any England team in the past, had played the best game of their life, having annihilated probably the best rugby team ever. They had to prepare themselves to play in the final against South Africa. They were a very good team and a very tough team to beat, but they were not nearly as good as New Zealand.

In top professional sport generally, but I think in rugby particularly, it is a relatively extremely physically and mentally tough hard sport to engage in, the extreme of which is at international level.

The England team/players/coaches were presented with a very challenging tricky situation to embrace and to prepare themselves and England for successfully. They needed to play in the oncoming final in the required emotionally conditioned state from which they would be able to win against a team that had become an extremely formidable challenge.

I would say that the standard of the England players' physical preparation, their power, stamina, confidence and their rugby technique and their collected confidence in this range of attributes were second to none. I think that this has increasingly been the case, particularly under Eddie Jones's tenure. However, the crucial area of their emotional and mental status, i.e. **the condition and state of their mind, was, I believe, not as it should have been to prepare to win this oncoming World Cup final. This was compounded by the failure to be made aware of the empowered state of the minds of their opposition.**

SUBCHAPTER 7.16.3: How I believe that the England team should have been prepared emotionally, psychologically and tactically to stand the best chance of winning the final.

a) At the start of the week leading up to the final, after the finish of the nice compliments etc., about the win against New Zealand, I would recommend Eddie Jones said this to the team.

"I am asking each of you here to think very carefully, deeply and honestly to search in the depth of your mind and answer this question. Do you think that, with your involvement as it may be, our team will win the World Cup? It is vitally important that you try and search out your answer from the depth of your mind and not at the surface/expected response that you know you should give. Take your time, think about it, and maybe your honest answer might be that you don't really know how you are feeling deep down. This is not a trick question. There are no brownies points on offer. I am desperate to know how you all feel so we can all move as individuals and therefore as a team/unit into the state at which we are best prepared mentally to beat South Africa.

"When you have each arrived at your individual answer, please turn your palm over. When all palms are up, I will go around the room, starting with our Captain Owen. Please believe me that I only want your honest answer as best as you can give it. Any answer is acceptable apart from one, and that is you telling me what you think I want to hear and not what you actually think. Therefore, you are being dishonest with me and your team. I will ask one of the coaches to make a note of what each of your answers is."

b) I would then review, with the whole team, each of the aspects about their opponents as detailed in 7.16.1 using someone who is best suited to lead this exercise, along with Eddie Jones adding his comments at times. It is vital that each of the England players fully understood and believed the weight of importance and the cumulative effect that these conditioning factors were having on the South African team. They needed to recognise that these player's minds, attitudes, confidence and determination were being bolstered. These players had the total, utter belief that **they** had to and would actually win the World Cup.

It was only from this clear understanding that they could be prepared to meet the onslaught they would face. From this, they would be aware of the required nullifying counter-attack they would have to generate in opposition to initially withhold the oncoming tidal onslaught from South Africa and then to turn it back against and go on to beat them.

It is extremely important that any required discussion about this topic is encouraged to fully understand each of these emotionally charging factors.

c) Discuss with all of the team's coaches and others as normal what the optimum tactics are of how best to play against and beat South Africa. Utilise the strengths of the England team and select the best team from the available fit players.

d) Explain all of these planned tactics to the whole of the England squad, present the planned team and the players on the bench. Discuss these tactics with those in attendance, as appropriate.

e) Repeat the exercise in **a)** above, except, ask each player to explain why he has come to his answer, whether it's the same as the first time or not. Again, it must be honest and from the depth of their mind. Again, have each person's answer recorded. Go round and ask every player who does not actually/deeply believe or doesn't know/feel that England will win, "Why are you saying that?"

f) Resolve any issues that **e)** throws up, which might result in a change of some tactics, for example.

SUBCHAPTER 7.16.4: The reasons why I believe England didn't achieve their goal of winning the final and lost in the manner that prevailed.

a)   The England players were clearly not made aware of all of the cumulative reasons detailed in 7.16.1 that created the state of the minds of the players and the resultant mindset of the South African team as they walked out to face England in the final. It was absolutely crucial that the England team were fully prepared and thus able to withstand the physical, emotional and playing onslaught that awaited them from the off. I believe that the attack they experienced was probably the most extreme, intense, emotionally and physically brutal that any rugby team had ever been exposed to. The makeup of the South African side made them a team who were so ultra-inspired they were, and realistically so, possibly unbeatable on that day.

I believe that the only way England could have been in with a good chance of winning the final was if they had very clearly understood beforehand and accepted the mindset of the South African team. This would have fully prepared them for the onslaught they were to be bombarded with from the start. Also, if they had been reminded a number of times of the enormity of their performance against the All Blacks, this would crucially have fortified and bolstered up their confidence and therefore ability to withstand the forthcoming ferocity of play and attitude from South Africa. With this dual preparation, based on the whole team's confidence from it and the placebo effect initiated, I believe that England could have coped with South Africa's emotion and play. Very gradually, they would have got South Africa to run down their adrenalin, confidence and stamina to come out in the second half and turn the tables to win.

b) I am sure that the point was made to the England team by Eddie and others that they must put the glorious win against New Zealand behind them. They would have been warned not to feel that because they had completely outplayed the best team in the world, the final against South Africa was going to be almost an expected, assumed, entitlement to win. No doubt, the players replied saying no, they didn't think like that, they realised that South Africa were a very good side etc. But, underneath these comments, my belief is that a significant number of players deep down did think, to some dangerous degree, they were going to win because of the way they had trounced New Zealand.

If Eddie and his coaches had focused upon this most crucial of topics re preparing the England team's psychological attitude towards the final as detailed in Subchapter 7.16.3, he would have gradually prepared the players' minds correctly.

c) The second of the two most important topics of preparation of the minds of the England team in order to win was to analyse, discuss and fully understand all of 7.16.1. Only when this had been fully achieved would the England players have fully understood the awesome rugby challenge that awaited them from South Africa. Then they could comprehend the reflective attitude that the England players had to feel and display to withstand South Africa's extreme emotional and physical power, determination and absolute and utter will to win.

My guess is that the England team did not carry out such a detailed analysis of the South African team to understand all of the accumulative reasons that created their immense focus, determination and their absolute will to win. Therefore, this was the other factor that combined with a) above to create the relatively poor state of the England team's minds, fundamentally contributing to the very poor way they played.

d) The third reason why I feel the England team did not play anywhere near as well as it was capable of was that Eddie and his coaches, very surprisingly, didn't appear to assess the strengths and weaknesses of the South African team. They sent out the same team to play the same way as they had so successfully against New Zealand. Because these two teams played in a totally different way in this World Cup, this was a big mistake.

e) The consequences of the combination of **a)**, **b)**, **c)** and **d)** created the states of mind and the style and playing plan that created England's performance. In combination with the states of mind of the South African team and their playing ability, this resulted in England being completely outplayed.

People sometimes forget that their every thought and action comes from within their own mind. If the emotional and psychological state of their mind is not good, their thoughts and inevitably their resultant actions will not be good. Concentrating primarily upon the physical conditioning and playing techniques and playing strategies of the England team are all vitally important. Yet also of absolute, crucial importance is the appropriate conditioning of the players' minds towards each game.

f) Two other aspects that contributed negatively to England's poor performance were that Kyle Sinckler, who had been one of England's popular stars, was badly concussed in the early minutes of the game. This lost the team a very valuable member of the scrum, which was of such importance for England in this match. Kyle was unconscious, prone on the ground for many minutes receiving medical treatment. Consequently, there is always the inevitable worry by his teammates. Is he going to be all right? Will he recover? How will the crucial game aspect of the England scrum fare without him? The psychological combination of these two factors a few minutes into the game would have very likely lowered the England team's mind-set even more that it was before this accident.

g) It was at this crucial point of the game, up to which, from the start, South Africa had clearly displayed their fired up state of mind and play against which England were continuing to struggle to contain, let alone combat. Therefore, it was so vital that the game's balance changed, which, from the start, had been totally in South Africa's favour. The longer it remained in their favour, the increasingly more difficult it is to be able to change it towards England's favour.

This is the absolute key moment when the England team's captain should have stood up and been counted for all that he was worth. He needed to show that when the chips are down and his team is seriously struggling mentally, physically and functionally, he is the man to rally the whole team around. It would have required the correct choice of words, the appropriate tone, emotional energy, some necessary degree of anger and some appropriate, tactical advice towards particular players, mixing raw constructive emotion with some encouragement.

You could plainly see that Owen Farrell was desperately trying to ignite and rally his troops, unfortunately without sufficient success. I must state very clearly and strongly that I have been a staunch supporter of Owen's world level standard of play and kicking, plus his general, constructive and fearless play as a player, captain, and overall contribution to England's cause.

In any sport, when one player or team is playing, it requires an immense continual mental effort to raise your emotional attitude and resultant and required standard of play from your current level up to your opponent's level. Then you have to raise it again to be able to start dominating them and therefore begin to change the tide of the game from how it started and continued, as in this final.

This change for the team can be sparked and developed by some utterly brilliant piece of play and achieving points etc., thus creating a seed of doubt in your opponent's minds for the first time. Their sleeping giant of an opponent has awoken and is now on the rampage. The last major potential opportunity for the England team to regroup and compete in this game and possibly claw their way to winning was at half-time. Eddie and his coaches had time to speak to the team and maybe make some player and tactical changes. But alas, this potential was not realised.

SUBCHAPTER 7.16.5: The aftermath of England's defeat in the final.

Following England's defeat in the final, due to how it was lost and because the team had not yet debriefed where they could have unearthed any root cause or causes for their failure, the following things occurred:

a)   The team disbanded from the World Cup and went home with extremely heavy hearts and a good degree of confusion as to why they had failed so miserably at the very last hurdle. This package of conditions will pretty certainly have left most if not all of the England players suffering from a significant degree of P.T.S.D. – Post Traumatic Stress Disorder. The degree of emotional hurt, anxiety and emotional stress they will have suffered due to all of these conditions mentioned is still residing in their memories at a very high degree of rawness. This is particularly the case because they can't understand the underlying cause or causes of why they played so badly.

They are therefore facing, in their minds, a whirlpool of negative thoughts, swirling around in the quiet periods of their days and whilst asleep without being able to process them tidily. They are unable to rationalise them into understandable and to a degree acceptable conditions and reasons. Extremely importantly, they are unable to at least learn from the underlying root causes as a team, as coaches and as individuals not to make the same mistakes ever again until they unearth the causes.

b) Eddie Jones said that the players would hold the hurt from this defeat for years to come. This is fundamentally true, until they de-brief as a complete team/squad and the coaches to identify the underlying cause/s. Until they carry out this vitally important process, they will be unable to commence gradually and fully coming to terms with this defeat.

During this analysis process, it is vital that they discuss openly, constructively and honestly how they felt during the game, afterwards and now. This will all contribute to beginning the emotional healing process to gradually reduce the levels of P.T.S.D., including a degree of confidence loss they will continue to suffer until they can emotionally move on from this defeat.

c) It is not just the players who will have suffered from the above situation. It will have negatively affected Eddie Jones and his team of specialist coaches. More so, Eddie Jones, I would guess, because I judge him to be an immensely proud man who had put his very heart and soul into the team that he had created and nurtured to win the World Cup.

Also, Eddie will have been hurting because he sits on the top of the pyramid he built and within which the entire management and operation of the England squad resides and functions. He will have to wait for four years to have another chance, providing he wishes to carry on and whether he is requested to carry on. **I do hope that Eddie continues into the next World Cup and that we win.**

d) **A very serious offer to Eddie Jones from Jan De Vinter.**

Eddie, it is now a long time since your World Cup loss. My book is out and I was so, so pleased for you and your squad that you remained in charge to kick the can until the next opportunity. I would like to make you a very serious offer to come and meet you and your team, if you wish, to discuss your view of my view/s about how and why you, your playing squad and your squad of lieutenants did everything so perfectly last time, except up to and in the final game.

I am prepared to do this without payment and I am not after employment from you – I have no spare time. However, I would love to compare my views with yours and hopefully find we have some degree of agreement, but who knows? Hopefully, the collective learning we create will spin off into benefiting you and yours, such that you win the next final, to which I will expect a number of free tickets, mate – I was born in Cronulla, by the way. The very best of luck to you, Eddie. You're a man after my own sporting, competitive heart.

CHAPTER 8.0 – THE COVID-19 PANDEMIC: A DIFFERENT OVERALL VIEW, WITH A SERIOUS PERSPECTIVE AND QUESTIONS I WOULD LIKE TO PRESENT FOR YOUR CONSIDERATION.

OVERVIEW: Over a very short period of time, from near the end of 2019 to a few months later, the whole world had been literally ravaged by the presence of the COVID-19 virus, which had made its appearance in all corners of our planet. Countries primarily responded in their own way to its presence, the resultant deaths and, in many cases, long-term damage to people's health. They enforced many major changes to people's working and social lives to contain and reduce the spread of the virus to prevent the otherwise inevitable increasing rate towards exponential growth, of the rise of infection cases, hospitalisations and deaths.

SUBCHAPTER A) A list of this particular virus's worst features of danger to our health compared to possibly all previous viruses.

a)   **A significantly high percentage of people who become infected are "asymptomatic."** This means that they can be highly infected with the virus but suffer absolutely no symptoms. Consequently, they don't know they are infected so no one else they come into the locality of knows they have it either.

b) **These "asymptomatic" people are mentally and physically normally fit,** which means they are able to get out of bed and continue their normal life practices within the new anti-virus rules, as they wish.

c) **This virus is not normally spread as most previous viruses were by coughs and sneezes. These "asymptomatic" virus carriers go out and about, and with each breath, they exhale a stream of very small and light virus particles which float around.** These particles are carried by air currents outside and inside. They do not drop to the ground around 2 metres from being exhaled as normal coughs and sneezes do. This means that, particularly when people are inside in pubs etc., when masks aren't worn, each "asymptomatic" carrier will be breathing out virus particles with every exhaled breath. They will float around in the normal air currents that travel around the room, be inhaled by the people who are inside, and subsequently become infected. The two-metre separation rule only protects you by reducing the degree of a direct transmission infection of the virus if you are too close to an infected person. It does nothing to protect you from being infected by virus particles travelling around and being inhaled by you while sitting still or walking off to the toilet and passing through a cloud of particles. When inside, the only ways the risk of being infected can be reduced are by wearing a mask and with the inside infected air being replaced regularly/continually by clean un-infected air. Otherwise, the density of infected particles floating in the air will continue increasing the longer these "asymptomatic" people are inside, breathing them out.

d) **The degree and ease of transmission from this virus, particularly its later variants, is much higher than the original version.** This is causing it to go out of control more rapidly if people don't follow the prevailing rules to minimise its transmission. Once the daily infection rate becomes too high, it disproportionately increases towards an exponential condition. Hospital personnel become overwhelmed and run out of beds, equipment and required treatments. This leads to experiencing increased death rates and doctors and nurses who just can't cope, with infected people waiting outside in ambulances, etc. This overloading of hospitals' treatment capacity for dealing with COVID-19 patients inherently creates consequential deaths and other complications for patients waiting for lifesaving treatments for cancer and many other illnesses and difficulties.

SUBCHAPTER B) The consequences upon countries of the ravages of the virus and their actions to try and contain and minimise its devastating effects.

Each country has dealt with their virus in their own way, with each leader or governing body enforcing rules and regulations that they decided were best for them. These enforcements normally affected most of their businesses, all of their populations and people's working and social lives. The consequences of these rules generally, apart from a small percentage of businesses that continued operating financially as before, was to have devastatingly negative effects overall. Countries suffered very significantly from a very long list of:

1) Governments' astronomical financial costs of subsidising jobs, businesses job losses, minimising redundancies and the large loss of income from taxes not being paid.

2) The total cost to modify businesses of all types and all education premises to make them COVID safe was astronomically expensive. This was caused by the cost of the modifications and with businesses suffering massively reduced incomes due to a large reduction of customers allowed on their premises.

3) Education across the whole age range at schools, including further education, suffered extreme difficulties. Schools closed for very long periods of time, with pupils falling behind on their learning and going backwards on previously learnt skills. Estimating pupils' level of knowledge presented extreme difficulties for all schools particularly.

4) The huge increase in people working from home resulted in a significant reduction in footfalls for many cities and large town centres. This caused many businesses to shut down from virtually no customers, thus causing many other

centre shops to close, further accelerating the demise of centre shopping.

The other extremely negative consequences of people working from home becoming the norm for most people are:

a) Spending nearly all of your waking time in your home, particularly if it is in a fairly small house/apartment, is physically and mentally unhealthy. You live the majority of your life in the same location with far less actual face-to-face contact with other human beings, particularly in connection with topics associated with your work.

b) This isolated, remote and removed method of working is not conducive to the development of young and inexperienced people. They inherently learn a huge amount about so many aspects of the work they are required to carry out for their company simply by being around experienced people within their company. Watching what they do and don't do. How they develop and consider options of decisions. How they relate and connect to other people emotionally, physically and psychologically. How they chair meetings, etc.

c) When people work in the same large office or office complexes, they automatically congregate in an ad-hock group or in a pre-arranged group or formal meeting to discuss and finalise some important decisions that are required. The collective power of decision-making from experienced brains is immense. The emotional buzz created amongst focused people who are connected in reality is way more the sum of the parts.

d) Most of the knowledge passed on and gathered by this format of working is natural but nonetheless so efficient and effective. Actually working with and amongst real people with real-world connections and contact creates immensely strong human bonds. They can be between those who work within the same company and when working among other companies on common projects. These relationships remain for life quite often, even when people move to other organisations.

5) The total number of deaths from the virus, in addition to the usual numbers of deaths from other normal causes, was extremely high, both in hospitals and care homes. The backlog of patients with serious health problems continued to grow as hospitals focused on treating virus patients. Also, many people would not go to the hospital for normal checks and problems because they were frightened of catching the virus.

6) A very large percentage of people across a wide range of ages, professions and in all categories of life have suffered from significant mental health issues caused by very high levels of anxiety. This is due to the 1001 stresses and strains that the anti-virus enforced rules have created and the consequences of difficulties mentioned above.

The consequences of the rules laid down by governments to contain the growth of the virus transmissions meant that the natural human nature practices were removed for more than a year, without even a clear end in sight. These included enjoying regular close physical and therefore close emotional contact within all of your extended family groups living in other locations, with friends and to a lesser extent within changed work-related arrangements, plus being unable to visit family in care homes, etc.

There also existed a daily concern, particularly for people working, that they brought the virus home and infected their own families. This quite extreme and unnatural way of living created immense emotional stress on everyone, the resultant and full consequences of which, I believe, are yet to be seen.

7) Day after day, month after month, the ultra-brave, ultra-dedicated and ultra-medically competent NHS nurses, doctors, ambulance paramedics and cleaners, worked on the frontline with increasing workloads and emotional stresses due to the growing numbers of deaths, with physically tired bodies and emotionally drained minds. The long term consequences of these working conditions will manifest themselves in a very high percentage of them suffering from long term P.T.S.D.

8) Virtually everyone's lives have been changed for the worse. In the earlier months, with no end in sight, people's view of their future tended to change. Rather than thinking some years ahead to retiring, a couple of years to become married, and a few months of going on a much-longed-for holiday, etc., they were looking ahead fourteen days. That was the time within which they would have known that they had

become infected with COVID! They questioned, "Will I survive, and if I do, what long-term state will I be in with potentially possible long COVID serious disabilities? Just stop and chew over for a second and consider, could this fundamentally frightening, awful change of any one's future view be worse than this?

9) Some countries that had dealt with the virus very well initially thought they had won the battle. They let their guard down far too early and started to make a return to normality too quickly and too soon. They suffered disastrous consequences with the virus returning with a vengeance. This meant that they had lost all of the ground they had gained in minimising the daily numbers of infections, hospitalisations and deaths. They almost had to start again, having already suffered a huge number of deaths, thus facing going through it all again.

SUBCHAPTER C) The good aspects that were achieved from the bad, created by the virus.

1) When the ravages of the virus caused it to be classified as a pandemic, and it became clear how devastating it was in all of its elements, the expert's advice was that the only way to get total control of and defeat it was to create a vaccine or vaccines, to fight and guard against its devastating effect. All

of these experts predicted from similar historical experiences this would take a period of years rather than months.

As soon as possible, various suitably capable laboratories around the world embarked upon this exercise with great gusto and expertise, including UK ones. Meanwhile, the various anti-virus vaccine design-creating laboratories, as is the case with top experts in this field, readily collaborated, when appropriate, with other laboratories, sharing their ideas, expertise and findings.

The consequences of these laboratories' activities, expertise, and ferocious 24/7 commitments in creating, testing and getting successfully validated and approved safe and effective for use **resulted in a few vaccines being available in early January 2021, approximately a year after commencing work to produce them.** They have since been proven extremely safe and effective in combating the early format of the virus and **represent an immense achievement by all of the people involved in creating them.**

2) The virus fundamentally presented itself to the whole world as a devastatingly disruptive, damaging, life-threatening and life-taking invisible enemy. It thrust its tentacles of ill-health and death into all corners of the world, as described in some detail above.

This inherently created quite a bonding effect amongst the countries of the world. They were each forced to face and deal with this common enemy that had an unlimited army of death-dealing warriors. It silently and invisibly searched out people of all creeds, faiths, races and colours to enter their bodies to mete out as much harm and death as possible, particularly to the elderly and infirm.

Some of the poorer, less developed countries in some aspects struggled to deal with the virus, particularly with their vaccine program. The world realised that until all countries were safe, none of them would be safe from the virus rearing up again.

With this virus inherently forcing countries to communicate with each other, increasingly more and more will hopefully lead to this increased cooperation continuing long after the virus has been brought under permanent control. Therefore, the whole world will collectively and individually benefit commercially and with a much-reduced risk of another serious war occurring. More frequent contact between country leaders, particularly face-to-face, should maintain at least reasonably respectful relationships.

3) Before the vaccines were available, some countries had been struggling to fight their way through, having imposed another lockdown or similar. They were additionally concerned that new, more virulent variants had been created that were in circulation in different countries. It was predicted that the vaccines would not offer much, if any, protection against them. The plan was for the laboratories to create a booster vaccine that was given in addition to the vaccines already received. This booster would target giving protection against these new variants.

The arrival of these vaccines was seen as a much-needed aid to fight off the virus. A greater effort was required to distribute them around the world, where needed, to begin making better progress in bringing the Virus to heel, particularly in poorer countries and in countries that were short of vaccines and required COVID-19 treatments.

SUBCHAPTER D) A serious perspective I would like to present for your consideration.

<u>My serious perspective throughout the COVID-19 pandemic</u>:

With many presentations, each by different people, held in different types of settings and all from religious leaders, the <u>unspoken question</u> has always been: *Why has their God brought all of this misery upon the whole of our world, with so many God-fearing, unarguably good human beings dying in great suffering from the COVID-19 virus?*

This unspoken question has been the immense elephant in the room, despite these times of such devastation suffered throughout the whole world, collectively worse in some assessment criteria than in previous wars.

SUBCHAPTER E) *Three serious questions I pose about the COVID-19 pandemic.*

The three serious questions I pose are:

Question 1: Has the Grand Creator brought all of this misery upon the world they created because of the way mankind has misused and abused this world they gave to us all?

Question 2: Is it a warning to conduct ourselves towards each other in a far, far, better manner than we have become accustomed to?

Question 3: If the answers to both of these questions are Yes and mankind continues without any efforts to improve both situations, what will be the consequences?

CHAPTER 9.0 – THE MANY SKILLS AND METHODS I USED TO UNLOCK THE FUNCTIONALITIES OF YOUR BRAIN.

This chapter covers a fairly simple list of the fundamental **skills, knowledge, experiences, decisions and basic methods.** I individually and collectively applied to gradually unlock and then tease open what I believe are the introductions to the most wondrous mysteries and workings of something we all have. It enables us to enjoy the precious lives we have all been given, and that is our **most wondrously powerful, wondrously capable BRAIN and its consciousness**.

OVERVIEW: To explain how this penultimate section came about, I was in the finishing stages of my book, and I started mulling over the different skills, knowledge, experiences etc., that I found I had employed whilst creating and developing it. I thought this might be of interest to some, so I include my thoughts here. Apart from number one, the rest are not in any particular order:

1.0 – Before I commenced writing my book in the form of a book, I spent the **first six months** just thinking about the general topic around – how does the whole of your brain function? Refer to the INTRODUCTION at the beginning of the book for a lot more details.

2.0 – I used the **immense, investigative power** of **appropriate questions,** as explained in **Chapter 10.0** and as highlighted in the **very detailed contents**, as a major tool in teasing out my beliefs and proposals throughout my book.

3.0 – I used the **explanatory power of examples,** as shown in the **very detailed contents,** which are commonly experienced in everyday life to most people. I utilised these to confirm to myself about the detailed functionality and validity of a particular process that I had never considered, certainly in-depth before. Additionally, these were to supplement or back up a **verbal description** of how the brain achieved some processing system or other.

These methods, in conjunction, normally achieve good understanding, particularly with some difficult concepts.

4.0 – I found my **extensive experience in my work** about the different types of **automatic and semi-automatic control systems** to be of immense value. I propose these are extensively utilised within our brain.

5.0 – Whilst developing my book, I utilised the **vast number of skills, techniques and knowledge I gained during my academic learning and from the extensive amount of project engineering and development work I carried out, managed and supervised over 50 years.** Refer in the book to the FOREWORD section.

6.0 – I made extensive use of searching out the functionality of the brain by creating notes of functionality. These were additionally supported by the use of **flow diagrams, multiple-category data spreadsheets, different categories of automation departments, storage times, and logic diagrams. Quite often, I also used a very simple diagram of the constituent parts** of a particular grouping of departments in, say, one of your M.C.'s Sections. I could paper the four sides of a large room with all of these notes and diagrams etc., most of which are dated.

7.0 – When you remove a millstream of swirling thoughts from your brain, **put them on paper in front of you** and study them from that totally different perspective, the **power of clarity of consideration and resultant understanding** always gives me great joy and satisfaction. This is whether the ideas are written in words, diagram form or sometimes in combined formats.

8.0 – My quite serious dyslexia has certainly caused me very significant difficulties in my life. However, it has also given me a greater balancing of some very great strengths, a lot of which I have utilised in developing this book. Refer to the FOREWORD for more details.

9.0 – I have enjoyed pretty close contact with a vast amount of different types of people throughout my life, from different walks of life, from other countries, across quite an age range and a wide range of hierarchy within companies. This has been during my working life, during my academic life, during the vast amount of sports that I played, including coaching. Continuing into my retirement, it has come from working on cruise ships for eight years with my wife, dancing with thousands of passengers, teaching them how to dance, and running dancing sessions with our music in the vast entertainment lounges every evening.

9.a – During all of these times, I have learnt a huge amount about the **psychology of the human being and about myself.** This was in order to achieve my prevailing objectives with these individuals when appropriate, and also to enjoy their company even more. From my mid-teens, I was always, and increasingly so, **fascinated by the behaviour of us human beings.** Despite my age, I continue to try and improve my own behaviour to maximise my strengths and minimise the weaknesses that I was born with.

9.b – Another area of knowledge and experiences I have acquired during all of these human connections, has related to **many people experiencing mental ill-health, their treatments and related consequences** of this most unfortunately rapidly accelerating aspect of everyday life.

10.0 – **Playing a lot of sports** at a very good level with one at a **very high level** enabled me to employ my **actual experience and understanding of:**

10.a – **How incredibly fast your brain works at processing the numerous different departments in your brain** for controlling all of your muscles, sinews, limbs, toes and joints, etc., for your required safe and effective movement and balance. This is all to achieve precisely what your brain's prevailing sporting objectives are in every moment of time. For example, participating in particularly some very highly active sports occasionally requires extremely complex balances and bodily movements with sudden changes of movement and direction etc. They always require an end product such as hitting/controlling a ball/shuttle with extreme accuracy and power to win a point.

All of this has to be done without damaging your highly complex human body in the process. Your brain controls all of these very many separate departments you have developed with thousands of hours of practice. Additionally, your brain's Master Conductor is constantly monitoring your opponent's position and deciding where best to hit that shot to win the rally, etc.

The utter sheer complexity of the sum total of all of the vast number of departments that your Brain is independently controlling during very short periods of time, represents a total brain processing performance of outstanding complexity and ultra-fast speed. It is carried out to a faultless performance every time, over very many thousands of hours of practice and play over many years of participation.

To cap it all, your M.C. is continually fine-tuning the control loops within the majority of these separate departments. It does this to accommodate the prevailing conditions, like wind, slippery conditions underfoot, opponents pushing you etc., achieving each department's prevailing sub-objective to accomplish its overall primary objective, for example, of scoring a goal in football or winning a rally in a tennis match.

I am completely and continually blown away in increasing admiration of your incredible brain's never-ending, continuing performance.

10.b – I have **played sport** with serious winning intent and carried out quite a lot of coaching, dance teaching and captaining teams. This has enabled me to experience the great importance of understanding and applying the resultant benefits of the **appropriate and correct psychology** and the **sheer power of the mind**. If done whilst engaging in sport, it achieves the best possible performance from yourself, your team, or from the people you are coaching. I believe these experiences also assisted me in fully understanding all of the multi-faceted aspects from which your **placebo effect is created.**

10.c – **Playing many sports** exposed me to experience a number of injuries, and I learnt how to deal with them and assist in the natural healing process required for a good recovery. It also crucially enabled me to experience how my brain helped me deal with the very serious chronic conditions of my lower back and both knee's difficulties.

Thirty years ago, upon studying the MRI scans of my lower back, the surgeon very pointedly said to me "If you continue to play these risky sports and suffer any more bad injuries to your lower back, we will not be able to operate/repair it. You will be stuck in a wheelchair for the rest of your life." So I decided to stop there and then. It took me two years to fully overcome the extreme feelings of bereavement because playing sport the whole year round had been one of the foundations of my life since I was five years old.

Upon studying the scans of my right knee sixteen years ago, the surgeon said he couldn't do anything for me, and it was so bad it had to be replaced. Sixteen years later, my left one is worse than my right knee. However, I am still keeping them both going with my developed regimes, and I can still enjoy vigorous dancing activities, whilst putting limits of physicality where required.

All of these challenges have given me the insight into understanding how precisely our brains use the tools of pain and dysfunctionality to assist in our dealing with both our physical and mental difficulties. Additionally, they have aided my deep understanding of how your placebo effect is created and how it works to benefit you significantly. Helping many other people deal with their physical and mental difficulties has further enforced and extended my overall and detailed understanding, which I have set out to share with the readers of my book.

11.0 – My driving focus was to theorise, seek and find functionalities of the brain for each area of functionality I was considering that **was a very simple method of achieving their objectives.** This was because your brain achieves so many processing activities, a lot of which are executed in parallel, at such astoundingly fast processing speeds, with zero failure rate. **Simplicity means maximum possible speed, plus faultless performance.**

12.0 – In the process of developing and writing this book, I did not work at any time with anyone else at all. Apart from the one book I mentioned in the **INTRODUCTION**, I also did not read any other books on the subject of my book. I did, though, read articles in newspapers and watch TV documentaries when the subjects related to my book came on. These were the collective sources of most of the topical everyday questions I listed in the last third of my book, along with the very many people I met during our time working on the cruise ships and from my life in general.

    12.a – I deliberately chose this method of a relative **"hermit approach"** because I wished to think about the whole of the brain's functionality with a totally virginal approach and not be biased or pushed in some direction or another by other people's ideas.

    12.b – I also chose this method because it appeared to me that, despite many people studying the topics, particularly of the human consciousness, for an awfully long time, very little progress had been made. I theorised that this was possibly due in part to a number of the thoughts and ideas that people held being **incorrect**.

There is nothing worse than believing fundamental, functional aspects about a particularly highly-complex, dynamic system, which are false. These false beliefs then merge into a bigger, cumulative whole which becomes increasingly wrong compared with the actual functional truth.

    12.c – I simply held a firm belief that I could present a book initially about these three topics (consciousness, mind and soul) with several beliefs and proposals that warranted some serious consideration from those whose opinions were highly respected on these matters.

It now remains for these others to pass their judgements.

CHAPTER 10.0 – THE DETAILED PROCESS I CREATED AT WORK AND USED TO HELP UNLOCK YOUR BRAIN'S WORKINGS.

This final chapter describes the detailed process I created and used whilst at work over very many years. I also used it to develop a significant percentage of my beliefs and proposals about the role and functionality of your brain, as presented in this book.

AN INTRODUCTION

The simple but extremely powerful process that I employed was one that I developed, used and refined during my forty years working as an industry Chartered Engineer. I used it to help resolve different kinds of difficulties on many types of systems, with each presenting very challenging conditions. I experienced a working life full of excitement, humour, stress, a high level of responsibility and extremely hard work but all with immense satisfaction, wonderful comradery and a sense of ultimate achievements throughout most of my working life.

It also entailed a lot of periods working with engineers in the UK and many countries around the world on large projects and process lines. At times, I worked with research and development laboratories, all as required for the nominally bespoke design and manufacture for the use within my company to satisfy its requirement for manufacturing process lines and manufacturing machines.

The general academic and engineering standard of competency, professionalism, experience and capability was immense. Whatever country I worked in, there prevailed a similar team spirit and sheer joy of working in a world of extremely hard work and commitment but one also of respect for your fellow engineer, despite what country and company you were each employed by.

My career included working on a top-secret project, in a tight race against two other competitors in the world to develop a new, extremely high-in-demand, high-in-profit aluminium alloy. I *and the* team I worked with had to design it from scratch and prove how to successfully and safely create and process it on a viable production processing line on the shop floor as part of the process to eventually sell it in its semi-fabricated state on to the world market. This was nominally working in the field of metallurgy, mechanical and electrical engineering work in industry. I worked with combinations of highly-complex electrical, mechanical, hydraulic systems and computer software, fully-automatically-controlled systems, and very large, high-power electrical machines and equipment on brand new projects and improving existing manufacturing processes and equipment.

One of the uses I employed this process for was establishing the root cause or causes of a system working incorrectly. The usual worst-case scenario was when the system was very occasionally faulty, with the potential status of the fault-related cause or occasional multiple root causes not always being easy to locate and/or accessible to monitor.

In addition to the above fault situations, the worst-case scenarios were when the list of root causes only occurred in a particular operating order or sequence within the operating process of the control system itself. This resulted in the extremely low frequency of the fault occurrence being sometimes three or four times *per year* despite a high 24/7 operational usage.

I also employed this process when experiencing extremely unusual and sometimes unseen before operational faults that occurred with standard and well-proven equipment where even the best and experienced experts in the particular field of this equipment were at times, initially totally stymied.

I believe that this process I employed could also be used to establish how <u>any</u> very complex processing system **actually functions**. This is even true when the process, with all of its elemental detailed conditions and steps, being active throughout the system itself, are all hidden from view/observation whilst the complete process is active in real-time, essentially as is the case with your brain.

So, despite your brain's incredible speed of logical processing performance and my belief about your brain's interrelated, interconnected, sequential and parallel processing functionality, and despite it quite possibly being the most powerful and capable single unit processing system in our universe, I decided to use this process as an important tool for me to begin developing my book, initially focusing on how the whole of your brain actually works.

My initial focus was on two of the three primary definitions I had very basically developed. Your consciousness had my main focus and attention because I just felt it was so foundational to your brain's overall functionality. I also worked equally on the individual development of your mind at this stage, focusing on its basic structure because I also felt that it was the other key player in your brain's overall functionality.

The following information is relatively minimal because I have attempted to keep it as such. I could have written a small book containing a lot more details and examples, but I didn't think this was appropriate within this book.

The process I used is not complex, so please don't expect it to be so because you will be disappointed. I believe that the simpler a system can be and still achieve the results you are after, the easier it will be to operate and diagnose. It is also liable to be more successful in a shorter time than a more complex system.

I use very conventional methods and terminology – each individual piece of **information or data, into** my senses (for example, a noise, a smell or something I had seen) going **into** my brain I would call an **input**. Each decision I would make, resulting in an action I would take, I would call an **output from my brain.**

My method was that for each different activity I was observing or considering, I would:

1.0 – In all of their variety of conditions and permutations, observe all **inputs,** noting all that I deemed to be relevant details prevailing *at that time.*

2.0 – Carefully study all of the **outputs from** my brain, in all of their variety of conditions and permutations, relating to all of these **inputs at the same/related period**.

3.0 – List all of the **facts** that I knew about to these **inputs** and **outputs**/actions/decisions that my brain had processed. This inevitably produces a list of questions, none of which you must ever ignore as irrelevant, thinking that this or that particular question does not relate to my objective, so there is no need to interrogate it.

4.0 – You then ask the question – how could each of, or sets of, these **outputs**, in relation to their **inputs**, have been achieved, i.e. what was my brain's internal process of functionality that received these **inputs** and resulted in it producing these **outputs?**

5.0 – Then combine with your noted facts, beginning to formulate some possible answers to this question. Start to form a possible picture of how the internal process is operating. More likely, or additionally, you produce more questions requiring answers and probably also a list of actions for further investigation.

6.0 – Continue this process above, each time, hopefully advancing towards your initial objective of arriving at a plausible understanding of how that part of the whole process actually functions at initially, a very basic level.

7.0 – If I got bogged down with struggling to achieve clarity of thought on a topic or area, I would take my thoughts or data out of my brain and put them down on paper where I could consider them with greater clarity and separation. I would put them into a spreadsheet, produce a flow diagram, a table of data and functionality or a combination of some or all of these for that topic. This, I find, always helps achieve at least some degree of progress. Whilst optional thoughts continue to remain in your brain, they tend to cycle repeatedly, without progress. Putting them onto paper stops this cycling, and some clarity of understanding and possibilities begin to emerge.

8.0 – Some of the most difficult sections where I struggled to begin writing, wondering where to start, were usually finally initiated by writing down four or five basic, fundamental and **extremely difficult and challenging questions** to answer for that section or topic.

I initially thought – how on earth am I going to be able to answer any of them? But, by, really taking these questions on, I nearly always achieved some quite surprisingly successful results.

9.0 – I am repeating this, but I have found time and time again that one of the most significant keys for unlocking the progressive knowledge you require is to **never ever to ignore any question you have unearthed** because you feel it is irrelevant. After all, the probable certainty is that it will not be irrelevant.

You must also never ignore any question you have because you feel it is too difficult to answer. Each question you flag up is a vital part of the process towards full understanding. Tackle each question and, if necessary, put your quest for a full answer to the side. Making progress upon some other piece or pieces of knowledge will connect into this initially difficult question which will further your progress to finally answering it.

10.0 – It is important to remember that most highly complex, extremely well-designed and operationally efficient systems comprise many sets of parts. Most of them interreact with many other parts, and when you get close to working out how different elements function, you will find that they very cleanly connect and interreact with other parts, just like pieces of a very intricate and complex jigsaw puzzle. The significant difference is that this jigsaw puzzle is alive, dynamic and is happening inside your brain that you are utilising to find out how it, itself, all works!

You will find that if your operational logic does not quite fit with other related parts, it is very likely that your theories are not quite correct and therefore require modifications. When you hopefully finally get things right, **you just know. That's it. It all fits**.

Why didn't I think of that aspect before, you may say?

I have found that the simplest solutions and answers to a question are nearly always the most difficult to arrive at.

11.0 – The progress towards final understanding is through related facts and knowledge. It is also *significantly and usually preceded by answering questions* produced during the above process. I have found that the essence and detail of a question is, by definition, inherently encapsulating the area of the knowledge and understanding that you are desperately trying to expose. Pushing to answer the question automatically focuses your mind upon the area/s in which lie your answers.

12.0 – Please forgive me for repeating this investigatory tool of questions. I would propose that most people dislike being faced with particularly extremely difficult probing questions, which they feel are virtually impossible to answer. I think there are a number of emotional and other categories of reasons for this, **but** I have always found, <u>without exception,</u> that posing extremely difficult but relevant questions are the primary keys to gradually and ultimately unlocking the doors to final and complete success. You can usually see the blank and non-supportive looks on most people's faces when you start making a list of questions in the middle of a discussion or investigation.

13.0 – Don't expect full answers just to appear quite soon. The more complex and difficult the process you are seeking answers to, the longer the journey will be. In my book's case, for several topics, it took many months of probing and probing, searching for the key to unlocking the understanding that finally made the whole of a particular area of functionality connect to all around it and within it. I found that I would sometimes write down quite a lot of logic and thoughts relating to a particular topic of functionality. I would finish it, re-read it and conclude that this is not correct. I was emphatically not happy with it. Sometimes though, I would write and nominally complete a page or so about a particular topic and read it through and conclude – I am just not comfortable about a key aspect here, or something is just not right, but I am not clear what.

I would sometimes leave it with a red note and date and return to it when I felt comfortable doing so. This would normally be after sufficient time has elapsed for me to be able to re-read it with a fresh and more open mind. Upon returning, I might spot what I need to change or maybe not, so I would have to leave it for yet another period of time again.

Sometimes, it was a very strange feeling if I was struggling to become very clear and confident about some aspect I was searching for. It was like I was travelling along a straight path and over a wall on my side was the solution to what I was searching for. When I finally found it, I felt I had passed through, not over, this wall to absorb the solution on its other side.

I find that the most difficult ones to crack produce the key unit of clarity of understanding from my brain, waking me up in the early hours. I have to rush downstairs and write non-stop about the particular explanation I have been desperately searching for, sometimes for months. Having solved my search, I usually say to my wife – it was normally **a no-brainer**.

They are always the most difficult ones to crack, but when this happens, I ride a surging tide of deep satisfaction for many days afterwards.

14.0 – The best tack is to not try and theorise the functionality of **all, or too much of the process,** at **the same time,** down to **a great depth of functionality** in **all of its parts**. This is just too difficult and is the road to permanent and probably increasing confusion. On the other hand, considering only one extremely small part of the whole process in isolation to all of the other parts will, I think, never lead to full process knowledge. If it did, it would pretty certainly take a lot longer!

15.0 – The best tack I have found is to continually consider the whole process initially and select one area of functionality that ideally is common to the whole or most of the whole process. Ideally, this area should have a large number of inputs and outputs which you have knowledge of. Consider this one area and apply the process detailed above. Initially, don't attempt to delve down to too great a depth of detail of functionality. Again, keep the whole process in mind on a continual basis. I refer to this technique as helicoptering around and in and out of the whole system.

When you have made progress in this area, you will undoubtedly have developed some ideas of functionality and questions relating to other areas. This is how the gradual progress towards full understanding continues and develops.

16.0 – To a large extent, try and keep to your own thoughts and ideas. Don't be deviated or biased away from this route, because other people's thoughts may come from other people's ideas, which may be from other people's opinions, which may all be fundamentally the same, **and they may all be wrong.** Try and think your thoughts/new thoughts/original thoughts, and you are probably more likely to find the road to the truth eventually.

17.0 – For the whole process, you will certainly not be able to theorise the entire **framework of principles of functionality** correctly initially, but you hopefully get a fair proportion approximately correct. The greater depth of functionality you initially theorise about will inevitably obtain a lower percentage of success.

18.0 – During the whole of the above process, as correct answers of functionality are hopefully arrived at for parts of the processing system (brain), these answers should fit snugly and comfortably together for each part or relate compatibly with other parts – as is appropriate. They should also fit with all of the prevailing answers for the other parts you have made progress with.

If this is not the case, you must note the questions that have arisen and deal with them. This sometimes means that you have to go backwards and review and modify some areas of previously perceived and finalised functionality.

19.0 – During my life, I have found that we have a tendency, particularly with large and very powerful systems which we are working with, to look for and expect complex answers and solutions to questions we seek to solve. But, in fact, we find that the answers and solutions are very often relatively simple. Also, I have found that paradoxically, the simpler the answer is, the more difficult the task is to solve it.

Despite this hermit-type approach with my book, I do believe, as I found at work, that there is great benefit in working in teams with other like-minded and capable people, providing various suitable individuals and working conditions are available, and the right attitudes and flexibilities prevail.

None of the above is rocket science – far from it. It is the application of common sense, with a very open-minded attitude and no pre-conceived ideas. In this case, I believe, for example, not assuming that the brain functions exactly the same as or predominantly like a computer.

You may think, how on earth can such a simple investigatory process unearth the workings of our brains? Well, I believe that it can because any system, no matter how complex and large in terms of, in this case, the number of cells, connections, data and interconnectivity, the vast number of processing systems working independently and also those working together, can be examined. It can be considered, initially in simple framework terms, then broken down into departments and subdepartments and worked away at, gradually unearthing more and more in-depth details.

CONCLUSION

I have put my absolute and utter heart, soul and an awful lot of my time over the last eight years into all of the thoughts, proposals and beliefs in this book, all of which I hold with honesty and hopefully useful purpose to my readers.

The more I have thought about your brain, what it does, and how it does it, I continue to become increasingly in awe of this most wondrous facility.

I do hope that my thoughts, comments and beliefs, when read by the honest, extremely hard-working people who study the workings of our brain, do not take any of my thoughts as being critical of them in any way directly or by implication.

I very much hope that all, or most of all who take the time to read it, do so with an open mind. I aspire that my proposals and beliefs provide pathways towards the eventual completion of full understanding of **the depth and breadth of** functionality **of this most wondrous thing we are all blessed with having,** the most astounding of the Grand Creator's creations – **our wonderful brain, in all of its magnificence**.

I have thoroughly enjoyed creating and then writing this book. I truly hope that you have enjoyed your journey through it and that it will enable you who have challenges in your life to deal with and manage them a lot easier.

With the rest of my time on this earth, I would love to continue this journey I have started. I want to advance from what feel like the end of the first part of my travels in and around my, your, all of our brains' majesty of functionalities and achievements. I would very much like to see someone take up my book and develop it, for example, by working on some of my proposals and developing them into their beliefs and maybe in other ways.

I look forward to meeting many of you on my future travels and hearing your thoughts. Till we connect/meet again, maybe in a book shop for a chat and to sign your book!

The very best of regards,

Look after yourself and keep safe!

Jan de Vinter

P.S. To those who are now most unfortunately unable to read my book, each of whom I would dearly liked to have received feedback from. Here they are, in absolutely no particular order: Tron, Mr Wolf, Gordon, Keith, Ted, Max, Bill, Dearest Dad, Dearest Mum, Dearest Grandma, Dearest Grandpa, Randy, Roger, Caribbean Min, John, Ron, John, Walter, Mr Garner, Hugh and Joan, Robert, Bill, Paddy, Maureen

DETAILED CONTENTS FOR QUICK LOCATION

Printed in Great Britain
by Amazon

84928818R00405